W9-CFB-046

Study Guide to Accompany

Foundations of Nursing
Third Edition

Study Guide to Accompany

Foundations of Nursing

Third Edition

Lois White, RN, PhD, Gena Duncan, MSEd, MSN, and Wendy Baumle, MSN

Prepared by
Cheryl Pratt, RN, MA, CNAA-BC
Regional Director of Nursing
School of Nursing
Rasmussen College

Previous editions prepared by
Kathleen Peck Schaefer, RNC, MSN, MEd
Brandy Coward, BSN

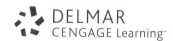

Australia • Brazil • Japan • Korea • Mexico • Singapore • Spain • United Kingdom • United States

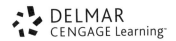

Foundations of Nursing Study Guide, Third Edition

By Lois White, RN, PhD, Gena Duncan, MSEd, MSN, and Wendy Baumle, MSN

Vice President, Career and Professional Editorial: Dave Garza

Director of Learning Solutions: Matt Kane

Executive Editor: Steven Helba

Managing Editor: Marah Bellegarde

Senior Product Manager: Juliet Steiner

Editorial Assistant: Meghan E. Orvis

Vice President, Career and Professional Marketing: Jennifer Ann Baker

Executive Marketing Manager: Wendy Mapstone

Senior Marketing Manager: Michele McTighe

Marketing Coordinator: Scott Chrysler

Production Director: Carolyn Miller

Production Manager: Andrew Crouth

Senior Content Project Manager: James Zayicek

Senior Art Director: Jack Pendleton

© 2011, 2005, 2001 Delmar, Cengage Learning

ALL RIGHTS RESERVED. No part of this work covered by the copyright herein may be reproduced, transmitted, stored, or used in any form or by any means graphic, electronic, or mechanical, including but not limited to photocopying, recording, scanning, digitizing, taping, Web distribution, information networks, or information storage and retrieval systems, except as permitted under Section 107 or 108 of the 1976 United States Copyright Act, without the prior written permission of the publisher.

For product information and technology assistance, contact us at **Professional & Career Group Customer Support, 1-800-648-7450**

For permission to use material from this text or product, submit all requests online at **cengage.com/permissions**. Further permissions questions can be e-mailed to **permissionrequest@cengage.com**.

Library of Congress Control Number: 2010920753
ISBN-13: 978-1-4283-1777-2
ISBN-10: 1-4283-1777-5

Delmar
5 Maxwell Drive
Clifton Park, NY 12065-2919
USA

Cengage Learning products are represented in Canada by Nelson Education, Ltd.

For your lifelong learning solutions, visit **delmar.cengage.com**
Visit our corporate website at **cengage.com**.

NOTICE TO THE READER
Publisher does not warrant or guarantee any of the products described herein or perform any independent analysis in connection with any of the product information contained herein. Publisher does not assume, and expressly disclaims, any obligation to obtain and include information other than that provided to it by the manufacturer. The reader is expressly warned to consider and adopt all safety precautions that might be indicated by the activities described herein and to avoid all potential hazards. By following the instructions contained herein, the reader willingly assumes all risks in connection with such instructions. The publisher makes no representations or warranties of any kind, including but not limited to, the warranties of fitness for particular purpose or merchantability, nor are any such representations implied with respect to the material set forth herein, and the publisher takes no responsibility with respect to such material. The publisher shall not be liable for any special, consequential, or exemplary damages resulting, in whole or part, from the readers' use of, or reliance upon, this material.

Printed in the United States of America
2 3 4 5 6 7 14 13 12 11

Contents

Preface . . . . *vii*

SECTION 1   BASIC NURSING

UNIT 1: FOUNDATIONS

1 Student Nurse Skills for Success 1

2 Holistic Care 7

3 Nursing History, Education, and
   Organizations 13

4 Legal and Ethical Responsibilities 19

UNIT 2: THE HEALTH CARE ENVIRONMENT

5 The Health Care Delivery System.......... 29

6 Arenas of Care.................................... 35

UNIT 3: COMMUNICATION

7 Communication.................................... 41

8 Client Teaching................................... 47

9 Nursing Process/Documentation/
   Informatics 53

UNIT 4: DEVELOPMENTAL AND PSYCHOSOCIAL CONCERNS

10 Life Span Development 65

11 Cultural Considerations 73

12 Stress, Adaptation, and Anxiety 81

13 End-of-Life Care 87

UNIT 5: HEALTH PROMOTION

14 Wellness Concepts 95

15 Self Concept.................................... 101

16 Spirituality..................................... 105

17 Complementary/Alternative
   Therapies....................................... 109

18 Basic Nutrition............................... 115

19 Rest and Sleep 125

20 Safety/Hygiene............................... 131

UNIT 6: INFECTION CONTROL

21 Infection Control/Asepsis................. 137

22 Standard Precautions and
   Isolation 145

23 Bioterrorism................................... 151

UNIT 7: FUNDAMENTAL NURSING CARE

24 Fluid, Electrolyte, and Acid–Base
   Balance 155

25 Medication Administration and IV
   Therapy.. 165

26 Assessment 175

27 Pain Management 183

28 Diagnostic Tests 193

UNIT 8: NURSING PROCEDURES

29 Basic Procedures............................. 201

30 Intermediate Procedures................... 205

31 Advanced Procedures....................... 211

SECTION II   ADULT HEALTH NURSING

UNIT 9:   ESSENTIAL CONCEPTS

32 Anesthesia 215

33 Surgery 221

34 Oncology 229

UNIT 10: NURSING CARE OF THE
CLIENT: OXYGENATION AND
PERFUSION

35 Respiratory System 237

36 Cardiovascular System 247

37 Hematologic and Lymphatic
    Systems 257

UNIT 11: NURSING CARE OF THE
CLIENT: DIGESTION AND ELIMINATION

38 Gastrointestinal System 265

39 Urinary System 273

UNIT 12: NURSING CARE OF THE
CLIENT: MOBILITY, COORDINATION,
AND REGULATION

40 Musculoskeletal System 283

41 Neurological System 293

42 Sensory System 305

43 Endocrine System 315

UNIT 13: NURSING CARE OF THE
CLIENT: REPRODUCTIVE AND SEXUAL
HEALTH

44 Reproductive System 325

45 Sexually Transmitted Infections 333

UNIT 14: NURSING CARE OF THE
CLIENT: BODY DEFENSES

46 Integumentary System 339

47 Immune System 349

UNIT 15: NURSING CARE OF THE
CLIENT: PHYSICAL AND MENTAL
INTEGRITY

48 Mental Illness 357

49 Substance Abuse 365

UNIT 16: NURSING CARE OF THE
CLIENT: OLDER ADULT

50 The Older Adult 373

UNIT 17: NURSING CARE OF THE
CLIENT: HEALTH CARE IN THE
COMMUNITY

51 Ambulatory, Restorative, and Palliative
    Care in Community Settings 379

UNIT 18: APPLICATIONS

52 Responding to Emergencies 383

53 Integration 391

SECTION III   MATERNAL &
PEDIATRIC NURSING

UNIT 19: NURSING CARE OF THE
CLIENT: CHILDBEARING

54 Prenatal Care 399

55 Complications of Pregnancy 409

56 The Birth Process 419

57 Postpartum Care 429

58 Newborn Care 437

UNIT 20: NURSING CARE OF THE
CLIENT: CHILDREARING

59 Basics of Pediatric Care 445

60 Infants with Special Needs: Birth
    to 12 months 451

61 Common Problems: 1–18 years 459

ANSWER KEY 467

Preface

This Study Guide is designed to accompany *Foundations of Nursing*, Third Edition, by Lois White, Gena Duncan, and Wendy Baumle. Each of the 61 chapters in this guide was created to facilitate student learning and refine student skills. By using this guide at home and in the clinical setting you will work with important concepts and begin to apply them to real-life situations.

To facilitate your learning, each chapter in this guide includes the following components:

- *Key Terms Review*: a matching exercise designed to enhance your understanding of new terms presented in the text.
- *Abbreviation Review*: exercise to test your knowledge of abbreviations, acronyms, and symbols used in the text.
- *Exercises and Activities*: short scenarios with related questions to test your understanding and application of concepts.
- *Self-Assessment Questions*: multiple-choice questions that draw on the key ideas in the chapter and prepare you to succeed in your examinations.

Student Nurse Skills for Success

Key Terms

Match the following terms with their correct definitions.

____ 1. Ability

____ 2. Accountability

____ 3. Anxiety

____ 4. Assignment

____ 5. Attitude

____ 6. Attribute

____ 7. Critical thinking

____ 8. Delegation

____ 9. Disciplined

____10. Encoding

____11. Judgment

____12. Learning

____12. Learning disability

____14. Learning style

____15. Mnemonic

____16. Opinion

a. System to help meet goals through problem solving.

b. Method to aid in association and recall; a memorable sentence created from the first letters of a list of items to be used to recall the items later.

c. Act or process of acquiring knowledge and/or skill in a particular subject.

d. Physiological response of the autonomic nervous system to a perceived stressful situation.

e. A level or degree of quality.

f. Intentionally putting off or delaying something that should be done.

g. Subjective beliefs.

h. Characteristic that belongs to an individual.

i. Heterogeneous group of disorders manifested by significant difficulties in the acquisition and use of listening, speaking, reading, writing, reasoning, or mathematical abilities.

j. The disciplined intellectual process of applying skillful reasoning, imposing intellectual standards, and using self-reflective thinking as a guide to a belief or an action.

k. Overwhelming expectation of being able to get everything done.

l. Individual preference for receiving, processing, and assimilating information about a particular subject.

m. Laying down tracks in areas of the brain to enhance the ability to recall and utilize information.

n. Manner, feeling, or position toward a person or thing.

o. Competence in an activity.

p. Conclusions based on sound reasoning and supported by evidence.

___17. Perfectionism

q. Trained by instruction and exercise.

___18. Procrastination

r. Use of the elements of thought to solve a problem or settle a question.

___19. Reasoning

s. Responsibility for actions and inactions performed by oneself or others.

___20. Standards

t. The transfer of activities from one person to another.

___21. Time management

u. Process of tranferring a select nursing task to a licensed individual who is competent to perform that specified task.

Abbreviation Review

Write the meaning or definition of the following abbreviations/acronyms.

1. BP _____

2. CAI _____

3. NCLEX-PN _____

4. ATT _____

5. UAP _____

6. NCSBN _____

7. CNA _____

Exercises and Activities

1. In the first column, list the abilities and skills you believe are useful or necessary to be a competent nurse. In the second column, list the abilities and skills you will need to be a successful student.

Nurse	*Student*

2. Using the list of skills in the first column, write at least three examples of how each skill might be used in nursing in the second column (skills may be combined in an example).

Skills	*Examples in Nursing*
Reading	
Mathematics	
Writing	
Listening	
Speaking	

3. Rewrite each of these negative statements into positive ones that encourage problem solving and goal-oriented behavior.

   a. "I can't understand math equations."

   _____

   b. "I have too much homework to do."

   _____

   c. "I can't stay awake in that class."

   _____

   d. "I don't understand what the teacher is saying."

   _____

   e. "The teacher goes through the material too fast."

   _____

   f. "I'm never going to be able to learn all of this."

   _____

   g. "I know I'm going to do poorly on this exam."

   _____

4. Reread the descriptions of the two classroom settings in your core text in the section entitled "Develop Your Learning Style." Professor A uses a variety of teaching techniques, and Professor B relies on a straight lecture format. Now imagine that you are a student in Professor B's class. List several strategies that you could use to enhance your learning in this class. Include ideas that relate to different learning styles.

   _____

   _____

   _____

   _____

5. Use the following time graph and personalize it for your class and clinical schedule. Don't forget to include class time, lecture and clinical work, religious activities, family commitments, study time, and transportation.

	Sunday	*Monday*	*Tuesday*	*Wednesday*	*Thursday*	*Friday*	*Saturday*
7 A.M.							
8 A.M.							
9 A.M.							
10 A.M.							

continued

	Sunday	Monday	Tuesday	Wednesday	Thursday	Friday	Saturday
11 A.M.							
12 P.M.							
1 P.M.							
2 P.M.							
3 P.M.							
4 P.M.							
5 P.M.							
6 P.M.							
7 P.M.							
8 P.M.							
9 P.M.							
10 P.M.							
11 P.M.							

What is your best study time? _____ Is that reflected in your schedule?

List three of your own personal time wasters and a strategy for each that could help you reclaim some of that time.

Time Waster	**Strategy**
(1) _____	_____
(2) _____	_____
(3) _____	_____

List two activities that you could delegate to others.

(1) _____

(2) _____

6. As a new (licensed practical/vocational nurse), you are caring for your client, Mrs. Thompson, a new mother who delivered her first baby yesterday evening. You note that Mrs. Thompson appears to be somewhat tired this morning, but very excited about her new baby. Although somewhat nervous about caring for her new baby, she asks you to show her how to give her baby a bath. The baby is awake but quiet—this is the perfect time. What teaching strategy could you include for each of the following learning styles to help Mrs. Thompson learn how to bathe her baby?

    Visual: _____

    _____

Auditory: _____

_____

Kinesthetic: _____

_____

7. The process of critical thinking is based on developing the following four skills: critical reading, critical listening, critical writing, and critical speaking.

    a. List two tactics that will help you to develop critical reading skills.

        (1) _____

        (2) _____

    b. Write two suggestions to improve your critical listening skills.

        (1) _____

        (2) _____

    c. List two critical thinking standards that evaluate the quality of your critical writing technique.

        (1) _____

        (2) _____

    d. Give two actions that should be avoided in critical speaking.

        (1) _____

        (2) _____

Self-Assessment Questions

Circle the letter that corresponds to the best answer.

1. Mild anxiety may cause a student to
    a. be more easily distracted.
    b. focus on small or scattered details.
    c. feel alert and motivated.
    d. lose a sense of the "whole."

2. It is crucial for a student who may have a learning disability to
    a. focus on application of information.
    b. develop alternative learning styles.
    c. become a kinesthetic learner.
    d. get professional testing.

3. Being able to summarize a writer's message shows evidence of
    a. basic competency.
    b. accuracy.
    c. comprehension.
    d. metacognition.

4. A student who has practiced testing skills for the NCLEX-PN will
   a. attempt to identify priorities correctly.
   b. infer additional data from experiences.
   c. first scan questions to determine difficulty level.
   d. establish agreement or disagreement with the question.

5. A nurse caring for several ill patients with multiple needs may rely primarily on
   a. skill building.
   b. time management skills.
   c. help from colleagues.
   d. goal setting.

6. A student who is learning to give an injection demonstrates a kinesthetic learning strategy by
   a. studying injection techniques with a small group of students.
   b. watching a nurse give an injection to a client.
   c. demonstrating an injection on a laboratory mannequin.
   d. developing a chart on various types of injection techniques.

7. Select the strategy not suited to getting the most from class.
   a. Write definitions and mathematical formulas exactly as you heard them.
   b. Pick an abbreviation system and stick to it.
   c. Condense the amount of actual writing.
   d. Take notes with the intent of writing them over.

8. Which of the following is *not* a trait of a disciplined thinker?
   a. Courage
   b. Sympathy
   c. Integrity
   d. Perseverance

9. Which of the five rights of delegation deals with the availability of resources?
   a. Right task
   b. Right circumstance
   c. Right person
   d. Right direction/communication
   e. Right supervision

10. Who cannot perform a task that falls within the protected scope of practice of any licensed profession?
    a. RN
    b. NP
    c. VN
    d. UAP

Holistic Care

Chapter 2

Key Terms

Match the following terms with their correct definitions.

____ 1. Attitude

____ 2. Body mechanics

____ 3. Culture

____ 4. Health

____ 5. Health continuum

____ 6. Holistic

____ 7. Homeostasis

____ 8. Intellectual wellness

____ 9. Maslow's Hierarchy of Needs

____10. Physical wellness

____11. Psychological wellness

____12. Self-awareness

____13. Self-concept

____14. Sociocultural wellness

____15. Spiritual wellness

____16. Wellness

a. Inner strength and peace.

b. Enjoyment of creativity, satisfaction of the basic need to love and be loved, understanding of emotions, and ability to maintain control over emotions.

c. Whole; includes physical, intellectual, sociocultural, psychological, and spiritual aspects as an integrated whole.

d. Theory of behavioral motivation based on needs; includes physiological, safety and security, love and belonging, self-esteem, and self-actualization needs.

e. A feeling about people, places, or things that is evident in the way one behaves.

f. Consciously knowing how the self thinks, feels, believes, and behaves at any specific time.

g. Balance or stability that the body strives to achieve with mind and spirit.

h. Behavior, customs, and beliefs of the family, extended family, tribe, nation, and society.

i. Use of the body to move or lift objects.

j. How a person thinks or feels about himself.

k. A healthy body that functions at an optimal level.

l. Ability to function as an independent person capable of making sound decisions.

m. State of an organism performing its vital functions normally and properly.

n. Ability to appreciate the needs of others and to care about one's environment and the inhabitants of it.

o. Highest potential for personal health.

p. Range of an individual's health, from highest health potential to death.

7

Abbreviation Review

Write the meaning or definition of the following abbreviations.

1. AHNA _____
2. CDC _____
3. NIH _____
4. OAM _____
5. WHO _____
6. NCCAM _____

Exercises and Activities

1. Describe the term *holistic health.*

   _____
   _____
   _____

2. List three ways in which the LP/VN assists clients in holistic health care.

   (1) _____
   (2) _____
   (3) _____

3. What role does client education play in helping individuals achieve wellness?

   _____
   _____
   _____

4. In what ways does a positive self-concept contribute to an individual's health/wellness?

   _____
   _____
   _____

5. List several healthy behaviors that you practice in your own life.

   (1) _____
   (2) _____
   (3) _____
   (4) _____
   (5) _____

6. How do you deal with anxiety or stress?

   _____
   _____
   _____

7. What changes would you like to make in your own physical/psychological wellness?

_____

_____

_____

8. Using the following image, draw a line from the term on the left to the appropriate location on the image.

   Love and belonging needs

   Physiological needs

   Self-actualization needs

   Self-esteem needs

   Safety and security needs

Courtesy of Delmar Cengage Learning

9. For each of the preceding levels of need, list two specific ways it would apply to your own life.

   Love and belonging needs (1) _____

   (2) _____

   Physiological needs (1) _____

   (2) _____

   Self-actualization needs (1) _____

   (2) _____

   Self-esteem needs (1) _____

   (2) _____

   Safety and security needs (1) _____

   (2) _____

10. Read the following scenario and answer the questions:

    J.W., a 32-year-old paraplegic who runs a small computer consulting business, sought help from a mental health clinic because of recurrent depression. His most recent episode seems to have been precipitated by his girlfriend "dumping" him. Prior to his injury, he was an ambulance driver. His injury occurred 5 years ago in a work-related accident when the ambulance he was driving was hit by a driver who failed to stop at a stop sign. He had been an avid hiker, rock climber, and mountain bike enthusiast prior to his injury. In the past couple of years, he has become involved in a para-basketball league. He was working out at a local gym three times a week until about 6 weeks ago, when the depression worsened.

a. Using the following blank image, identify the five parts of wellness.

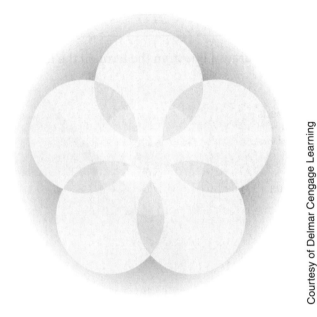

Courtesy of Delmar Cengage Learning

b. Within each circle, identify the client's issues as they relate to each of the five parts of wellness.

c. As an LPN/VN, what would your role and responsibilities be regarding the care of this client?

_____

_____

_____

Self-Assessment Questions

Circle the letter that corresponds to the best answer.

1. Homeostasis can best be described as the
    a. middle range of the health–illness continuum.
    b. integration of holistic modalities into client care.
    c. organism's attempt to balance body, mind, and spirit.
    d. highest level of wellness possible for an individual.

2. The nursing student explains that which is true according to Maslow's Hierarchy of Needs?
    a. Basic physiological needs must be met before higher-level needs.
    b. All physiological and psychosocial needs must be met to maintain life.
    c. An individual moves steadily up the hierarchy toward self-actualization.
    d. Nursing care plans should focus on clients' physiological needs.

3. A client's ability to maintain a positive attitude while being treated for a serious illness is an indication of
    a. self-awareness.
    b. spiritual wellness.
    c. intellectual adaptation.
    d. psychological wellness.

4. The individual whose posture demonstrates good alignment, with shoulders back and head held up, conveys
    a. self-confidence.
    b. aggression.
    c. domination.
    d. curiosity.

5. The most effective way to teach wellness to a client is to
    a. assist the client in developing self-awareness.
    b. be a positive example by practicing good health habits.
    c. explain to the client what can be done to improve health.
    d. explain the concept of wellness in terms the client can understand.

6. An individual's place on the health continuum
    a. does not require constant effort.
    b. can be maintained easily.
    c. demonstrates good physical self-care at a lower level.
    d. can change daily or even hourly.

7. Which of the following needs is not within Maslow's physiological level?
    a. Food
    b. Activity
    c. Shelter
    d. Sex

8. Which of the following best describes self-concept?
    a. It is how others perceive an individual.
    b. It begins forming in infancy.
    c. It is formed solely by negative experiences.
    d. It is not affected during the developing years.

9. One life-cycle consideration for a client's nutritional need is that
    a. proper food choices are more important than quantity of food eaten.
    b. the amount of food eaten increases in the elderly person.
    c. children's appetites do not vary.
    d. healthy eating habits should be established during adulthood.

10. Which of the following best describes spirituality?
    a. It is the concept of religion.
    b. It is not a major healing force.
    c. It involves one's relationship with self, others, the natural order, and a higher power.
    d. It cannot be understood.

Chapter

3

Nursing History, Education, and Organizations

Key Terms

Match the following terms with their correct definitions.

___ 1. Accreditation

___ 2. Autonomy

___ 3. Clinical

___ 4. Didactic

___ 5. Empowerment

___ 6. Health maintenance organization

___ 7. Morbidity

___ 8. Mortality

___ 9. Nursing

___10. Primary care provider

___11. Primary health care

___12. Staff development

a. Systematic presentation of information.

b. Process by which a voluntary, nongovernmental agency or organization appraises and grants accredited status to institutions and/or programs or services that meet predetermined structure, process, and outcome criteria.

c. Client's point of entry into the health care system; includes assessment, diagnosis, treatment, coordination of care, education, prevention services, and surveillance.

d. Death.

e. Prepaid health plan that provides primary health care services for a preset fee and focuses on cost-effective treatment methods.

f. Delivery of instruction to assist the nurse in achieving the goals of the employer.

g. Illness.

h. Observing and caring for living clients.

i. Health care provider whom a client sees first for health care.

j. An art and a science that assists individuals to learn to care for themselves whenever possible; also involves caring for others when they are unable to meet their own needs.

k. Self-direction.

l. Process of enabling others to do for themselves.

Abbreviation Review

Write the meaning or definition of the following abbreviations/acronyms.

1. ADN _____

2. *AJN* _____

3. ANA _____

4. APRN _____

5. BSN _____

6. CEPN-LTC _____

7. CEU _____

8. CLTC_____

9. CPNP _____

10. GED _____

11. HMO _____

12. ICN _____

13. JCAHO _____

14. LPN _____

15. LP/VN _____

16. LVN _____

17. NAPNES _____

18. NCLEX _____

19. NCSBN _____

20. NFLPN _____

21. NLN _____

22. NLNAC _____

23. OBRA _____

24. RN _____

25. TEFRA _____

26. USDHHS _____

Exercises and Activities

1. Describe four nursing leaders who have had a significant impact on nursing and health care.

    a. _____

    _____

    b. _____

    _____

    c. _____

    _____

    d. _____

    _____

2. Briefly describe how each of these events affected the nursing profession in the United States.

    a. Nightingale's service in Crimea: _____

    _____

    _____

b. The founding of the American Red Cross: _____
_____
_____

c. The founding of the Ballard School: _____
_____
_____

d. Flexner Report: _____
_____
_____

e. The establishment of the American Nurses Association: _____
_____
_____

f. Goldmark Report: _____
_____
_____

g. The establishment of the National Association for Practical Nurse Education and Service: _
_____
_____

h. The establishment of insurance plans: _____
_____
_____

i. Visiting Nurses Associations: _____
_____
_____

j. Brown Report: _____
_____
_____

k. The establishment of the National League for Nursing: _____
_____
_____

Insert dates and place each of the preceding events on the following time line:

2003

3. Refer to the Nursing Practice Standards for LPNs (Table 3-2) to decide which of the following topics addresses each activity listed.
   a. Education
   b. Legal/ethical status
   c. Practice
   d. Continuing education
   e. Specialized nursing practice

   _____ Participates in peer review and evaluation processes
   _____ Successfully passes the NCLEX for Practical Nurses
   _____ Does not accept or perform professional activities for which she is not competent
   _____ Applies nursing knowledge and skills to promote health
   _____ Determines new career goals
   _____ Requires completion of at least 1 year's experience in nursing
   _____ Completes an orientation program for employment
   _____ Maintains a current license to practice nursing

Self-Assessment Questions

Circle the letter that corresponds to the best answer.

1. The process of enabling others to do for themselves is called
   a. competency.
   b. autonomy.
   c. empowerment.
   d. endorsement.

2. Florence Nightingale promoted the use of
   a. public health agencies.
   b. rural nursing services.
   c. nursing organizations.
   d. environmental modifications.

3. The women's rights movement in the 1800s advanced nursing by
   a. supporting university education for women.
   b. effecting federal and state health care legislation.
   c. extending the right to vote to women.
   d. founding professional nursing organizations.

4. Florence Nightingale can be credited with
   a. establishing the Kaiserswerth Institute.
   b. lowering morbidity and mortality rates.
   c. promoting public health nursing.
   d. providing nursing care to indigent people.

5. Which of the following outcomes could be attributed to the Goldmark Report?
   a. Provision of autonomy of practice to home health care nurses
   b. Establishment of nursing research and publications
   c. Identification of inadequacies in nursing education
   d. Enactment of federal funding for nursing education

6. Who organized the Red Cross in the United States?
   a. Dorothea Dix
   b. Clara Barton
   c. Isabel Hampton Robb
   d. Lillian Wald

7. The Mary Mahoney Award is bestowed in recognition of individuals who have made contributions in
   a. nursing leadership.
   b. public health nursing.
   c. nursing education.
   d. improving relationships among cultural groups.

8. Standards for the licensed practical/vocational nurse in legal/ethical status include
   a. knowing the scope of nursing practice.
   b. participating in continuing education activities.
   c. observing, recording, and reporting changes that require intervention.
   d. maintaining the highest possible level of professional competence at all times.

9. Which nursing organization restricts its membership to registered nurses only?
   a. National League for Nursing
   b. National Association for Practical Nurse Education and Service, Inc.
   c. American Nurses Association
   d. National Council of State Boards of Nursing, Inc.

10. Title III of the Health Amendment Act of 1955 resulted in
    a. an alternative to private health insurance.
    b. the establishment of practical nursing.
    c. different levels of nursing.
    d. a deficit in the supply of nurses.

Legal and Ethical Responsibilities

Key Terms

Match the following terms with their correct definitions.

_ss_ 1. Active euthanasia

_d_ 2. Administrative law

_g_ 3. Advance directive

_h_ 4. Assault

_ww_ 5. Assisted suicide

aaa 6. Autonomy

_t_ 7. Battery

_xx_ 8. Beneficence

_mm_ 9. Bioethics

_vv_ 10. Client advocate

_x_ 11. Civil law

_cc_ 12. Confidential

a. Civil wrong committed by a person against another person or property.

b. Wrong that results from a deliberate deception intended to produce unlawful gain.

c. A legal document designating who may make health care decisions for a client when that client is no longer capable of decision making.

d. Law developed by those persons who are appointed to governmental administrative agencies and who are entrusted with enforcing the statutory laws passed by the legislature.

e. Contract that recognizes a relationship between parties for services.

f. Obligation one has incurred or might incur through any act or failure to act.

g. Written instruction for health care that is recognized under state law and is related to the provision of such care when the individual is incapacitated.

h. Situation wherein a person is made to wrongfully believe that he cannot leave a place.

i. Negligent acts on the part of a professional; relates to the conduct of a person who is acting in a professional capacity.

j. Statute that is enacted by the legislature of a state and that outlines the scope of nursing practice in that state.

k. Enforcement of duties and rights among individuals independent of contractual agreements.

l. Laws that provide protection to health care providers by ensuring them immunity from civil liability when care is provided at the scene of an emergency and the caregiver does not intentionally or recklessly cause the client injury.

hh 13. Constitutional law

m 14. Contract law

U 15. Criminal law

ce 16. Defamation

bbb 17. Deontology

s 18. Durable power of attorney for health care

qq 19. Ethical dilemna

ddd 20. Ethical principles

nn 21. Ethical reasoning

t t 22. Ethics

e e e 23. Euthanasia

W 24. Expressed contract

h 25. False imprisonment

V 26. Felony

h hh 27. Fidelity

O 28. Formal contract

b 29. Fraud

L 30. Good Samaritan Laws

dd 31. Impaired nurse

m. Enforcement of agreements among private individuals.

n. Threat to do something that may cause harm or be unpleasant to another person.

o. Written contract that cannot be changed legally by an oral agreement.

p. A competent client's ability to make health care decisions based on full disclosure of the benefits, risks, potential consequences of a recommended treatment plan, and alternate treatments, including no treatment, and the client's agreement to the treatment as indicated by the client's signing a consent form.

q. Risk-management tool used to describe and report any unusual event that occurs to a client, visitor, or staff member.

r. Law that deals with an individual's relationship to the state.

s. Guidelines established to direct nursing care.

t. Unauthorized or unwanted touching of one person by another.

u. Law concerning acts of offense against the welfare or safety of the public.

v. Crime of a serious nature that is usually punishable by imprisonment in a state penitentiary or by death.

w. Conditions and terms of a contract given in writing by the concerned parties.

x. Law that deals with relationships between individuals.

y. Offense that is less serious than a felony and may be punished by a fine or by sentence to a local prison for less than 1 year.

z. Words that are communicated verbally to a third party and that harm or injure the personal or professional reputation of another.

aa. Law enacted by legislative bodies.

bb. Written words that harm or injure the personal or professional reputation of another person.

cc. Private or secret.

dd. Nurse who is habitually intemperate or is addicted to the use of alcohol or habit-forming drugs.

ee. Use of words to harm or injure the personal or professional reputation of another person.

_e_ 32. Implied contract

_q_ 33. Incident report

_p_ 34. Informed consent

_uu_ 35. Justice

_gg_ 36. Law

_f_ 37. Liability

_bb_ 38. Libel

_kk_ 39. Living will

_ll_ 40. Malpractice

fff 41. Material principle of justice

_y_ 42. Misdemeanor

_jj_ 43. Negligence

iii 44. Nonmaleficence

_j_ 45. Nursing Practice Act

ggg 46. Passive euthanasia

_ff_ 47. Peer assistance program

jjj 48. Privacy

_r_ 49. Public law

_ii_ 50. Restraint

_z_ 51. Slander

_s_ 52. Standards of practice

ff. Rehabilitation program that provides an impaired nurse with referrals, professional and peer counseling support groups, and assistance and monitoring to get back into nursing.

gg. That which is laid down or fixed.

hh. Law that defines and limits the power of government.

ii. Any device used to restrict movement.

jj. General term referring to careless acts on the part of an individual who is not exercising reasonable or prudent judgment.

kk. Legal document that allows a person to state preferences about the use of life-sustaining measures should she be unable to make her wishes known.

ll. Individual's collection of inner beliefs that guides the way the person acts and helps determine the choices the person makes.

mm. Application of general ethical principles to health care.

nn. Process of thinking through what one ought to do in an orderly, systematic manner based on principles.

oo. Principles that influence the development of beliefs and attitudes.

pp. Calling attention to unethical, illegal, or incompetent actions of others.

qq. Situation wherein there is a conflict between two or more ethical principles.

rr. Ethical theory that states that the value of a situation is determined by its consequences.

ss. Process of taking deliberate action that will hasten a client's death.

tt. Branch of philosophy concerned with determining right from wrong on the basis of a body of knowledge.

uu. Ethical principle based on the concept of fairness extended to each individual.

vv. Person who speaks up for or acts on behalf of the client.

ww. Situation wherein another person provides a client with the means to end his own life.

xx. Ethical principle based on the duty to promote good and prevent harm.

yy. Process of analyzing one's own values to better understand those things that are truly important.

zz. Ethical principle that states that an act must result in the greatest degree of good for the greatest number of people involved in a given situation.

aa 53. Statutory law

vv 54. Teleology

a 55. Tort

k 56. Tort law

zz 57. Utility

ll 58. Value system

oo 59. Values

yy 60. Value clarification

cc 61. Veracity

pp 62. Whistle-blowing

aaa. Ethical principle based on the individual's right to choose and the individual's ability to act on that choice.

bbb. Ethical theory that considers the intrinsic significance of an act as the criterion for determination of good.

ccc. Ethical principle based on truthfulness (neither lying to nor deceiving others).

ddd. Widely accepted codes, generally based on the humane aspects of society, that direct or govern actions.

eee. Intentional action or lack of action that causes the merciful death of someone suffering from a terminal illness or incurable condition; derived from the Greek word *euthanatos,* which means "good or gentle death."

fff. Rationale for determining those times when there can be unequal allocation of scarce resources.

ggg. Process of cooperating with the client's dying process.

hhh. Ethical concept based on faithfulness and keeping promises.

iii. Ethical principle based on the obligation to cause no harm to others.

jjj. The right to be left alone, to choose care based on personal beliefs, to govern body integrity, and to choose how sensitive information is shared.

Abbreviation Review

Write the meaning or definition of the following abbreviations/acronyms.

1. ADA _____
2. AHA _____
3. AMA _____
4. ANA _____
5. CPR _____
6. DNR _____
7. DPAHC _____
8. ED _____
9. FCA _____
10. HIPAA_____
11. HIPDB _____
12. HIV _____
13. ICN _____
14. IM _____
15. JCAHO _____
16. LP/VN _____

17. NCLEX _____

18. NFLPN _____

19. PHI _____

20. RN _____

21. VA _____

Exercises and Activities

1. Give examples of how each of the following may directly affect your practice as an LP/VN.

   a. Statutory law: _____

   _____

   b. Administrative law: _____

   _____

   c. Contract law: _____

   _____

   d. Good Samaritan Acts: _____

   _____

   e. Nursing Practice Act: _____

   _____

2. Match each situation with the probable type of tort involved.
   a. Assault and battery
   b. False imprisonment
   c. Invasion of privacy
   d. Defamation, libel
   e. Defamation, slander
   f. Negligence
   g. Malpractice

   _____ A student nurse is overheard talking in the cafeteria with fellow students about a client and his recent bout of depression.

   _____ A nurse asks a client why she chose Dr. Smith for her physician, saying, "He treats his patients like they were children and is always so rude to the staff."

   _____ The nurse caring for a client with a new leg cast fails to routinely check the foot for adequate circulation. The client requires additional treatment and loses some function as a result.

   _____ The nurse is preparing to administer an intravenous antibiotic to the client. Because of a failure to check the armband, the wrong client receives the medication.

   _____ The nurse misreads an order for "2u of insulin" as "20 units of insulin," resulting in harm to the client.

   _____ A nurse fails to obtain an order for restraints that were initiated on a client who had become confused.

   _____ A client is told he must pay the remainder of his medical bill before he can leave the facility.

   _____ The names of the clients in a hospital unit are displayed on an assignment board.

   _____ Although the client is showing signs of an adverse reaction to a medication, the physician orders the medication to be continued. The nurse follows the physician's order.

3. Describe correct documentation in terms of timing of the entries, legibility, and thoroughness. In what ways can documentation support a nurse's actions?

  _____

  _____

4. What is the difference between a durable power of attorney for health care and a living will?

  _____

  _____

  _____

  a. Describe in your own words what you might include in your own health care directive or living will. Who would you designate to make health care decisions? What treatments would you want to have withheld?

    _____

    _____

    _____

  b. How is a DNR order different from a living will?

    _____

    _____

    _____

5. P.L. is being treated for a fracture of his right hip. The nurse assigned to care for him is reviewing his chart for information. Because there is no advance directive, the nurse asks P.L. if he would like information or assistance to complete one. P.L. is uncomfortable and tells the nurse to let his wife sign any papers because she is the one who would make the decisions anyway.

  a. How could you explain an advance directive to P.L. and his wife? Can his wife sign the forms for him?

    _____

    _____

  b. P.L. is scheduled for surgery and the nurse is asked to witness the surgical consent form. In what circumstances should the nurse refuse to witness the form?

    _____

    _____

  c. The nurse believes that P.L. does not understand the surgical procedure or the risks involved. What should the nurse do?

    _____

    _____

  d. This nurse was actually assigned to a pediatric unit but was "floated" to P.L.'s unit for the day. The nurse feels unfamiliar with the equipment and medications used with the clients on this unit. What is her responsibility?

    _____

    _____

e. Could the nurse be held liable if P.L. suffers as a result of improper nursing care? How might personal malpractice or liability insurance help the nurse in this situation?

_____

_____

Exercises and Activities

1. Address the following concerning why ethical dilemmas occur in health care.
   a. Write your values or beliefs about each of the following issues:
      Passive euthanasia: _____

      _____

      Active euthanasia: _____

      _____

      Assisted suicide: _____

      _____

      Refusal of treatment: _____

      _____

      Organ donation and selection of organ recipients: _____

      _____

   b. How is the process of values clarification helpful to you?

      _____

      _____

2. Differentiate each of the following terms:
   a. Ethics vs. values

      _____

      _____

   b. Ethical vs. legal

      _____

      _____

   c. Nonmaleficence vs. negligence

      _____

      _____

   d. Teleology vs. deontology

      _____

      _____

3. Complete each of the following statements:

   a. Understanding ethical principles is important for the nurse because _____
   _____

   b. The nurse bases the care of clients on ethical behavior because _____
   _____

   c. The Code for Licensed Practical/Vocational Nurses is important because _____
   _____

   d. If faced with an ethical dilemma, the nurse should _____
   _____

4. A.N. gave birth to her fourth child 10 months ago. She received no prenatal care. The baby was diagnosed at birth with a serious genetic disorder that causes severe retardation, facial and skull abnormalities, and heart defects. Survival past a few months of age is rare. A.N. had originally been advised to withhold feedings and allow the infant to die. Instead, she chose to feed and care for her child at home in addition to her other children. Since then, however, A.N. has repeatedly brought the child back to the hospital for medical treatment, at great expense to the hospital. Members of the health care team have asked A.N. to meet with them to discuss her child's medical issues.

   a. For this situation, what are the ethical issues involved?
   _____
   _____

   b. In what way are each of the following ethical principles involved?

   Autonomy: _____
   _____

   Nonmaleficence: _____
   _____

   Justice: _____
   _____

   Veracity: _____
   _____

   c. What are the consequences of providing or withholding care?
   _____
   _____

   d. Who should represent the interests of the child in this situation?
   _____

   e. Should the costs of providing care be a factor in any decisions?
   _____

   f. What is the nurse's role in this process?
   _____

Self-Assessment Questions

1. An intentional tort differs from an unintentional tort. A nurse fails to verify a questionable order with the physician, resulting in harm to the client. This is an example of
   a. battery.
   b. negligence.
   c. malpractice.
   d. misdemeanor.

2. A client who resides in a facility that receives Medicare funding must
   a. forgo life-prolonging procedures.
   b. complete a living will document.
   c. initiate a durable power of attorney for health care.
   d. have the opportunity to complete an advance directive.

3. An incident or variance report is most useful in any health care institution to help
   a. clarify in the client's chart what happened in an incident.
   b. identify problem areas for possible lawsuits.
   c. prevent a lawsuit from being initiated.
   d. document poor professional activities.

4. A nurse is asked by a neighbor to look at her child who is ill. In this situation, the nurse would be
   a. liable for any harm caused by misdiagnosis or treatment.
   b. protected by his employer's liability policy.
   c. protected by the Good Samaritan Act.
   d. violating the Nursing Practice Act.

5. The first priority for the nurse who suspects a colleague is using habit-forming drugs is to
   a. determine what laws may have been broken.
   b. document any incidences and report to a supervisor.
   c. report the colleague to the State Board of Nursing.
   d. confront the colleague with any suspicions.

6. The ethical foundation of the nurse–client relationship is the
   a. duty to promote good and prevent harm.
   b. principle of nonmaleficence.
   c. Patient's Bill of Rights.
   d. concept of fidelity.

7. The principle that an act must result in the greatest degree of good for the greatest number of people involved in a given situation is called
   a. utility.
   b. beneficence.
   c. client advocacy.
   d. situational theory.

8. The Patient's Bill of Rights is most useful
   a. to guide health care workers in treatment decisions.
   b. to outline clients' responsibilities and ways they will be treated in the hospital.
   c. as a legally binding contract between health care workers and clients.
   d. to provide a framework for ethical dilemmas.

9. If you are caring for a client whose value system conflicts with your own, you should first attempt to
   a. be aware of your own values.
   b. ask the client to clarify her values.
   c. engage in a meaningful dialogue with the client.
   d. determine which nursing actions you are willing to do.

10. The first step in ethical decision making is to
    a. examine the values involved.
    b. recognize the ethical dimension of the issue.
    c. discuss the issue with relevant others.
    d. check the legal and organizational policies.

The Health Care Delivery System

Chapter 5

Key Terms

Match the following terms with their correct definitions.

d 1. Capitated rate

a 2. Comorbidity

e 3. Exclusive provider organization (E.P.O.)

j 4. Fee-for-Service

p 5. Health care delivery system

i 6. Health maintenance organization (H.M.O.)

b 7. Managed care

8. Medicaid

9. Medical model

10. Medicare

11. Medigap insurance

12. Preferred provider organization (P.P.O.)

a. Simultaneous existence of more than one disease process within an individual.

b. System of providing and monitoring care wherein access, cost, and quality are controlled before or during delivery of services.

c. Care focused on promoting wellness and preventing illness.

d. Preset fee based on membership rather than services provided; payment system used in managed care.

e. Organization wherein care must be delivered by the plan in order for clients to receive reimbursement for health care services.

f. Health care provider whom a client sees first for health care, typically a family practitioner (physician/nurse), internist, or pediatrician.

g. Predetermined rate paid for each episode of hospitalization based on the client's age and principal diagnosis and the presence or absence of surgery or comorbidity.

h. Health care delivery model wherein the government is the only entity to reimburse.

i. Prepaid health plan that provides primary health car services for a preset fee and focuses on cost-effective treatment methods.

j. System in which the health care recipient directly pays the provider for services as they are provided.

k. Traditional approach to health care wherein the focus is on treatment and cure of disease.

l. Legal recognition of the ability to prescribe medications.

___ 13. Prescriptive authority

___ 14. Primary care

___ 15. Primary care provider

___ 16. Primary health care

___ 17. Prospective payment

___ 18. Secondary care

___ 19. Single-payer system

___ 20. Single point of entry

___ 21. Tertiary care

m. Care focused on diagnosis and treatment after the client exhibits symptoms of illness.

n. Plan that covers inpatient hospital care, home health care, and hospice care for individuals over the age of 65, as well as those who are permanently disabled and those with end-stage renal disease.

o. Client's point of entry into the health care system; includes assessment, diagnosis, treatment, coordination of care, education, preventive services, and surveillance.

p. Mechanism for providing services that meet the health-related needs of individuals.

q. Type of managed care model wherein member choice is limited to providers within the system.

r. A common feature of health maintenance organizations wherein the client is required to enter the health care system through a point designated by the plan.

s. Care focused on restoring the client to the state of health that existed before the development of an illness; if unattainable, then care directed to attaining the optimal level of health possible.

t. Pays for health services for low-income families with dependent children, the aged poor, and the disabled.

u. Policies purchased from private insurance companies to pay for costs not covered by Medicare.

Abbreviation Review

Write the meaning or definition of the following abbreviations/acronyms.

1. ADAMHA ___
2. AHCPR ___
3. AHRQ ___
4. AIDS ___
5. AMA ___
6. ANA ___
7. APRN ___
8. ATSDR ___
9. CDC ___
10. CHIP ___
11. CNM ___
12. CNO ___
13. CNS ___

14. DDS _____

15. DMD _____

16. DRG _____

17. EPO _____

18. FDA _____

19. HCFA _____

20. HMO _____

21. HRSA _____

22. IHS _____

23. LP/VN _____

24. MD _____

25. NFLPN _____

26. NIH _____

27. NLN _____

28. NP _____

29. OT _____

30. PA _____

31. PCP _____

32. PPO _____

33. PT _____

34. RD _____

35. RN _____

36. RPh _____

37. RT_____

38. SW_____

39. USDHHS _____

40. USPHS _____

41. VA _____

Exercises and Activities

1. What factors have contributed to the increased number of clients now receiving care in outpatient clinics and in-home settings?

   _____

   _____

   _____

2. Explain the nursing roles of:

   a. Caregiver: _____

   _____

b. Teacher: _____

_____

c. Advocate: _____

_____

d. Team member: _____

_____

3. L.C. is a 73-year-old client in your long-term care facility. She was admitted 2 weeks ago to continue her recovery from a hip fracture. Prior to her injury, she had been living alone in a small apartment in a retirement community not far from her married daughter. She rejects her daughter's offer to move into their home but is now willing to accept some help with cleaning and cooking if it allows her to remain independent.

List activities or referrals for L.C. that would be examples of each level of care.

Primary care: _____

_____

Secondary care: _____

_____

Tertiary care: _____

_____

Self-Assessment Questions

Circle the letter that corresponds to the best answer.

1. While participating in an immunization clinic for influenza, the nurse is providing
   a. primary care.
   b. secondary care.
   c. tertiary care.
   d. early intervention.

2. The system for financing health care services in the United States is based on
   a. a single-payer system.
   b. a managed care model.
   c. an exclusive provider model.
   d. a private insurance model.

3. The primary goal of managed care is to
   a. provide preventive services by a primary care provider.
   b. provide health education and disease prevention services to clients.
   c. deliver service in the most cost-efficient manner possible.
   d. set fees and determine reasonable reimbursement for medical and surgical treatment.

4. Conducting research and education related to specific diseases is a function of the
   a. Agency for Health Care Policy and Research.
   b. Centers for Disease Control and Prevention.
   c. National Institutes of Health.
   d. Health Resources and Services Administration.

5. The nurse providing care in the hospital setting knows that as a result of the Prospective Payment System and diagnosis-related groups
   a. clients may be discharged sooner.
   b. clients' response to treatment is less important.
   c. clients are less likely to be critically ill.
   d. clients are receiving higher-quality care.

6. A major challenge facing the U.S. health care system is the (USHCS)
   a. lack of prescriptive authority for advanced-practice nurses.
   b. decreased use of hospitals and its impact on quality of care.
   c. greater availability of outpatient facilities and services.
   d. cultural beliefs of a diverse population and their effect on health care.

7. Which health care team member works with clients who have functional impairments and teaches skills for activities of daily living?
   a. Physician's assistant
   b. Social worker
   c. Physical therapist
   d. Occupational therapist

8. Which role is *not* a nursing role?
   a. Caregiver ✓
   b. Therapist
   c. Teacher ✓
   d. Manager ✓

9. A cultural belief or value that may prevent an individual from seeking health care is
   a. refusal of care on holy days. ✓
   b. that illness is a result of sins committed in a previous life. ✓
   c. that one should trust in divine healing. ✓
   d. any of the above.

10. A trend affecting delivery of health care service is
    a. an aging U.S. population.
    b. a decreasing number of single-parent families.
    c. fewer states using managed care to provide services.
    d. a diminished interest in quality improvement.

Arenas of Care

Chapter

6

Key Terms

Match the following terms with their correct definitions.

_b_ 1. Accreditation

_i_ 2. Adult day care

_g_ 3. Assisted living

_a_ 4. Certification

_f_ 5. Hospice

_c_ 6. Licensure

_h_ 7. Long-term care facility

_d_ 8. Rehabilitation

_e_ 9. Respite care

_j_ 10. Subacute care

a. Voluntary process that establishes and evaluates standards of care; mandatory for any health care service receiving federal funds.

b. Process by which a voluntary, nongovernmental agency or organization appraises and grants accredited status to institutions and/or programs or services that meet predetermined structure, process, and outcome criteria.

c. Mandatory system of granting licenses according to specified standards.

d. Process designed to assist individuals to reach their optimal level of physical, mental, and psychosocial functioning.

e. Care and service that provides time off to caregivers and is utilized for a few hours a week, an occasional weekend, or longer periods of time.

f. Humane, compassionate care provided to clients who can no longer benefit from curative treatment and have 6 months or less to live.

g. Combination of housing and services for people who require assistance with activities of daily living.

h. Health care facility that provides services to individuals who are not acutely ill, have continuing health care needs, and cannot function independently at home.

i. Provision of a variety of services in a protective setting for adults who are unable to stay alone but who do not need 24-hour care.

j. Health care designed to provide services for clients who are out of the acute stage of illness but still require skilled nursing, monitoring, and ongoing treatments. (20-30 days)

Abbreviation Review

Write the meaning or definition of the following abbreviations/acronyms.

1. ADL _____
2. AHCA _____
3. AIDS _____
4. ALFA _____
5. APRN _____
6. CARF _____
7. CCRC _____
8. CCU _____
9. CEPN-LTC™ _____
10. CHAP _____
11. CLTC _____
12. CT _____
13. ECF _____
14. ECG _____
15. ED _____
16. EEG _____
17. EMG _____
18. HCFA _____
19. HMO _____
20. IADL _____
21. ICF _____
22. ICU _____
23. IHCT _____
24. JCAHO _____
25. MRI _____
26. OBRA _____
27. OR _____
28. RPCH _____
29. RR _____
30. SBC _____
31. SNF _____

Exercises and Activities

1. List and explain three nonacute health care services.

   _____
   _____
   _____

2. List several "rights" provided by the resident's rights document that directly affect your nursing care of clients in long-term care facilities.

   (1) _____

   (2) _____

   (3) _____

   (4) _____

   (5) _____

   (6) _____

3. How would you compare Medicare and Medicaid for the type of assistance they provide?

   _____

   _____

   _____

4. Describe the goal of rehabilitation for the client. When does rehabilitation begin?

   _____

   _____

   _____

5. What skills are important for the nurse working in the field of rehabilitation?

   _____

   _____

   _____

6. Identify services that might be used in home health care for the client or family.

   _____

   _____

   _____

7. What are the nurse's responsibilities in the home health care setting?

   _____

   _____

   _____

8. Compare each of the following types of assistance for clients.

   Extended-care facility: _____

   _____

   Subacute care: _____

   _____

   Assisted living: _____

   _____

   Respite care: _____

   _____

Adult day care: _____

_____

Hospice: _____

_____

10. T.P. is a 38-year-old insurance agent who enjoys writing short stories as a hobby. Last week during a storm, a car coming toward him crossed into his lane, hitting him head-on. T. P. was tossed around in the car and thrown out through the windshield. Rescue workers arrived and transported him to the trauma center. After stabilization of the injury and further assessment, it was determined that T. P. had sustained a T8 injury and is paraplegic. Next week he will be transferred to a rehabilitation facility with a spinal cord injury program. An IHCT will focus on assisting T.P. to regain as much independence as possible.

a. Describe the importance of the IHCT for this client in rehabilitation.

_____

_____

_____

b. How would the nurse function as a member of this team?

_____

_____

_____

_____

c. Why is the early assessment and intervention of psychological well-being essential in the rehabilitation process?

_____

_____

_____

_____

d. How can the nurse and the IHCT support T. P.'s efforts toward independence?

_____

_____

_____

_____

e. One month after his transfer to rehabilitation, T. P. appears to be doing well. He has some function of his upper body, including his hands. His immediate learning needs are a.m. care, feeding and grooming, intermittent self-catheterization, and bowel training. List several long-term goals for this client.

(1) _____

(2) _____

(3) _____

(4) _____

(5) _____

f. Why will good nutrition and skin care be lifelong issues for this client?

_____

_____

_____

_____

g. T. P. has limited insurance coverage for the rehabilitation facility. He is now being discharged home and will be seen as an outpatient for 3 hours a day. He is divorced, and he will be moving into his parents' home at least until he has completed his rehabilitation program. How can home health care support his transition to independence?

_____

_____

_____

_____

_____

_____

Self-Assessment Questions

Circle the letter that corresponds to the best answer.

1. In what setting is hospice care not provided?
   a. Rehabilitation ✓
   b. Acute care ✓
   c. Home care
   d. Outpatient care ✓

2. A home health care nurse has been assigned to care for a client with a chronic illness following discharge from the hospital. A major priority for this nurse will be to
   a. educate the client and family.
   b. maintain accurate documentation.
   c. obtain Medicare/Medicaid funding.
   d. determine the most appropriate placement for long-term care.

3. A primary effect of the Omnibus Budget Reconciliation Act of 1987 on long-term care was to
   a. determine funding for long-term care facilities.
   b. regulate the reporting of client abuse.
   c. provide accreditation for long-term care facilities.
   d. develop the resident's rights document.

4. The increase in nonacute health care services over the past 10 years is related to all but which of the following factors?
   a. Change in costs of health care
   b. Decline in hospital-bed availability
   c. Longer life span of clients with health problems
   d. Early discharge of clients from acute care settings

5. A 68-year-old widowed client, who has just had abdominal surgery for cancer, is expected to do well. There are no family members able to care for the client following early discharge. The most appropriate short-term placement for this client is
   a. hospice.
   b. respite care.
   c. subacute care.
   d. assisted living.

6. All are examples of resident's rights except
   a. right to vote.
   b. right to choose an attending physician.
   c. right to limited access to family of relatives.
   d. right to remain in the facility except in certain circumstances.

7. A voluntary process that indicates that the delivery of care and services is above minimum standards is called
   a. accreditation.
   b. certification.
   c. licensure.
   d. compliance.

8. Health care facilities must be _____ to be reimbursed by government funds, Medicare, and Medicaid.
   a. accredited
   b. certified
   c. licensed
   d. compliant

9. A facility designed to provide services for clients who are out of the acute stage of their illness but still require ongoing treatments, skilled nursing, and monitoring is called
   a. a nursing home.
   b. an adult day care center.
   c. a rest home.
   d. a subacute care facility.

10. Higher-level tasks such as household and money management are part of
   a. ADLs.
   b. PROM.
   c. IADLs.
   d. respite care.

Communication

Chapter 7

Key Terms

Match the following terms with their correct definitions.

_g_ 1. Active listening

_p_ 2. Aphasia

_m_ 3. Communication

_q_ 4. Congruent

_e_ 5. Dysarthria

_l_ 6. Dysphasia

_r_ 7. Empathy

_f_ 8. Feedback

_o_ 9. Hearing

_v_ 10. Interpersonal communication

_u_ 11. Intrapersonal communication

_j_ 12. Listening

_d_ 13. Nonverbal communication

_a_ 14. Professional boundaries

_n_ 15. Proxemics

_k_ 16. Rapport

_s_ 17. Shift report

a. The limits of the professional relationship that allow for a safe, therapeutic connection between the professional and the client.

b. Permits physicians to provide care through a telecommunication system.

c. Communication that is purposeful and goal directed, creating a beneficial outcome for the client.

d. Sending a message without words; sometimes called body language.

e. Difficult and defective speech due to a dysfunction of the muscles used for speech.

f. Response from the receiver of a message so that the sender can verify the message.

g. Process of hearing spoken words and noting nonverbal behaviors.

h. Use of communications technology to transmit health information from one location to another.

i. Using words, either spoken or written, to send a message.

j. Interpreting the sounds heard and attaching meaning to them.

k. Relationship of mutual trust and understanding.

l. Impairment of speech resulting from damage to the speech center in the brain.

m. The sending and receiving of a message.

n. Study of the space between people and its effect on interpersonal behavior.

o. Act or power of receiving sounds.

p. Inability to communicate, as a result of a brain lesion.

q. Agreement between two things.

_h_ 18. Telehealth

_b_ 19. Telemedicine

_t_ 20. Telenursing

_c_ 21. Therapeutic communication

__ 22. Verbal communication

_r._ Capacity to understand another person's feelings or perception of a situation.

_s._ Report about each client between shifts.

_t._ Permits nurses to provide care through a telecommunication system.

_u._ Self-talk of internal thoughts and discussions with oneself.

_x._ Basic level of communicating between nurse and client.

Abbreviation Review

Write the meaning or definition of the following abbreviations.

1. ANA _American Nursing Assosiation_.
2. CPR _Computer Pt. record_
3. HIV _Human immunodeficency virus_
4. IOM _Institute of medicine_
5. WPM _words per minute_

Exercises and Activities

1. Look at each of these photographs and describe what types of nonverbal communication are present.
   a. Are they positive or negative?

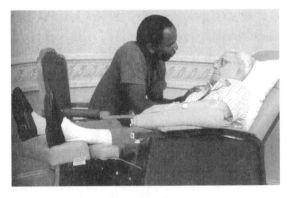

Courtesy of Delmar Cengage Learning

b. What nonverbal communication does the nurse convey?

_____
_____
_____
_____
_____
_____
_____
_____
_____
_____

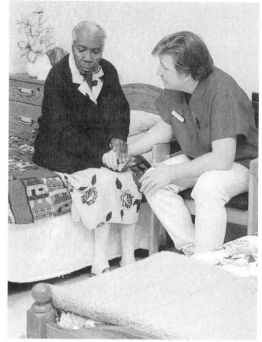

Courtesy of Delmar Cengage Learning

c. What nonverbal communication do you observe in this client?

_____
_____
_____
_____
_____
_____
_____
_____
_____
_____

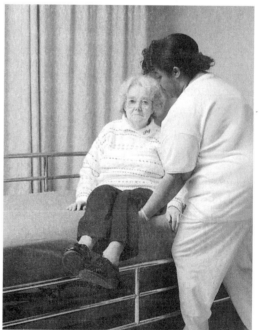

Courtesy of Delmar Cengage Learning

2. If you were having a conversation with a client right now, how might each of the following factors influence your communication style?

 a. Your age: _____

_____

 b. Your education: _____

_____

 c. Your emotions: _____

_____

 d. Your culture: _____

_____

 e. Your language: _____

_____

 f. Your attention: _____

_____

 g. Your surroundings: _____

_____

3. For each of the following statements, give the communication technique being demonstrated. Does it have a positive or a negative effect? If it is negative, rewrite it in a way that might be therapeutic.

Nurse's Statement	Technique or Barrier Demonstrated	Rewrite If Necessary
a. "Tell me about your surgery last month."		
b. "You know the rules about visitors. They'll have to leave."		
c. "Well, I don't believe you should be doing that in your condition."		
d. "You look uncomfortable. Do you need more pain medication?"		
e. "Earlier you talked about feeling light-headed. Tell me more about that."		
f. "Every cloud has a silver lining."		
g. "Under the circumstances, it was the only thing you could do."		
h. "What did you learn in the class this morning?"		

4. V.S. is a 42-year-old client recently diagnosed with lung cancer. He is facing surgery tomorrow and appears very worried. At home, his wife is caring for their two children, ages 11 and 14. When you enter his room at the start of your shift, he is sitting quietly in bed and doesn't seem to hear you.

   a. What behaviors or attitudes might help you to communicate with V.S. in a caring manner?

_____

_____

   b. How could you begin a conversation with him using one or more of the therapeutic communication techniques?

_____

_____

   c. How could you use silence in this situation?

_____

_____

Self-Assessment Questions

Circle the letter that corresponds to the best answer.

1. The nurse caring for a client states, "A minute ago, you said you were sleeping poorly at night. Could you tell me more about that?" This is an example of
   a. reflecting.
   b. restating.
   c. focusing.
   d. paraphrasing.

2. The nurse practicing therapeutic communication will avoid
   a. giving advice.
   b. procedural touch.
   c. using gestures.
   d. silence.

3. The goals of therapeutic communication include
   a. self-disclosure, validation, and empathy.
   b. obtaining information, developing trust, and showing caring.
   c. offering assistance, showing acceptance, and reducing communication blocks.
   d. active listening, data gathering, and developing a communication style.

4. Imposing a personal set of values while caring for a client is a barrier to communication that is called
   a. value sharing.
   b. validating.
   c. giving advice.
   d. judgmental response.

5. To communicate with a client with dysphasia, the nurse will remember to
   a. speak normally.
   b. use slightly exaggerated word formation.
   c. ask a family member to assist.
   d. touch the client's arm before speaking.

6. During a conversation, a client reveals to you that she may be in an abusive relationship. As the nurse, you realize that
   a. you can demonstrate caring by encouraging the client to share her fears.
   b. nurse–client communication is privileged and should be kept confidential.
   c. a client care conference will help determine what steps the client should take.
   d. you have a responsibility to share the information with health care team members.

7. All are forms of verbal communication except
   a. speaking.
   b. listening.
   c. writing.
   d. tone of voice.

8. The statement "Don't worry, I'm sure everything will be fine" is an example of
   a. a cliché.
   b. false reassurance.
   c. belittling.
   d. defending.

9. The statement "Yes, everyone feels like that" is an example of
   a. a cliché.
   b. false reassurance.
   c. belittling.
   d. defending.

10. A person whose style of communication puts his own feelings, needs, and rights first is using a style best described as
    a. aggressive.
    b. assertive.
    c. passive.
    d. judgmental.

Client Teaching

Key Terms

Match the following terms with their correct definitions.

___ 1. Affective domain

___ 2. Auditory learner

___ 3. Cognitive domain

___ 4. Formal teaching

___ 5. Informal teaching

___ 6. Kinesthetic learner

___ 7. Learning

___ 8. Learning plateau

___ 9. Learning style

___10. Motivation

___11. Psychomotor domain

___12. Readiness for learning

___13. Self-efficacy

___14. Teaching

___15. Teaching-learning process

a. Planned interaction that promotes a behavioral change that is not a result of maturation or coincidence.

b. Technique to promote learning.

c. Teaching that takes place any time, any place, and whenever a learning need is identified.

d. Area of learning that involves performance of motor skills.

e. Person who learns by processing information through seeing.

f. Belief in one's ability to succeed in attempts to change behavior.

g. Area of learning that involves attitudes, beliefs, and emotions.

h. Teaching that takes place at a specific time, in a specific place, and on a specific topic.

i. Peak in the effectiveness of teaching and depth of learning.

j. Active process wherein one individual shares information with another as a means to facilitate learning and thereby promote behavioral changes.

k. Person who learns by processing information through hearing.

l. Person who learns by processing information through touching, feeling, and doing.

m. Area of learning that involves intellectual understanding.

n. Process of assimilating information, resulting in behavioral change.

o. Evidence of willingness to learn.

___16. Teaching strategy

    p. Manner whereby an individual incorporates new information.

___17. Visual learner

    q. Forces acting on or within organisms that initiate, direct, or maintain behavior.

Abbreviation Review

Write the meaning or definition of the following abbreviations.

1. AEB _____

2. JCAHO _____

3. NPO _____

4. R/T _____

Exercises and Activities

1. Describe the role that client teaching plays to help you provide nursing care.

   _____

   _____

   _____

   How are formal and informal teaching different? Give an example of each.

   _____

   _____

   _____

2. Give examples from your own nursing education program for each of the three learning domains.

   a. Cognitive: _____

   _____

   b. Affective: _____

   _____

   c. Psychomotor: _____

   _____

3. You have been assigned to care for G.R., a 68-year-old woman who was diagnosed with breast cancer. She is now in the hospital recovering from surgery to remove her right breast tissue and lymph nodes. She will need to perform exercises at home to promote healing and maintain circulation and function in her right arm. As you are caring for her, you note that she has a hearing loss and understands some English, but is not fluent. G.R. shares a semiprivate room with another client, and you note that they both have a lot of visitors. One of the visitors is G.R.'s sister, who will be helping her at home during her recovery.

   a. In what ways will your teaching be important to G.R.?

   _____

   _____

b. How would you determine her readiness to learn?

_____

_____

c. Write in the following diagram what learning barriers might be present for G.R. Give two interventions that might help overcome each type of learning barrier.

Type of Barrier	Findings	Interventions
External Barriers		
Environmental		
Sociocultural		
Internal Barriers		
Psychological		
Physiological		

4. You have decided that G.R. will need to know how to perform the exercises at home after she is discharged.

a. What are her specific learning needs?

_____

_____

b. What types of teaching methods could you use?

_____

_____

c. List two ways you can evaluate whether G.R. has learned this skill.

(1) _____

(2) _____

d. Unfortunately, G.R. is having difficulty remembering how you demonstrated the exercises. She appears frustrated and tired. List three ideas that you could use to help with her learning.

(1) _____

(2) _____

(3) _____

e. Why would it be helpful to discuss community resources with G.R.?

_____

_____

Self-Assessment Questions

Circle the letter that corresponds to the best answer.

1. In today's health care setting, a major goal of client teaching is to
    a. facilitate and enhance the nurse–client relationship.
    b. assess for psychological and physiological barriers to learning.
    c. determine which clients will benefit most from teaching.
    d. promote wellness and prevent illness.

2. The nurse is teaching a new mother breastfeeding techniques. Which of the following teaching strategies will promote learning in the affective domain?
    a. The nurse determines how much the client already knows about breastfeeding.
    b. The nurse has the client demonstrate how to hold her newborn for feeding.
    c. The nurse encourages the client to discuss her family's attitude toward breastfeeding.
    d. The client explains why breast milk is the most beneficial for her newborn.

3. When teaching a client who is hearing impaired, an effective approach would include
    a. using repetition of the materials.
    b. providing large-print education materials.
    c. using short sentences and words that are easily understood.
    d. determining the client's self-care abilities.

4. Client teaching is mandated by JCAHO and the Patient's Bill of Rights because
    a. informed consent is essential to health care.
    b. more patients are being discharged sooner from hospitals.
    c. an educated client is able to achieve higher levels of wellness.
    d. the client develops positive feelings toward health care providers.

5. Which of the following teaching methods would promote learning in the cognitive domain?
    a. Demonstration and supervised practice
    b. Games and computer activities
    c. Discussion and role play
    d. Visual stimuli and return demonstration

6. Formal teaching includes
    a. instruction on a specific topic, at a specific time.
    b. unscripted answers to a question.
    c. explaining the care being given to a client at the time of care.
    d. instruction at any time or place.

7. That clients must believe that they need to learn the information before learning can occur is an example of which learning principle?
    a. Maturation
    b. Readiness
    c. Motivation
    d. Relevance

8. That clients should be able and willing to learn is an example of which learning principle?
   a. Maturation
   b. Readiness
   c. Motivation
   d. Relevance

9. Retention of material is reinforced by
   a. checking literacy.
   b. maturation.
   c. organization.
   d. repetition.

10. The visual learner would prefer information in the form of
    a. question-and-answer sessions.
    b. handouts.
    c. lectures.
    d. discussion sessions.

Nursing Process/ Documentation/Informatics

Key Terms

Match the following terms with their correct definitions.

____ 1. Actual nursing diagnosis

____ 2. Analysis

____ 3. Assessment

____ 4. Assessment model

____ 5. Charting by exception

____ 6. Comprehensive assessment

____ 7. Critical pathway

____ 8. Data clustering

____ 9. Defining characteristics

____10. Dependent nursing intervention

____11. Discharge planning

____12. Documentation

____13. Etiology

a. Continuous updating of the client's plan of care.

b. Review of the client's functional health patterns prior to the current contact with the health care agency.

c. Process of putting data together in order to identify areas of the client's problems and strengths.

d. Cause of or contributor to a problem.

e. Written guide that organizes data about a client's care into a formal statement of the strategies that will be implemented to help the client achieve optimal health.

f. Order written in a client's medical record or nursing care plan by a physician or nurse especially for that individual client; not used for any other client.

g. Putting data together in a new way.

h. Clinical judgment by the physician that identifies or determines a specific disease, condition, or pathological state.

i. Fifth step in the nursing process; involves determining whether client goals have been met, partially met, or not met.

j. Second step in the nursing process; a clinical judgment about individual, family, or community (aggregate) responses to actual or potential health problems/life processes.

k. Nursing diagnosis that indicates the client's expression of a desire to obtain a higher level of wellness in some area of function; composed of the diagnostic label preceded by the phrase "potential for enhanced."

l. Data source other than the client; can include family members, other health care providers, or medical records.

m. Fourth step in the nursing process; involves the execution of the nursing plan of care formulated during the planning phase.

_____14. Evaluation

n. Framework that provides a systematic method for organizing data.

_____15. Expected outcome

o. Nursing diagnosis that indicates that a problem exists; composed of the diagnostic label, related factors, and signs and symptoms.

_____16. Focus charting

p. Planning that involves critical anticipation and planning for the client's needs after discharge.

_____17. Focused assessment

q. Nursing action that is implemented in a collaborative manner with other health care professionals.

_____18. Goal

r. Observable and measurable data that are obtained through standard assessment techniques performed during the physical examination and through laboratory and diagnostic tests.

_____19. Health history

s. Type of assessment that is limited in scope in order to focus on a particular need or health care problem or on potential health care risks.

_____20. Implementation

t. Third step of the nursing process; includes both the formulation of guidelines that establish the proposed course of nursing action in the resolution of nursing diagnoses and the development of the client's plan of care.

_____21. Incident report

u. First step in the nursing process; includes systematic collection, verification, organization, interpretation, and documentation of data.

_____22. Independent nursing intervention

v. Type of assessment that includes systematic monitoring and observation related to specific problems.

_____23. Initial planning

w. Comprehensive, standard plan of care for specific case situations.

_____24. Interdependent nursing intervention

x. Nursing action that requires an order from a physician or other health care professional.

_____25. Kardex

y. Major provider of information about a client.

_____26. Long-term goal

z. Objective that outlines the desired resolution of the nursing diagnosis over a short period of time, usually a few hours or days (less than a week).

_____27. Medical diagnosis

aa. Elements that should be in clinical records and abstracted for studies on the effectiveness and costs of nursing care.

_____28. Narrative charting

bb. Collected data; also known as signs and symptoms, subjective and objective data, or clinical manifestations.

_____29. Nursing care plan

cc. Action performed by a nurse that helps the client achieve the results specified by the goals and expected outcomes.

___30. Nursing diagnosis

dd. Standardized intervention written, approved, and signed by a physician that is kept on file within health care agencies to be used in predictable situations or in circumstances requiring immediate attention.

___31. Nursing intervention

ee. Development of a preliminary plan of care by the nurse who performs the admission assessment and gathers the comprehensive admission assessment data.

___32. Nursing Intervention Classification (NIC)

ff. Type of assessment that provides baseline client data, including a complete health history and current needs assessment.

___33. Nursing Minimum Data Set (NMDS)

gg. Detailed, specific statement that describes the methods through which a goal will be achieved and that includes aspects such as direct nursing care, client teaching, and continuity of care.

___34. Nursing Outcomes Classification (NOC)

hh. Objective that outlines the desired resolution of the nursing diagnosis over a longer period of time, usually weeks or months.

___35. Nursing process

ii. Nursing diagnosis indicating that a problem does not yet exist but that specific risk factors are present; composed of the diagnostic label followed by the phrase "Risk for" and a list of the specific risk factors.

___36. Objective data

jj. Statement written in objective format and demonstrating an expectation to be achieved in resolution of the nursing diagnosis over a long period of time, usually weeks or months.

___37. Ongoing assessment

kk. Data from the client's point of view, including feelings, perceptions, and concerns.

___38. Ongoing planning

ll. Systematic method of providing care to clients, consisting of five steps: assessment, diagnosis, outcome identification and planning, implementation, and evaluation.

___39. PIE charting

mm. Breaking down the whole into parts that can be examined.

___40. Planning

nn. Nursing action initiated by the nurse that does not require direction or an order from another health care professional.

___41. Point-of-care charting

oo. Written evidence of the interactions between and among health care professionals, clients and their families, and health care organizations; the administration of tests, procedures, treatments, and client education; and the result of or client's response to diagnostic tests and interventions.

___42. Primary source

pp. Standardized language for nursing outcomes.

___43. Problem-oriented medical record

qq. Documentation of an unusual occurrence or an accident in delivery of client care.

___44. Risk nursing diagnosis

rr. Documentation method that requires the nurse to document only deviations from preestablished norms.

___45. Secondary source

ss. Documentation method focusing on the client's problem and using a structured, logical format to narrative charting, categorized by subjective data, objective data, assessment, and plan.

___46. Short-term goal

tt. Reporting method used when members of the care team walk to each client's room and discuss care with each other and with the client.

___47. SOAP charting

uu. Goals not met or interventions not performed according to the time frame; also called variances.

___48. Source-oriented charting

vv. Documentation system that allows health care providers to gain immediate access to client information at the bedside.

___49. Specific order

ww. Standardized language for nursing interventions.

___50. Standing order

xx. Documentation method using a column format to chart data, actions, and responses.

___51. Subjective data

yy. Documentation method using the problem, intervention, evaluation format.

___52. Synthesis

zz. Narrative recording by each member (source) of the health care team on a separate record.

___53. Variance

aaa. Documentation method using subjective data, objective data, assessment, and plan.

___54. Walking rounds

bbb. Summary worksheet reference of basic client care information.

___55. Wellness nursing diagnosis

ccc. Story format of documentation that describes the client's status, the interventions and treatments, and the client's response to treatments.

Abbreviation Review

Write the meaning or definition of the following abbreviations, acronyms, and symbols.

1. AEB _____
2. ANA _____
3. CBE _____
4. DAR _____
5. DNR _____
6. DRG _____

7. HIS _____

8. JCAHO _____

9. L _____

10. MAR _____

11. NANDA _____

12. NIC _____

13. NIS _____

14. NMDS _____

15. NOC _____

16. PIE _____

17. POMR _____

18. PPS _____

19. PRO _____

20. RN _____

21. ROM _____

22. R/T _____

23. SOAP _____

24. SOAPIE _____

25. SOAPIER _____

26. t.o. _____

27. UMLS _____

Exercises and Activities

1. Write a short definition for each phase of the nursing process: Assessment, Planning, Intervention, and Evaluation.

   _____

   _____

   _____

   _____

2. Differentiate the three types of nursing diagnoses: actual, risk (potential problem), and wellness.

   _____

   _____

   _____

   _____

   a. How does a three-part statement of a diagnosis differ from a two-part statement?

      _____

      _____

b. Give one example of a two-part statement for each type of nursing diagnosis.

Actual: _____

Risk (potential problem): _____

Wellness: _____

3. In what ways does a nursing diagnosis differ from a medical diagnosis?

_____

_____

a. For each of the following medical diagnoses, write two nursing diagnoses that might apply to a client.

Medical Diagnosis	*Nursing Diagnosis*
Myocardial infarction	(1) _____
	(2) _____
Anorexia	(1) _____
	(2) _____
Fracture of the pelvis	(1) _____
	(2) _____

b. Choose one of your nursing diagnoses from the preceding table and write it as a three-part statement.

_____

_____

4. Where do you find each of these items in a nursing care plan?
   a. Assessment
   b. Diagnoses
   c. Planning and outcome identification
   d. Implementation
   e. Evaluation

_____ "Take blood pressure every 3 hours."
_____ "Instruct client to self-administer medication."
_____ "Exercises three times a week to relieve stress."
_____ "I have been having headaches for the past week."
_____ "Client will eat 75% of meal with assistance."
_____ "Vitals signs will remain stable."
_____ "Anxiety related to hospitalization."
_____ "Sleep pattern disturbance."
_____ "Assess and document patient's sleeping pattern."
_____ "Goal met: client able to select appropriate foods for low-sodium diet."
_____ "Client was able to state signs and symptoms of infection."

5. Review the following client health history. O.N. was diagnosed 2 years ago with type II diabetes and takes metformin (Glucophage) 500 mg b.i.d. (twice a day) with meals. She is being seen in the clinic for her 6-month visit. She says, "I hardly have the energy to get up and dress in the morning. I am thirsty all day and awaken several times during the night, having to go to the bathroom." She does not work outside the home and has not been involved in community activities for the past 5 years since her youngest child graduated from high school. Her daily routine involves cooking for her husband and brother, reading, and watching TV for 6 to 8 hours. She says, "I eat because I have nothing else to do." She is concerned about her eating habits and her recent weight gain.

a. Using the list of NANDA-approved nursing diagnoses, list several actual and potential (risk) diagnoses for this client. Include a diagnosis related to O.N.'s teaching needs, as learning about diet, blood glucose testing, medication, and activity will contribute to her health and sense of well-being.

(1) _____

(2) _____

(3) _____

(4) _____

(5) _____

Is there a wellness diagnosis that may be appropriate?

_____

_____

b. Now rank your diagnoses according to Maslow's Hierarchy of Needs. Physiological diagnoses have highest priority, followed by safety and security needs and self-esteem.

(1) _____

(2) _____

(3) _____

(4) _____

(5) _____

c. Choose two of your nursing diagnoses for O.N. Write long- and short-term goals and possible interventions.

Diagnoses	Short-Term Goals—Client will	Long-Term Goals—Client will	Interventions—Nurse will
_____	(1) _____ (2) _____	(1) _____ (2) _____	(1) _____ (2) _____
_____	(1) _____ (2) _____	(1) _____ (2) _____	(1) _____ (2) _____

6. In what ways is the evaluation phase of the nursing process important to the nurse and the client?

_____

_____

    a. O.N., your client with diabetes, has returned to your clinic 3 weeks later. How will you determine if O.N. has met her goals?

_____

_____

    b. Your assessment indicates that O.N. did not meet a goal of losing weight; in fact, she has gained 2 pounds. In what way will you use this information to reevaluate your goals and interventions?

_____

_____

7. What information could you obtain from documentation tools that could help you provide appropriate nursing care for your client?

_____

_____

_____

    a. In what ways can accurate and complete documentation help you to communicate information to other members of the health care team?

_____

_____

    b. List three ways documentation helps communication in the health care setting.

       (1) _____

       (2) _____

       (3) _____

    c. List two ways documentation supports nursing/health education.

       (1) _____

       (2) _____

    d. How does documentation support nursing/health care research?

_____

_____

    e. How can documentation help or hurt the nurse in legal situations?

_____

_____

8. On October 12 of this year, you are caring for a 42-year-old female client who is recovering from abdominal surgery. You are now responsible for documentation of her care.

    a. Using the sample flowsheet, enter the following information using military time for entries.

Your nursing care included assisting the client with a bed bath and perineal care, but she was able to brush her teeth. You note that she took less than half of her clear liquid diet this morning. Her vital signs at 7:30 A.M. were a temperature of 97.4°F, a pulse of 88, a respiratory rate of 14, and a blood pressure of 128/84.

By the end of your shift, you have noted that her fluid intake included 225 cc po at 8:30 A.M., 50 cc at 11 A.M., and another 320 cc at 1 P.M. She is also receiving IV fluids; by 11 A.M. she had received approximately 500 cc, and another 450 cc by 3 P.M. You emptied her Foley catheter bag for urine twice on your shift; at 11 A.M. there were 350 cc of urine, and at 3 P.M., another 425 cc. She became nauseated and had an emesis of approximately 75 cc after breakfast.

b. Now document in the Nurse's Progress Record (nurse's notes) the following information on your client.

At 9:15 in the morning, your client said she felt uncomfortable because of a sharp, burning sensation at her surgical incision site. You check her MAR and decide to administer Demerol 50 mg by intramuscular (IM) injection. Thirty minutes later, she tells you she is feeling less pain but is now feeling a little nauseous.

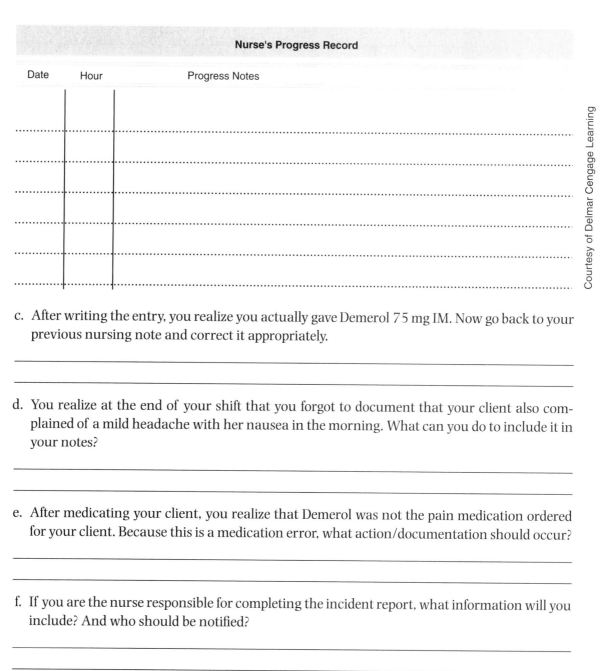

Courtesy of Delmar Cengage Learning

c. After writing the entry, you realize you actually gave Demerol 75 mg IM. Now go back to your previous nursing note and correct it appropriately.

_____

_____

d. You realize at the end of your shift that you forgot to document that your client also complained of a mild headache with her nausea in the morning. What can you do to include it in your notes?

_____

_____

e. After medicating your client, you realize that Demerol was not the pain medication ordered for your client. Because this is a medication error, what action/documentation should occur?

_____

_____

f. If you are the nurse responsible for completing the incident report, what information will you include? And who should be notified?

_____

_____

Date:

Nutrition:		Hygiene:		7-3			3-11			11-7		
Diet ☐	NPO ☐	Bath ☐ Sitz ☐		self ☐ assist ☐ total			self ☐ assist ☐ total			self ☐ assist ☐ total		
Hyperal ☐ Tube Fed ☐		Shower ☐		refused ☐ ☐			refused ☐ ☐			refused ☐ ☐		
Breakfast:		Oral Care		self ☐	assist ☐	total ☐	self ☐	assist ☐	total ☐	self ☐	assist ☐	total ☐
All >1/2 <1/2 0		Shave		self ☐	assist ☐	total ☐	self ☐	assist ☐	total ☐	self ☐	assist ☐	total ☐
☐ ☐ ☐ ☐		Peri Care		self ☐	assist ☐	total ☐	self ☐	assist ☐	total ☐	self ☐	assist ☐	total ☐
Lunch:		Other:										
All >1/2 <1/2 0		Comments:										
☐ ☐ ☐ ☐												
Dinner:												
All >1/2 <1/2 0												
☐ ☐ ☐ ☐												
Snacks:												
All >1/2 <1/2 0												
☐ ☐ ☐ ☐												

Tube Feeding Residuals		Intake						Output			
Time	Amount	7-3	PO	IV	NG & Flush	Enteral	Other	Urine	Ng/Emesis	Stool	Drains
		7-3 Total									
Weight		3-11									
Today:											
Previous:											
Vital/Signs											
Time	T	P	R	B/P	3-11 Total						
					11-7						
					11-7 Total						
					24° Total						

SPOHN HEALTH SYSTEM
SPOHN HOSPITAL
CORPUS CHRISTI, TEXAS 78404

FLOW SHEET—24 HOUR RECORD
PATIENT CARE SERVICES

2705066

NEW: 07/94
REV: 06/26/98
.FM2

4010

Courtesy of Spohn Health System, Corpus Christi, TX

Self-Assessment Questions

Circle the letter that corresponds to the best answer.

1. The primary source of data for the nursing assessment is
    a. the client.
    b. the health history.
    c. nursing observations.
    d. the medical/health record.

2. Which finding is an example of subjective data?
    a. Pain
    b. Weight loss
    c. Diarrhea
    d. Frequency of urination

3. Analysis and synthesis of data occur in which phase of the nursing process?
    a. Planning and outcome identification
    b. Assessment
    c. Evaluation
    d. Diagnosis

4. The nurse determines the priority of the patient diagnoses in the
    a. assessment phase.
    b. diagnosis phase.
    c. planning and outcome identification phase.
    d. evaluation phase.

5. Which statement best describes a primary function of the nursing process?
    a. The nursing process can evaluate and predict patient outcomes.
    b. The nursing process is an organized method of planning and delivering health care.
    c. The nursing process helps the nurse to prioritize care for multiple patient tasks.
    d. The nursing process helps to develop critical-thinking, problem-solving, and decision-making skills.

6. A student shows understanding of the importance of documentation by stating:
    a. "I will avoid using abbreviations to eliminate any confusion."
    b. "I need to be timely and accurate when I write."
    c. "I can save time by telling the next nurse what I did instead of writing it."
    d. "Taking care of the clients is more important than documenting it."

7. Your client has an adverse response to a medication that was ordered for him. You would document this outcome in the
    a. nurse's progress notes.
    b. medication administration record.
    c. incident report.
    d. nursing plan of care.

8. The primary advantage that computerized documentation systems have over written methods is that they
   a. cost less than paper systems.
   b. decrease documentation time.
   c. protect patient confidentiality.
   d. allow alteration of documentation errors.

9. Which of the following statements regarding incident or occurrence reports is incorrect?
   a. Incident reports are most frequently filed due to client falls.
   b. Incident reports are filed to protect the client.
   c. An incident report can alert the facility's insurance company to a possible claim.
   d. When an incident report is filed, it should be documented in the nurse's notes.

10. Oral reporting is most effective when it
   a. includes all laboratory results.
   b. summarizes the entire care of the client.
   c. is structured and organized.
   d. takes place at the bedside.

Life Span Development

Key Terms

Match the following terms with their correct definitions.

___ 1. Accommodation

    a. Onset of the first menstrual period.

___ 2. Adaptation

    b. Component of cognitive development that allows for readjustment of the cognitive structure (mindset) in order to take in new information.

___ 3. Adolescence

    c. Component of cognitive development that involves taking in new experiences or information.

___ 4. Assimilation

    d. Developmental stage that occurs during the first 2 to 8 weeks after fertilization of a human egg.

___ 5. Bonding

    e. Developmental stage from the ages of 21 years through approximately 40 years.

___ 6. Critical period

    f. Developmental stage from the ages of 3 years to 6 years.

___ 7. Development

    g. Developmental stage from the ages of 40 years to 65 years.

___ 8. Developmental tasks

    h. Component of cognitive development that refers to the changes that occur as a result of assimilation and accommodation.

___ 9. Embryonic phase

    i. Time of the most rapid growth or development in a particular stage of the life cycle during which an individual is most vulnerable to stressors of any type.

___10. Fetal phase

    j. Developmental stage from the end of the first month to the end of the first year of life.

___11. Germinal phase

    k. Developmental stage beginning at approximately 12 to 18 months of age, when a child begins to walk, and ending at approximately age 3 years.

___12. Growth

    l. Individual's perception of self; includes self-esteem, body image, and ideal self.

___13. Infancy

    m. Ability to decide for oneself what is "right."

___14. Learning

    n. Certain goals that must be achieved during each developmental stage of the life cycle.

___15. Maturation

    o. Developmental stage that begins with conception and lasts approximately 10 to 14 days.

___16. Menarche

___17. Middle adulthood

___18. Moral maturity

___19. Neonatal stage

___20. Older adulthood

___21. Polypharmacy

___22. Preadolescence

___23. Prenatal stage

___24. Preschool stage

___25. Puberty

___26. School-age stage

___27. Self-concept

___28. Sexuality

___29. Spirituality

___30. Teratogenic substance

___31. Toddler stage

___32. Young adulthood

p. First 28 days of life following birth.

q. Developmental stage beginning with conception and ending with birth.

r. Quantitative (measurable) changes in the physical size of the body and its parts.

s. Developmental stage from the ages of approximately 10 years to 12 years.

t. Emergence of secondary sex characteristics that signals the beginning of adolescence.

u. Relationships with one's self, with others, and with a higher power or divine source.

v. Developmental stage from the ages of 12 years to 20 years that begins with the appearance of the secondary sex characteristics (puberty).

w. Developmental stage from the ages of 6 years to 10 years.

x. Behavioral changes in functional abilities and skills.

y. Intrauterine developmental period from 8 weeks to birth.

z. Process of becoming fully grown and developed; involves physiological and behavioral aspects.

aa. Formation of attachment between parent and child; begins at birth when neonate and parents make eye contact.

bb. Process of assimilating information, resulting in a change in behavior.

cc. Substance that can cross the placental barrier and impair normal growth and development.

dd. Developmental stage occurring from the age of 65 years until death.

ee. Recognition of or emphasis on sexual matters.

ff. The use of multiple drugs to treat singular conditions.

Abbreviation Review

Write the meaning or definition of the following abbreviations, acronyms, and symbols.

1. AIDS _____

2. BSE _____

3. CDC _____

4. CNS _____

5. FAS _____

6. PKU _____

7. STD _____

8. Td _____

9. TSE _____

Exercises and Activities

1. What is the difference between growth and development?

   _____

   _____

   _____

   a. How do each of the following factors influence growth and development?

   Heredity: _____

   _____

   Life experiences: _____

   _____

   Health status: _____

   _____

   Cultural expectations: _____

   _____

   b. Why is it important for the nurse to understand principles of growth and development?

   _____

   _____

2. According to the following theorists, at what stage would you find each of these individuals?

Age	Freud	Erikson	Piaget	Sullivan
Infant				
Toddler, age 2				
Adolescent, age 12				
Adult, age 40				

   a. What is your own developmental stage according to Erikson's stages of psychosocial development? Why did you select that stage?

   _____

   _____

   Describe yourself in terms of the task to be achieved.

   _____

   _____

   b. What is your stage of cognitive development according to Piaget?

   _____

   _____

How are you achieving the tasks for this stage?

_____

_____

3. Using the diagram, fill in at least one characteristic for each dimension of development (physiological, spiritual, moral, cognitive, psychosocial) for each individual.

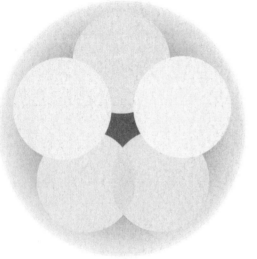

Preschooler, age 4

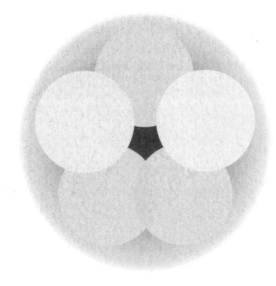

Young adult, age 21

Courtesy of Delmar Cengage Learning

List three nursing implications for each individual:

(1)_____   (1) _____

(2)_____   (2) _____

(3)_____   (3) _____

4. List two safety issues for each of the following age groups. Describe two interventions that you could discuss with parents.

Age Group	Safety Issues	Interventions
Newborn (first 4 weeks)	1. 2.	1. 2.
Infant (1 month to 1 year)	1. 2.	1. 2.
Toddler (12 months to 3 years)	1. 2.	1. 2.
Preschool (3–6 years)	1. 2.	1. 2.
School-age child (6–10 years)	1. 2.	1. 2.
Preadolescence (10–12 years)	1. 2.	1. 2.

5. Respond to the following scenarios.

   a. A.M. is a 16-year-old client who is being seen in the clinic for a sports physical examination. A.M.'s mother, however, expresses concern about her daughter's weight loss over the past several weeks and a change in eating patterns. A.M.'s height and weight are below normal for her age.

   What physiological and psychosocial changes might be particularly important for A.M.?

   _____

   _____

   _____

   _____

   If A.M. were to become your client in a hospital setting, what nursing implications would be important to consider in planning her care?

   _____

   _____

   How can you develop a trusting relationship with A.M.?

   _____

   _____

   What can you do to promote wellness with your adolescent client?

   _____

   _____

   b. T.O., a 2½-year-old child, was brought to the clinic for an immunization. His mother mentions to you that T.O. "still isn't toilet trained" and has become "really picky about what he'll eat." She is worried that he is not getting enough protein and vitamins now.

   Using your knowledge of growth and development for a toddler, how would you address his mother's concerns?

   _____

   _____

   What are the nursing implications for a toddler who is hospitalized?

   _____

   _____

   Why should wellness promotion begin in the early years?

   _____

   _____

6. L.C., a 53-year-old construction worker, comes to the clinic for a routine physical. What physiological changes occur during middle adulthood?

   _____

   _____

   _____

a. Why is maintaining physical activity important for L.C.at this point in his life?

_____

_____

b. It has been seven years since L.C.'s last tetanus shot. L.C. wonders if he should get another one since he is here. How should the nurse reply?

_____

_____

c. He also wonders about receiving a flu vaccination. How should the nurse respond?

_____

_____

d. What safety concerns should the nurse address with L.C. since he is middle-aged?

_____

_____

Self-Assessment Questions

Circle the letter that corresponds to the best answer.

1. The principles of growth and development include all but which of the following?
    a. Some stages are more critical than others.
    b. Development occurs in a head-to-toe direction.
    c. The pattern is continuous, orderly, and predictable.
    d. Development occurs in a distal to proximal manner.

2. An individual's ability to adapt effectively to stressors results primarily from
    a. life experiences.
    b. hereditary factors.
    c. a positive self-concept.
    d. moral maturity and spirituality.

3. The nurse encourages early and frequent parent–infant interaction to facilitate
    a. parenting skills.
    b. bonding and trust.
    c. anticipatory guidance.
    d. cognitive development.

4. The nurse caring for a toddler understands that the greatest source of stress in the hospital relates to the
    a. separation from the parents.
    b. lack of familiar surroundings.
    c. symptoms of the illness or injury.
    d. anxiety over medical procedures.

5. The nurse anticipating a teaching procedure for a 60-year-old client would include health screening recommendations, exercise and weight control, and
    a. coping with loss.
    b. suicide prevention.
    c. acceptance of aging.
    d. time management skills.

6. A 5-year-old child would be in Erikson's stage of
   a. autonomy vs. shame and doubt.
   b. initiative vs. guilt.
   c. industry vs. inferiority.
   d. identity vs. role confusion.

7. Which of these methods for bottle-feeding should *not* be avoided?
   a. Using the bottle as a pacifier
   b. Using the microwave to heat bottles
   c. Propping the bottle for feeding
   d. Placing the baby in a semireclining position

8. The nurse would teach a toddler's parent that
   a. using food as a reward is beneficial.
   b. serving large portions will ensure that the toddler eats.
   c. the toddler may have sporadic eating patterns.
   d. snacks are not necessary to meet dietary requirements.

9. In preadolescent boys, the first signs of puberty include
   a. testicular enlargement.
   b. pubic hair growth.
   c. thickening of the scrotum.
   d. both a. and b.

10. While assessing an adolescent, a nurse notices a neglect of personal hygiene and loss of interest in pleasurable activities. These can be signs of
    a. suicide risk.
    b. pain.
    c. rebelling.
    d. impulsive behavior.

Cultural Considerations

Key Terms

Match the following terms with their correct definitions.

_____ 1. Acculturation

_____ 2. Agnostic

_____ 3. Atheist

_____ 4. Cultural assimilation

_____ 5. Cultural diversity

_____ 6. Culture

_____ 7. Dominant culture

_____ 8. Ethnicity

_____ 9. Ethnocentrism

_____ 10. Minority group

_____ 11. Oppression

_____ 12. Race

_____ 13. Religious support system

a. Opposing forces that, when in balance, yield health.

b. Group of ministers, priests, rabbis, nuns, or laypersons who are able to meet clients' spiritual needs in the health care setting.

c. Cultural group's perception of itself or a group identity.

d. Process of learning norms, beliefs, and behavioral expectations of a group.

e. Process whereby individuals from a minority group are absorbed by the dominant culture and take on the characteristics of the dominant culture.

f. Dynamic and integrated structures of knowledge, beliefs, behaviors, ideas, attitudes, values, habits, customs, languages, symbols, rituals, ceremonies, and practices that are unique to a particular group of people.

g. Assumption of cultural superiority and an inability to accept other cultures' ways of organizing reality.

h. Condition wherein the rules, modes, and ideals of one group are imposed on another group.

i. Recognition of spiritual needs and the assistance given toward meeting those needs.

j. Individual who believes that the existence of God cannot be proved or disproved.

k. Differences among people that result from racial, ethnic, and cultural variables.

l. Group of people who constitute less than a numerical majority of the population and who, because of their cultural, racial, ethnic, religious, or other characteristics, are often labeled and treated differently from others in the society.

m. Individual's desire to find meaning and purpose in life, pain, and death.

____14. Spiritual care

n. Individual who does not believe in God or any other deity.

____15. Spiritual needs

o. Group whose values prevail within a society.

____16. Stereotyping

p. Grouping of people based on biological similarities such as physical characteristics.

____17. Yin and yang

q. Belief that all people within the same racial, ethnic, or cultural group act alike and share the same beliefs and attitudes.

Abbreviation Review

Write the meaning or definition of the following abbreviations.

1. WASP _____

2. WHO _____

Exercises and Activities

1. How do the terms *ethnicity* and *race* differ in meaning?

_____

_____

_____

a. How would you explain the term *cultural diversity* to another student?

_____

_____

b. In what ways does cultural diversity of health care workers, clients, and community populations affect you and your clients in today's health care settings?

_____

_____

2. Describe your own cultural background using the Cultural Assessment Guide.

_____

_____

_____

_____

_____

_____

CULTURAL ASSESSMENT GUIDE

Name _____

Other names or nicknames _____

Date of birth _____ Place of birth _____

Primary language _____ Other languages _____

Religious affiliation _____

Describe how you identify with your cultural group. _____

Define your ethnic group. _____

Describe your beliefs or customs about:

    Life _____

    Health _____

    Illness _____

    Death _____

How do you best learn?　Seeing (Visual) _____　Hearing (Auditory) _____
Doing (Kinesthetic) _____

What foods are forbidden by your religion or culture? _____
_____

What are your food preferences? _____

Give examples of your family's dietary habits. _____
_____

How do your religious practices and beliefs affect your life when in good health? _____
_____

When in poor health? _____

Who provides your health care services? _____
_____

What cultural health practices are you aware of, and which do you utilize? _____
_____

List cultural restrictions that your caregiver needs to know. _____
_____

Describe how your family members relate to and communicate with each other. _____
_____

What or who is your primary source of health information? _____
_____

What other cultural beliefs would you like to share? _____
_____

a. Choose two cultural groups different from your own. Compare and contrast your beliefs/customs concerning each of the following topics with what you know about those beliefs/customs of the other cultural groups.

Your Beliefs/Customs   *Cultural Group:*_____   *Cultural Group:*_____

Family structure

Time orientation

Religion

What causes disease

Who provides health care

Special healing practices

b. How might each of the following affect health care practices?

Religious beliefs: _____

_____

Family structure: _____

_____

Time orientation: _____

_____

Nutritional preferences: _____

_____

3. In which cultural or religious group would you find each of the following beliefs or health practices?

_____ Cupping may be used to draw out evil or illness.

_____ A talisman worn around the wrist or neck wards off disease.

_____ A healing ritual called the Blessingway ceremony may be performed.

_____ Traditional healers include the *curandero* and *yerbero*.

_____ Prayers to Allah may be offered five times a day.

_____ Traditional healers include the shaman.

_____ Illness can be eliminated through prayer and spiritual understanding.

_____ Male circumcision is a religious custom performed 8 days after birth.

_____ Blood and blood products are usually refused.

_____ A special undergarment may be worn that symbolizes dedication to God.

a. Describe how you might feel about caring for each of the following clients.

A client who relies on folk remedies and healers: _____

_____

A client who responds to pain in a different way than you: _____

_____

A client who is using healing rituals and ceremonies: _____

_____

b. In what ways does each of the following religions support the spiritual needs of an ill client?

Christian Science: _____

_____

Judaism: _____

_____

Islam: _____

_____

Protestantism: _____

_____

Roman Catholicism: _____

_____

4. You are assigned to care for Y.H., a 68-year-old client who has been admitted to your hospital for congestive heart failure. She and her husband have been in the United States for 2 months to visit their son and had planned on returning home before Y.H. became ill. As you enter her room to do a physical assessment, you note that she is wearing traditional clothing with only her face and hands exposed, rather than her hospital gown. Her husband, who speaks limited English, sits next to her. Y.H. appears anxious and uncomfortable but doesn't respond to your questions about pain. You want to help your client but are unfamiliar with her culture and religion.

a. In what ways can health care givers support Y.H.'s religious beliefs while she is hospitalized?

_____

_____

b. List two nursing diagnoses with cultural implications that might be appropriate for your client.

(1) _____

(2) _____

c. How can members of Y.H.'s family assist you in providing culturally sensitive nursing care?

_____

_____

d. If you are caring for a client of a cultural or religious group with which you are unfamiliar, how could you determine the special needs/support for your client?

_____

_____

e. Y.H. speaks very little English. How does the nurse explain care and treatment to Y.H.?

_____

_____

f. Y.H. family wishes to bring her food from home. She is on a general diet. How should the nurse respond to the request?

_____

_____

5. Nurses are expected to deliver culturally competent care. What does this statement mean?

_____

_____

_____

6. The nurse cares for a new refugee from Haiti. The client smiles and nods her head as if she is in agreement with the plan of care. How does the nurse validate that the client understands the treatments?

_____

_____

_____

   a. The client clutches an amulet tightly while the nurse is in the room. How should the nurse respond to this foreign object?

_____

_____

7. The nurse admitting M.K. to the unit for leukemia notes that M.K. is of the Jehovah's Witness faith. Explain how the usual treatment plan may have to be altered to accommodate M.K.'s faith.

_____

_____

_____

   a. What dietary accommodations should the nurse consider for M.K.?

_____

_____

8. J.B., an elderly Roman Catholic male patient, has pneumonia and is very ill. The priest visiting with him asks if J.B. may receive communion. How should the nurse respond?

_____

_____

   a. J.B.'s family asks for "last rites." Explain what this means.

_____

_____

   b. What should the nurse do if presented with the request for the Sacrement of the Sick?

_____

_____

Self-Assessment Questions

Circle the letter that corresponds to the best answer.

1. The first priority for the nurse providing culturally sensitive care is to
   a. accommodate differences when possible.
   b. identify the client's cultural/religious group.
   c. examine one's own cultural and personal beliefs.
   d. listen for cues in the client's conversation about ethnic beliefs.

2. A time orientation to the past may be demonstrated by which of the following cultural groups?
   a. Asian American
   b. Native American
   c. African American
   d. Hispanic American

3. The process of learning the norms, beliefs, and behaviors of a culture is referred to as
   a. ethnocentrism.
   b. cultural assimilation.
   c. socialization.
   d. acculturation.

4. The nurse is caring for an Asian American client who refuses ice water and the cold foods served for her meal. The nurse recognizes that because of the client's cultural background, her refusal is most likely due to her
   a. acceptance of a supernatural cause for disease.
   b. belief in a yin and yang etiology of disease.
   c. preference for her own family's foods.
   d. attempt to cleanse her body of unhealthy organisms.

5. Which of the following statements is true concerning cultural influence on health care?
   a. All cultures value health and good medical practice.
   b. Response to health and illness varies according to cultural origin.
   c. Knowing a client's cultural identity allows the nurse to make certain assumptions.
   d. Clients from all cultures respond positively to the nurse's caring touch.

6. An area not affected by culture is
   a. attitude.
   b. beliefs.
   c. values.
   d. All are affected by culture.

7. Labeling people according to cultural preconceptions is called
   a. oppression.
   b. stereotyping.
   c. cultural characteristics.
   d. ethnocentrism.

8. An inability to accept another culture's ways is called
    a. oppression.
    b. stereotyping.
    c. cultural characteristics.
    d. ethnocentrism.

9. Which statement is *not* an identified cultural characteristic?
    a. Culture is learned.
    b. Culture is integrated.
    c. Culture is inherited.
    d. Culture is dynamic.

10. Agnostics believe
    a. that the existence of God cannot be proved or disproved.
    b. that God does not exist.
    c. that a believer will reach an age of understanding.
    d. in reincarnation.

Stress, Adaptation, and Anxiety

Key Terms

Match the following terms with their correct definitions.

___ 1. Adaptation

___ 2. Adaptive energy

___ 3. Adaptive measure

___ 4. Anxiety

___ 5. Burnout

___ 6. Catharsis

___ 7. Change

___ 8. Change agent

___ 9. Conditioning

___10. Cognitive reframing

___11. Crisis

___12. Crisis intervention

___13. Defense mechanism

___14. Depersonalization

___15. Distress

a. State of physical and emotional exhaustion that occurs when caregivers deplete their adaptive energy.

b. Ongoing process whereby individuals use various responses to adjust to stressors and change.

c. Person who intentionally creates and implements change.

d. Measure used to avoid conflict or stress.

e. Teaching a person a behavior until it becomes an automatic response; method of conserving adaptive energy.

f. Inner forces that an individual uses to adapt to stress (phrase coined by Selye).

g. Stress that results in positive outcomes.

h. Any situation, event, or agent that produces stress.

i. Physiological response to a stressor (e.g., trauma, illness) affecting a specific part of the body.

j. Acute state of disorganization that occurs when the individual's usual coping mechanisms are no longer effective.

k. Measure for coping with stress that requires a minimal amount of energy.

l. Specific technique used to assist clients in regaining equilibrium.

m. State wherein the body becomes physiologically ready to defend itself by either fighting or running away from the danger.

n. Nonspecific response to any demand made on the body (Selye, 1974).

o. Subjective response that occurs when a person experiences a real or a perceived threat to well-being; a diverse feeling of dread or apprehension.

___16. Endorphins

p. Process of talking out one's feelings; "getting things off the chest" through verbalization.

___17. Eustress

q. Unconscious operation that protects the mind from anxiety.

___18. Fight-or-flight response

r. Dynamic process whereby an individual's response to a stressor leads to an alteration in behavior.

___19. General adaptation syndrome

s. Subjective experience that occurs when stressors evoke an ineffective response.

___20. Homeostasis

t. Physiological response that occurs when a person experiences a stressor.

___21. Local adaptation syndrome

u. Treating an individual as an object rather than as a person.

___22. Maladaptive measure

v. Balance or equilibrium among the physiological, psychological, sociocultural, intellectual, and spiritual needs of the body.

___23. Stress

w. Group of opiate-like substances produced naturally by the brain, which raise the pain threshold, produce sedation and euphoria, and promote a sense of well-being.

___24. Stressor

x. Stress-management technique whereby the individual changes a negative perception of a situation or event to a more positive, less threatening perception.

Abbreviation Review

Write the meaning or definition of the following abbreviations and acronyms.

1. CVA _____

2. GAS _____

3. LAS _____

4. NANDA _____

Exercises and Activities

1. Differentiate stress and anxiety.

_____

_____

_____

a. How are low levels of anxiety helpful to an individual?

_____

_____

b. What can happen when stress intensifies or continues for a long period?

_____

_____

c. What role does client education play in helping to manage stress?

_____

_____

    d. Why are a healthy diet and physical exercise valuable for stress management?

_____

_____

2. Think of a stressful event that has occurred in your life. Briefly describe the event or situation that was a source of stress.

_____

_____

_____

    a. What manifestations of stress did you experience (physiological, psychological, cognitive, behavioral, and spiritual)?

_____

_____

    b. What coping mechanisms did you use?

_____

_____

    c. If a similar situation would occur in the future, in what ways might you respond differently?

_____

_____

3. A nurse is working the night shift in a busy unit at a large tertiary care center. Her nursing responsibilities, which once seemed like a challenge, are now overwhelming. Clients are sicker; it seems like there is a constant staff shortage; and once again, the unit will have a new nurse manager. The nurse volunteered to work on two important nursing committees and has often adjusted her schedule to accommodate other staff members' needs. She thought working the night shift would give her more time with her family, but she has never adapted to sleeping during the day and seldom feels well rested. With two teenagers and a 9-year-old at home, there never seem to be enough hours in the day. She is becoming short-tempered at work and at home.

    a. How does stress contribute to burnout in the nursing profession?

_____

_____

    b. What are the stressors in the nurse's life?

_____

_____

    c. Suggest two strategies that she could use at work to help her cope.

_____

_____

    d. What would you recommend to this nurse to help her manage stress in her life?

_____

_____

4. C.G. is a 31-year-old father of two children, ages 8 and 5, and has been enjoying a successful career working for a construction company. He has recently been diagnosed with multiple sclerosis following progressive muscle weakness and now also with some problems with a visual disturbance. In addition to his medical bills and physical needs, he is worried about his job and the ability of his wife to handle additional responsibilities at home.

   a. Write two nursing diagnoses for C.G.

   (1) _____

   (2) _____

   b. C.G. may experience long-term stress related to his illness and possible job loss. In what ways might this affect his illness or adaptation?

   _____

   _____

   c. What specific suggestions could you make to help C.G.?

   _____

   _____

   d. Why would it be important to involve family members in this situation?

   _____

   _____

5. Explain how a person who is healthy demonstrates adaptation.

   _____

   _____

   _____

6. What are the characteristcs of a crisis?

   _____

   _____

   _____

   a. Explain how a crisis is *not* mental illness.

   _____

   _____

7. Describe how a nurse might be a change agent.

   _____

   _____

   _____

8. Identify three traits necessary for a nurse to adapt to change.

   (1) _____

   (2) _____

   (3) _____

9. The owner of a small business is in the hosipital on bedrest with a fractured leg. He tripped over an electric cord at work. As the nurse is providing care to him, he admits that he is worried about how his business is operating without him. He is concerned that OSHA will investigate his fall and whether his insurance will cover the cost of his hospitalization. Additionally, his wife just lost her job at a local factory, and his 16-year-old daughter wants to get married and move out of the house. The nurse recognizes that he needs to verbalize his feelings. What are the effects of verbalization?

_____

_____

_____

   a. The nurse recognizes that the client needs less stress and external stimuli. How can this be accomplished?

_____

_____

   b. What are some stress management techniques that the nurse can use with this client?

_____

_____

Self-Assessment Questions

Circle the letter that corresponds to the best answer.

1. A client with chronic obstructive pulmonary disease who continues to smoke may be exhibiting a defense mechanism called
   a. denial.
   b. avoidance.
   c. suppression.
   d. rationalization.

2. An individual's ability to use problem-solving skills to cope with stress or change is
   a. behavioral change.
   b. cognitive reframing.
   c. cognitive adaptation.
   d. psychological adaptation.

3. An individual's response to stressors, according to the general adaptation syndrome, occurs in three stages, which include alarm, resistance, and
   a. exhaustion.
   b. adaptation.
   c. homeostasis.
   d. fight-or-flight response.

4. Your client appears tense and is complaining of headache and nausea. Because your client has been dealing with a stressful situation for some time, you realize that these may be symptoms of
   a. mild anxiety.
   b. moderate anxiety.
   c. severe anxiety.
   d. denial.

5. A primary nursing intervention for the client experiencing mild anxiety is to
   a. provide limits and structure.
   b. develop appropriate diagnoses.
   c. minimize environmental stimuli.
   d. use the opportunity for teaching.

6. The nurse caring for a client who is experiencing panic should first
   a. encourage catharsis.
   b. maintain client safety.
   c. teach coping methods.
   d. focus the client on specific tasks.

7. Which statement is *not* an aspect of a stressor?
   a. A stressor is neutral.
   b. A pleasant event cannot be a stressor.
   c. The individual's perception of a stressor will determine its effect.
   d. A stressor can be internal or external.

8. Physiological effects that occur in the first stage of GAS are
   a. relaxation of respiratory muscles, maintenance of blood pressure, and slowing of the digestive system.
   b. inflammatory suppression, dilated pupils, and exhaustion.
   c. fluid retention, gluconeogenesis, and increased energy.
   d. epinephrine secretion, decrease in heart rate, and fatigue.

9. Physiological effects that occur in the second stage of GAS are
   a. relaxation of respiratory muscles, maintenance of blood pressure, and slowing of the digestive system.
   b. inflammatory suppression, dilated pupils, and exhaustion.
   c. fluid retention, gluconeogenesis, and increased energy.
   d. epinephrine secretion, decrease in heart rate, and fatigue.

10. Outcomes of stress include
    a. personal growth.
    b. disorganization.
    c. distress.
    d. All can be outcomes of stress.

End-of-Life Care

Key Terms

Match the following terms with their correct definitions.

____ 1. Advance directive

____ 2. Algor mortis

____ 3. Anticipatory grief

____ 4. Autopsy

____ 5. Bereavement

____ 6. Breakthrough pain

____ 7. Cheyne-Stokes respirations

____ 8. Complicated grief

____ 9. Death rattle

____10. Disenfranchised grief

____11. Dysfunctional grief

____12. End-of-life care

____13. Grief

____14. Health Care Surrogate Law

a. Breathing characterized by periods of apnea alternating with periods of dyspnea.

b. Persistent pattern of intense grief that does not result in reconciliation of feelings.

c. Imagining the feeling of horror felt by a victim or reliving the terror of an incident.

d. Form of reminiscence wherein a client attempts either to come to terms with conflict or to gain meaning from life and die peacefully.

e. Loss that occurs as a result of moving from one developmental stage to another.

f. Period of grief following the death of a loved one.

g. Care given immediately after death before the body is moved to the mortuary.

h. Covering for the body after death.

i. Decrease in body temperature after death, resulting in lack of skin elasticity.

j. Grief associated with traumatic death such as death by homicide, violence, or accident; a survivor suffers emotions of greater intensity than those associated with normal grief.

k. Bluish purple discoloration of the skin, usually at pressure points, that is a by-product of red blood cell destruction.

l. Funeral home.

m. Occurrence of grief work before an expected loss actually occurs.

n. Care that relieves symptoms, such as pain, but does not alter the course of disease.

___15. Hospice

o. Stiffening of the body that occurs 2 to 4 hours after death as a result of contraction of skeletal and smooth muscles.

___16. Life review

p. Sudden, acute, temporary pain that is usually precipitated by a treatment, a procedure, or unusual activity of the client.

___17. Liver mortis

q. "Grief that is not openly acknowledged, socially sanctioned, or publicly shared" (Doka, Rushton, & Thorstenson, 1994).

___18. Loss

r. Law enacted by some states that provides a legal means for decision making in the absence of advance directives.

___19. Maturational loss

s. Support measures implemented to restore consciousness and life.

___20. Mortuary

t. Grief reaction that normally follows a significant loss.

___21. Mourning

u. Any situation, either actual, potential, or perceived, wherein a valued object or person is changed or is no longer accessible to the individual.

___22. Palliative care

v. Examination of a body after death by a pathologist to determine cause.

___23. Postmortem care

w. Breathing sound in the period preceding death caused by a collection of secretions in the larynx.

___24. Resuscitation

x. Care of the terminally ill founded on the concept of allowing individuals to die with dignity and surrounded by those who love them.

___25. Rigor mortis

y. Loss that occurs in response to external events that are usually beyond the individual's control.

___26. Shroud

z. Period of time during which grief is expressed and resolution and integration of the loss occur.

___27. Situational loss

aa. Series of intense physical and psychological responses that occurs following a loss; a normal, natural, necessary, and adaptive response to a loss.

___28. Traumatic imagery

bb. Nursing care of the terminally ill that focuses on the physical and psychological needs of the patient and family.

___29. Uncomplicated grief

cc. Any written instruction recognized under state law, including a durable power of attorney, for health care or living will.

Abbreviation Review

Write the meaning or definition of the following abbreviations and acronyms.

1. ANA _____

2. DNR _____

3. HMO _____

4. IM _____

5. MS _____

6. NANDA _____

7. OBRA _____

8. PSDA _____

9. PTSD _____

10. SIDS _____

11. TB _____

Exercises and Activities

1. Why is mourning an important process for an individual who is experiencing a loss?

_____

_____

_____

   a. Briefly describe each of the following types of loss.

   External object: _____

   Familiar environment: _____

   Aspect of self: _____

   Significant other: _____

   b. Give two examples of loss for each developmental stage.

   Childhood   (1) _____

                            (2) _____

   Adolescence   (1) _____

                            (2) _____

   Early adulthood   (1) _____

                            (2) _____

   Middle adulthood   (1) _____

                            (2) _____

   Late adulthood   (1) _____

                            (2) _____

2. Choose one type of loss that you have experienced. Briefly describe the loss and any feelings of grief that may have accompanied it.

_____

_____

_____

   a. Did your feelings of grief resolve? If so, how long did the process take?

   _____

   _____

   b. What actions or statements by others were most helpful?

   _____

   _____

   c. Were any actions or statements not helpful?

_____

_____

3. Differentiate dysfunctional and disenfranchised grief.

_____

_____

_____

   a. Why might an abortion cause an individual to experience disenfranchised grief?

_____

_____

   b. How might the grief response differ for parents who have lost an infant to sudden infant death syndrome versus a neonatal death for other reasons?

_____

_____

   c. Why is the loss of a child considered one of the most difficult?

_____

_____

4. One of your clients today is N.W., a 25-year-old woman who is terminally ill with ovarian cancer, diagnosed shortly after the birth of her second child a few months ago. She completed a round of chemotherapy that was extremely difficult for her and had little effect on the cancer. After much thought, she has made the decision not to continue therapy. Her primary concern now is her husband and the welfare of her children. P.W. appears to be in denial at times, or is angry with her physician for not diagnosing the disease earlier. There are many issues he needs to face, including taking over the care of both children.

   a. According to Kübler-Ross's stages of dying and death, what stage do you feel N.W. is in?

_____

     What stage is her husband in?

_____

   b. How might anticipatory grief be helpful for her husband?

_____

_____

     How might it be a disadvantage?

_____

_____

   c. N.W. and P.W. have a 4-year-old child at home. How does a child at that age perceive dying?

_____

_____

d. What role could hospice play in helping N.W. and her family cope with her impending death?

_____

_____

e. N.W. and her husband have finally discussed her wishes concerning terminal care. What documents should she complete?

_____

_____

f. List four physiological changes that occur as death becomes imminent, and signs or symptoms that accompany each.

(1) _____

(2) _____

(3) _____

(4) _____

g. You find yourself having difficulty dealing with N.W.'s death, as you had become fond of her and very involved in her care. What symptoms might indicate that you are in need of grief counseling? What actions might be helpful to deal with the loss?

_____

_____

_____

_____

5. G.H. has multiple sclerosis that no longer reponds to treatment. His condition has deteriorated to the piont he is unable to swallow liquids, talk, or care for himself. He will be entering a hospice unit. How are hospice and palliative care different?

_____

_____

_____

a. M.H., his wife, would like to know what the goals of treatment for him are now. How does the nurse explain this to her?

_____

_____

b. M.H. is concerned that G.H. has lost interest in food and drink. How should the nurse explain this?

_____

_____

c. G.H. complains of pain and rates his pain as an 8 out of 10. he has a prescription for morphine liquid 10 mg every 4 hours, but it does not seem to be working. What can the nurse do to increase G.H.'s comfort level?

_____

_____

d. Explain the World Health Organization's three-step ladder for pain control.

_____

_____

e. G.H. can hardly speak because of the multiple sclerosis. What nonverbal cues will the nurse observe for when assessing his comfort level?

_____

_____

f. Why might Fentanyl become the drug of choice for pain managment with G.H.?

_____

_____

g. M.H. wants to stay with her husband around the clock. She tells the nurse that they have been married for 58 years and have never been apart. How can the nurse accommodate M.H.'s request?

_____

_____

h. A student nurse has been assigned to care for G.H. today. The nurse asks the student nurse to identify the physical signs of death. How does the student nurse respond?

_____

_____

i. G.H. finally dies and the nurse notes the time of death. The nurse has explained to the student nurse that the postmortem cares must be completed. What does this mean?

_____

_____

j. The nurse says she is relieved that G.H.'s suffering is finally over. The student nurse asks the nurse how the nurse handles her emotions. How should the nurse respond to the student?

_____

_____

Self-Assessment Questions

Circle the letter that corresponds to the best answer.

1. Your client experienced the death of her spouse several months ago. She continues to talk about him and the death repeatedly and is having difficulty eating and sleeping. This client is experiencing
   a. absent grief.
   b. detachment.
   c. dysfunctional grief.
   d. loss of patterns of conduct.

2. When dealing with a child who is experiencing the loss of a parent or sibling, the nurse should
   a. avoid using euphemisms like the person is "gone to sleep" in reference to death.
   b. offer thoughtful explanations about abstract ideas like death.
   c. encourage the child to get over the loss as quickly as possible.
   d. protect the child from potentially frightening places like the mortuary.

3. The nurse is caring for a client with terminal cancer. Nursing interventions for this client that focus on relieving symptoms such as pain are called
   a. respite care.
   b. palliative care.
   c. adjuvant therapy.
   d. anticipatory support.

4. The nurse understands that a client with a living will and durable power of attorney
   a. is required to sign the Patient Self-Determination form.
   b. relinquishes the right to make health care decisions.
   c. has a life-threatening disease or terminal illness.
   d. still needs a "do not resuscitate" medical order.

5. According to Kübler-Ross, the fifth and final stage of dying experienced by an individual is
   a. life review.
   b. resignation.
   c. acceptance.
   d. hopefulness.

6. The first stage of grief is
   a. acceptance.
   b. recovery.
   c. shock.
   d. anger.

7. During the second stage of grief, a person may feel
   a. anger and guilt.
   b. emotional numbness.
   c. able to live again.
   d. a positive attitude.

8. The *inability* to conclude grieving is called
   a. masked grief.
   b. exaggerated grief.
   c. delayed grief.
   d. chronic grief.

9. What developmental disruption may occur in a school-age child experiencing the loss of a parent?
   a. Long-lasting psychosocial problems
   b. Belief that death was his/her fault
   c. Potential death-avoidance behavior
   d. Difficulty forming intimate relationships

10. Which type of death with a negative stigma may prohibit survivors from successfully resolving their guilt?
    a. Unexpected death
    b. Suicide
    c. Traumatic death
    d. Neonatal death

Wellness Concepts

Key Terms

Match the following terms with their correct definitions.

___ 1. Genogram

___ 2. Health

___ 3. Prevention

___ 4. Primary prevention

___ 5. Secondary prevention

___ 6. Tertiary prevention

___ 7. Wellness

a. Early detection, diagnosis, screening, and intervention, generally before symptoms appear, to reduce the consequences of a health problem.

b. State of optimal health wherein an individual moves toward integration of human functioning, maximizes human potential, takes responsibility for health, and has greater self-awareness and self-satisfaction.

c. According to the World Health Organization, the state of complete physical, mental, and social well-being, not merely the absence of disease or infirmity.

d. Hindering, obstructing, or thwarting a disease or illness.

e. Treatment of an illness or disease after symptoms have appeared so as to prevent further progression.

f. All practices designed to keep health problems from developing.

g. Method of visualizing family members, their birth and death dates or ages, and specific health problems.

Abbreviation Review

Write the meaning or definition of the following abbreviations and acronyms.

1. AIDS _____

2. BMI _____

3. CDC _____

4. ECG _____

5. EKG _____

6. Hgb _____

7. HIV _____

8. LDL _____

9. Pap _____

10. PHS _____

11. SPF _____

12. USDHHS _____

13. WHO _____

Exercises and Activities

1. Write your own definition of wellness as you believe it applies to you. Include behaviors in each of the seven areas of wellness: emotional, mental, intellectual, vocational, social, spiritual, and physical.

   _____

   _____

   _____

   _____

   _____

   a. Choose three of the areas of wellness and describe what you could do to promote wellness for yourself in each of those areas.

   (1) _____

   (2) _____

   (3) _____

   b. Describe your concept of wellness as it might apply to an elderly client.

   _____

   _____

2. List three overall goals for the Healthy People 2010 objective.

   a. _____

   b. _____

   c. _____

3. Review Table 14-1 in your text. Look at the objectives for physical activity and fitness, nutrition, and AIDS/HIV infection. Briefly describe each objective and state whether the objective met the year 2000 target. If the target was not met, give a possible reason.

   Physical activity and fitness _____

   _____

   Nutrition _____

   _____

   AIDS/HIV infection _____

   _____

4. In what ways can nurses be involved in helping to achieve the goals of Healthy People 2010?

   _____

   _____

   _____

5. Why are preconception and prenatal health important?

_____

_____

_____

6. List the four factors affecting health. Describe the role each factor plays in determining the health of an individual.

a. _____

b. _____

c. _____

d. _____

7. Define each type of prevention and give two examples.

	Definition	*Examples*
Primary		(1)
		(2)
Secondary		(1)
		(2)
Tertiary		(1)
		(2)

8. N.T. is a 20-year-old college student who is studying computer programming. Although she finds her courses interesting, she is becoming increasingly stressed about her class load and grades. Struggling to maintain a passing average, she has started smoking again, after quitting 6 months ago. She has regained several pounds that she had previously lost through diet and exercise. To pay for classes, N.T. has been working 25 hours a week at a restaurant. Her boyfriend, with whom she is sexually active, tries to be supportive. Because of her schedule she has little time for exercise, and she knows she shouldn't be smoking but can't stop.

a. What health problems might N.T. encounter if she continues with her present lifestyle?

_____

_____

b. What changes would be most helpful to N.T. at this time?

_____

_____

c. Recommend three methods of stress reduction for N.T.

_____

_____

d. At N.T.'s age, what routine exams would you suggest she have?

_____

_____

e. After reviewing a genogram with information regarding N.T.'s family, you determine that she is also at an increased risk for osteoporosis. What steps could you recommend to N.T. that might prevent or reduce her risk for this disease?

_____

_____

Self-Assessment Questions

Circle the letter that corresponds to the best answer.

1. Which of the following areas has the most factors affecting health and wellness?
   a. Genetics and human biology
   b. Environmental influences
   c. Personal behavior
   d. Health care

2. Monthly breast self-examination is an example of which of the following?
   a. Primary prevention
   b. Secondary prevention
   c. Tertiary prevention
   d. Early intervention

3. A major goal of Healthy People 2010 is to
   a. increase access to preventive services.
   b. provide more health care workers.
   c. establish health care guidelines.
   d. identify concepts of wellness.

4. An important part of tertiary prevention is
   a. screening.
   b. rehabilitation.
   c. health promotion.
   d. consumer awareness.

5. A client who is experiencing excessive stress is at risk for accidents, heart disease, and
   a. stroke.
   b. cancer.
   c. diabetes.
   d. atherosclerosis.

6. Health care employers are required to provide
   a. child care.
   b. hepatitis B vaccination.
   c. stress reduction.
   d. prophylaxis exams.

7. A genogram should include
   a. one generation.
   b. two generations.
   c. three generations.
   d. four generations.

8. A guideline to promote healthy living for the prevention of heart disease can include
   a. a low-fiber diet.
   b. weekly exercise.
   c. having a physical exam every 5 years.
   d. maintaining an appropriate weight.

9. A guideline to promote healthy living for the prevention of cancer can include
   a. limiting smoking.
   b. a low-fiber diet.
   c. limiting alcohol intake.
   d. going to sun-tanning booths.

10. Wellness encompasses
    a. prevention.
    b. early detection.
    c. treatment of health problems.
    d. All are factors of wellness.

Self-Concept

Chapter 15

Key Terms

Match the following terms with their correct definitions.

___ 1. Body image

___ 2. Empowerment

___ 3. Ideal self

___ 4. Identity

___ 5. Public self

___ 6. Real self

___ 7. Role

___ 8. Role performance

___ 9. Self-awareness

___10. Self-concept

___11. Self-esteem

a. How one really thinks about oneself.

b. What individuals think others think of them.

c. Consciously knowing how the self thinks, feels, believes, and behaves at a specific time.

d. One's perception of physical self.

e. A helping process and partnerships through which individuals are enabled to make change.

f. An individual's perception of self.

g. Specific behaviors that a person exhibits in each role.

h. An ascribed or assumed expected behavior in a social situation.

i. The person that the client would like to be.

j. One's personal opinion of oneself.

k. An individual's conscious description of who he or she is.

Abbreviation Review

Write the meaning or definition of the following abbreviations, acronyms, and symbols.

1. NANDA _____

Exercises and Activities

1. What are some characteristics of clients with positive self-concepts?

_____

_____

_____

2. Using the memory trick **I LIKE ME**, identify nursing interventions used to promote a positive self-concept.

I _____

L _____

I _____

K _____

E _____

M _____

E _____

3. Discuss how health-related factors may affect body image.

_____

_____

_____

4. How might nurses teach clients to increase their self-image?

_____

_____

_____

5. Explain how an individual's self-concept develops across the life span.

Infancy _____

Childhood _____

Adolescence _____

Adulthood _____

Self-Assessment Questions

Circle the letter that corresponds to the best answer.

1. The nurse assesses the client's vital signs and gathers data about the client's health history and psychological factors such as spirituality. These specific behaviors are known as
   a. role performance.
   b. real self.
   c. public self.
   d. ideal self.

2. Which of the following factors reinforces the development of a healthy self-concept?
   a. An individual accomplishes a goal.
   b. An individual experiences failure.
   c. Individuals avoid their cultural heritage.
   d. Individuals experience stress.

3. B.R., age 38, found a lump on her breast. Following a biopsy that confirmed the diagnosis of breast cancer, B.R. is scheduled for a mastectomy. She says that she will never look at such an ugly scar and that her husband will not love her anymore. Which of the following *nursing diagnoses* would be appropriate for the nurses to use?
   a. *Disturbed* **Body** *Image*
   b. *Impaired* **Coping**
   c. *Risk for* **Loneliness**
   d. *Impaired Public* **Image**

4. A 15-year-old male client tells the nurse, "I'm a scrawny, stupid loser." This statement best reflects the client's:
   a. real self
   b. other self
   c. public self
   d. ideal self

5. A 22-year-old female client is struggling with low self-esteem. Which of the following activities could the nurse teach the client to help increase her self-esteem?
   a. indulge her sweet tooth and eat a pint of ice cream
   b. make a list of all her flaws
   c. tell herself she's fine just as she is
   d. learn something new

Spirituality

Key Terms

Match the following terms with their correct definitions.

___ 1. Faith

___ 2. Hope

___ 3. Meditation

___ 4. Prayer

___ 5. Religion

___ 6. Spiritual distress

___ 7. Spirituality

___ 8. Transcendence

___ 9. Values

a. A state of being or existence above and beyond the limits of material experience.

b. Communication with spiritual and divine entities.

c. Activity that brings the mind and spirit in focus on the present.

d. Disruption in the life principle that pervades a person's entire well-being.

e. Looking forward with hope and confidence.

f. Principles, standards, or qualities considered worthwhile or desirable.

g. A system of organized beliefs, rituals, and wishes to be associated with.

h. Confident belief in the truth, values, or trustworthiness of a person, idea, or things.

i. Core of a person's being.

Abbreviation Review

Write the meaning or definition of the following abbreviations, acronyms, and symbols.

1. ANA _____

2. NANDA _____

Exercises and Activities

1. Explain the difference between prayer and meditation.

   _____

   _____

   _____

2. The client would like to learn about meditation. What are some of the basic steps to meditation?

   _____

   _____

   _____

3. Describe the four ways in which parents transmit values to their children.

   a. _____

   b. _____

   c. _____

   d. _____

4. Discuss some of the ANA responsibilities for nurses who deal with spirituality issues.

   _____

   _____

   _____

5. What are some of the defining characteristics of spiritual distress?

   _____

   _____

   _____

6. Fill in the concept map for spiritual distress.

Connection to self

Connection with others

Nursing diagnosis: Spiritual Well-Being, Readiness for Enhanced

Connection with power greater than self

Connections with art, music, literature, or nature

Courtesy of Delmar Cengage Learning

Self-Assessment Questions

Circle the letter that corresponds to the best answer.

1. The client is of the Jehovah's Witness faith. The nurse understands that which of the following options are contraindicated, as it would cause spiritual distress?
   a. Drinking coffee
   b. Receiving blood products
   c. Having surgery
   d. Eating pork products

2. An American Indian client uses cedar and sage as part of a ceremonial experience. How might the nurse make accommodations to the treatment plan in order to prevent spiritual distress with this client?
   a. Provide privacy for the ceremony.
   b. Ask to participate in the ceremony.
   c. Call the hospital chaplain for permission.
   d. Refuse to allow the ceremony to occur.

3. A new patient is being admitted to the nursing unit in the hospital. Which of the following questions helps the nurse determine if there are issues related to spirituality?
   a. When do you pray?
   b. Where do you pray?
   c. May I place your prayer beads in the bedside stand?
   d. What religious practices are important to you?

4. The client refuses to eat meat on certain days because of religious beliefs, yet the client needs protein for wound healing. How could the nurse resolve this dilemma?
   a. Insist the client eat the meat provided.
   b. Ask the dietician to help find other protein sources.
   c. Ask the family to bring food from home.
   d. Offer the client extra liquids on the special days.

5. The client who is dying of cancer states, " I wish God would just take me." This is an example of
   a. hope.
   b. values.
   c. spiritual distress.
   d. grief.

Complementary/ Alternative Therapies

Key Terms

Match the following terms with their correct definitions.

___ 1. Acupressure

___ 2. Acupuncture

___ 3. Allopathic

___ 4. Alternative therapies

___ 5. Antioxidant

___ 6. Aromatherapy

___ 7. Biofeedback

___ 8. Bodymind

___ 9. Complementary therapies

___ 10. Curing

___ 11. Energy therapy

___ 12. Free radical

___ 13. Healing

a. Ridding of disease.

b. Altered state of consciousness or awareness resembling sleep and during which a person is more receptive to suggestion.

c. Folk healer-priest who uses natural and supernatural forces to help others.

d. Therapies used instead of conventional or mainstream medical practices.

e. Nonnutritive, physiologically active compounds present in plants in very small amounts; store nutrients and provide structure, aroma, flavor, and color.

f. Technique of releasing blocked energy within an individual when specific points (Tsubas) along the meridians are pressed or massaged by the practitioner's fingers, thumbs, and heel of the hands.

g. Measurement of physiological responses that yields information about the relationship between the mind and body and helps clients learn the way to manipulate these responses through mental activity.

h. Energy-based therapeutic modality that alters the energy fields through the use of touch, thereby affecting physical, mental, emotional, and spiritual health.

i. Quieting of the mind by focusing the attention.

j. Relaxation technique of using the imagination to visualize a pleasant, soothing image.

k. Therapies used in conjunction with conventional medical therapies.

l. Therapeutic use of concentrated essences or essential oils that have been extracted from plants and flowers.

m. Technique of application of heat and needles to various points on the body to alter the energy flow.

___14. Healing touch

n. Inseparable connection and operation of thoughts, feelings, and physiological functions.

___15. Hypnosis

o. Amino acids produced in the brain and other sites in the body that act as chemical communicators.

___16. Imagery

p. Study of the complex relationship among the cognitive, affective, and physical aspects of humans.

___17. Meditation

q. Application of pressure and motion by the hands with the intent of improving the recipient's well-being.

___18. Neuropeptide

r. Unstable molecules that alter genetic codes and trigger the development of cancer growth in cells.

___19. Neurotransmitter

s. A technique of assessing alterations in a person's energy fields and using the hands to direct energy to achieve a balanced state.

___20. Phytochemical

t. Chemical substances produced by the body that facilitate nerve-impulse transmission.

___21. Psychoneuroimmunoendo-crinology

u. Means of perceiving or experiencing through tactile sensation.

___22. Shaman

v. Practice of entering altered states of consciousness with the intent of helping others.

___23. Shamanism

w. Substance that prevents or inhibits oxidation, a chemical process wherein a substance is joined to oxygen.

___24. Therapeutic massage

x. Techniques of using the hands to direct or redirect the flow of the body's energy fields and thus enhance balance within those fields.

___25. Therapeutic touch

y. Process that activates the individual's recovery forces from within.

___26. Touch

z. Traditional medical and surgical treatment.

Abbreviation Review

Write the meaning or definition of the following abbreviations.

1. AAT _____

2. CA _____

3. FDA _____

4. NCAAM _____

5. NHI _____

6. PMR _____

7. PNIE _____

Exercises and Activities

1. How would you describe a nurse's role in complementary/alternative therapy?

   _____

   _____

   _____

   a. How would you explain the concept of the bodymind to another student?

   _____

   _____

2. For each of the following cultures, write a short description of its health perception and specific examples of modern therapies.

Culture	Health Perception	Modern Therapies
Greek culture		
Far East		
China		
India		

3. Differentiate the following terms: therapeutic massage; therapeutic touch; healing touch.

   a. List a benefit of each complementary/alternative therapy.

   (1) _____

   (2) _____

   (3) _____

4. List two primary benefits of each of the following complementary/alternative therapies and the types of conditions they may help.

Therapy		Primary Benefits	Types of Conditions
Guided imagery	(1)		
	(2)		
Biofeedback	(1)		
	(2)		
Yoga	(1)		
	(2)		
Shiatsu/acupressure	(1)		
	(2)		

a. Using Table 17-3, Medicinal Value of Selected Herbs, name two herbs a holistic practitioner might use for each of these conditions.

Healing a wound: _____

Mild depression: _____

Headache: _____

Common cold/sinus congestion: _____

b. Why should nurses encourage their clients to reveal the use of herbs to their primary care provider?

_____

_____

5. You have been working as an LP/VN at a long-term care facility since your graduation 6 months ago. The facility is pleasant, nicely decorated, and home to 64 residents. You particularly enjoy caring for C.S., whose daughter and granddaughter visit twice a week. On her next visit, the daughter mentions how much her father enjoyed his dog at home, a black Labrador retriever. She asks if this facility ever thought about having a pet therapy program. Apparently, many long-term care facilities are using pet therapy with very good results. You mention it to the supervising nurse, who asks you to evaluate the idea.

a. In what ways might a pet therapy program benefit the clients in this facility?

_____

_____

b. What issues would you need to consider?

_____

_____

c. What other types of complementary therapies might you consider for this facility?

_____

_____

d. If this were a long-term care facility for sick children, what complementary therapies might be appropriate?

_____

_____

Self-Assessment Questions

Circle the letter that corresponds to the best answer.

1. The use of complementary/alternative therapies is increasing because most are
   a. noninvasive and inexpensive.
   b. covered by insurance.
   c. easy to learn at home.
   d. spiritual in nature.

2. Because it deals with physiological, psychological, sociological, intellectual, and spiritual aspects of the individual, nursing can be described as
   a. comprehensive.
   b. complemental.
   c. humanistic.
   d. holistic.

3. The nurse explains that the benefits of meditation for the client include
   a. decreased oxygen consumption and blood pressure.
   b. enhanced stamina, agility, and balance.
   c. restoration of sensation and function.
   d. increased heart rate and lactic acid.

4. Chiropractic therapy is an example of which category of complementary/alternative intervention?
   a. Energetic touch
   b. Manipulative body based
   c. Mind/body therapy
   d. None of the above

5. Reflexology is a complementary/alternative therapy based on the
   a. shamanistic tradition.
   b. human energy fields.
   c. ancient healing arts.
   d. Ayurvedic system.

6. The nurse understands that massage therapy
   a. is also called therapeutic touch.
   b. is useful with clients from all cultural backgrounds.
   c. may be contraindicated in hypertension and diabetes.
   d. is a treatment modality specified in the Nursing Practice Act.

7. Which statement is *not* an assumption of therapeutic touch?
   a. A human being is a closed energy system.
   b. Anatomically, a human being is bilaterally symmetrical.
   c. Illness is a balance in an individual's energy field.
   d. Human beings cannot transcend their conditions of living.

8. What complementary/alternative therapy employs proper breathing, posture, and movement?
   a. Yoga therapy
   b. Chiropractic therapy
   c. Energy therapy
   d. Touch therapy

9. Contraindications for massage therapy are
   a. necrosis and stiffness.
   b. immobility and phlebitis.
   c. varicose veins and dermatitis.
   d. inflammation and stress.

10. Reflexology is the art and science of
    a. correcting areas of vertebral subluxation.
    b. releasing blocked energy within Tsubas.
    c. enervating the nerves in the feet.
    d. using the hands to realign the energy flow.

Basic Nutrition

Key Terms

Match the following terms with their correct definitions.

_____ 1. Absorption

    a. Constructive process of metabolism whereby new molecules are synthesized and new tissues are formed, as in growth and repair.

_____ 2. Anabolism

    b. Vitamin requiring the presence of fats for its absorption from the gastrointestinal (GI) tract into the lymphatic system and for cellular metabolism: vitamins A, D, E, and K.

_____ 3. Anthropometric measurements

    c. Pancreatic hormone that aids in the diffusion of glucose into the liver and muscle cells and in the synthesis of glycogen.

_____ 4. Atherosclerosis

    d. Measurement used to ascertain whether a person's weight is appropriate for height; calculated by dividing the weight in kilograms by the height in meters squared.

_____ 5. Basal metabolism

_____ 6. Body mass index

    e. Protein containing all nine essential amino acids.

    f. Coordinated, rhythmic, serial contraction of the smooth muscles of the gastrointestinal tract.

_____ 7. Calorie

    g. Lipid compound consisting of three fatty acids and a glycerol molecule.

_____ 8. Catabolism

    h. Process whereby the end products of digestion pass through the epithelial membranes in the small and large intestines and into the blood or lymph system.

_____ 9. Cholesterol

_____10. Chyme

    i. Equivalent to 1,000 calories.

    j. Vitamin that must be ingested daily in normal quantities because it is not stored in the body: vitamins C and B-complex.

_____11. Complete protein

    k. Chewing food into fine particles and mixing the food with enzymes in saliva.

_____12. Deglutition

_____13. Dehydration

    l. Conversion of amino acids into glucose.

    m. Measurements of the size, weight, and proportions of the body.

_____14. Diet therapy

    n. Swallowing of food.

____15. Dietary prescription/order

____16. Digestion

____17. Empty calories

____18. Enriched

____19. Enteral nutrition

____20. Euglycemia

____21. Excretion

____22. Extracellular fluid

____23. Fat-soluble vitamin

____24. Fortified

____25. Gluconeogenesis

____26. Glycogenesis

____27. Glycogenolysis

____28. Hypergylcemia

____29. Hypoglycemia

____30. Incomplete protein

____31. Ingestion

____32. Insensible water loss

____33. Insulin

____34. Intracellular fluid

____35. Ketosis

____36. Kilocalorie

o. All of the processes (ingestion, digestion, absorption, metabolism, and elimination) involved in consuming and utilizing food for energy, maintenance, and growth.

p. Fingerlike projections that line the small intestine.

q. Sum total of all the biological and chemical processes in the body as they relate to the use of nutrients in every body cell.

r. Lack of fluid in the tissues.

s. Feeding method, meaning both the ingestion of food orally and the delivery of nutrients through a GI tube, but generally meaning the latter.

t. Descriptor for food in which nutrients not naturally occurring in the food are added to it.

u. Lipoid composed of glycerol, fatty acids, and phosphorus; the structural component of cells.

v. Condition wherein blood glucose levels become too high as a result of the absence of insulin.

w. Organic compound that is insoluble in water but soluble in organic solvents such as ether and alcohol; also known as fats.

x. Energy needed to maintain essential physiological functions such as respiration, circulation, and muscle tone, when a person is at complete rest physically, digestively, and mentally.

y. Weight that is 20% or more above the ideal body weight.

z. Feeling of fulfillment.

aa. Elimination of drugs or waste products from the body.

bb. Condition wherein blood glucose levels are exceedingly low.

cc. Acidic, semifluid paste found in the GI tract.

dd. Chemical process of combining with oxygen.

ee. Treating a disease or disorder with a special diet.

ff. Protein with one or more of the essential amino acids missing.

gg. Cardiovascular disease of fatty deposits on the inner lining, the tunica intima, of vessel walls.

hh. Quantity of heat required to raise the temperature of 1 gram of water 1°C.

ii. Condition wherein acids called ketones accumulate in the blood urine, upsetting the acid–base balance.

jj. Order written by the physician for food, including liquids.

___37. Kwashiorkor

___38. Lipid

___39. Marasmus

___40. Mastication

___41. Metabolic rate

___42. Metabolism

___43. Monounsaturated fatty acid

___44. Nutrition

___45. Obesity

___46. Oxidation

___47. Parenteral nutrition

___48. Peristalsis

___49. Phospholipid

___50. Polyunsaturated fatty acid

___51. Satiety

___52. Sensible water loss

___53. Triglyceride

___54. Villi

___55. Vitamin

___56. Water-soluble vitamin

kk. The taking of food into the digestive tract, generally through the mouth.

ll. Fluid outside the cells, including plasma fluid, lymph, cerebrospinal fluid, interstitial fluid, and GI fluids.

mm. Destructive process of metabolism whereby tissues or substances are broken into their component parts.

nn. Conversion of glucose into glycogen.

oo. Sterol produced by the body and used in the synthesis of steroid hormones.

pp. Mechanical and chemical processes that convert nutrients into a physically absorbable state.

qq. Conversion of glycogen into glucose.

rr. Fluid within the cells.

ss. Feeding method whereby nutrients bypass the small intestine and enter the blood directly.

tt. Normal blood glucose level.

uu. Descriptor for food in which nutrients that were removed during processing are added back in.

vv. Calories that provide few nutrients.

ww. Rate of energy utilization in the body.

xx. Fluids we are not conscious of losing, such as fluid lost through normal respiration.

yy. Fluids we are aware of losing, such as fluid lost through urine.

zz. A condition that results from sudden or recent lack of protein-containing foods that manifests in the client as edema, painful skin lesions, and changes in the pigmentation of skin and hair.

aaa. A condition that afflicts very young children who lack protein, energy foods, vitamins, and minerals, observable in a client who has an emaciated look, dull and dry hair, and thin and wrinkled skin.

bbb. Foods in this category are nuts, fowl, and olive oil.

ccc. Foods in this category are fish, sunflower seeds, and spybeans.

ddd. Substances that regulate body processes and are necessary for metabolism of fats, carbohydrates, and proteins.

Abbreviation Review

Write the meaning or definition of the following abbreviations and symbols.

1. AI _____
2. BMI _____
3. CHO _____
4. CHON _____
5. CI _____
6. CNS _____
7. dL _____
8. DNA _____
9. DRI _____
10. EAR _____
11. ECF _____
12. FDA _____
13. Fe _____
14. ft _____
15. g _____
16. GI _____
17. I&O _____
18. ICF _____
19. in _____
20. K^+ _____
21. kcal _____
22. kg _____
23. lb _____
24. Mg _____
25. mg _____
26. mL _____
27. Na _____
28. NG _____
29. NLEA _____
30. NPO _____
31. oz _____
32. P _____
33. RBC _____
34. RDA _____
35. RNA _____
36. S _____
37. TF _____

38. TPN _____
39. UL _____
40. USDA _____
41. WBC _____
42. Zn _____

Exercises and Activities

1. Label the food groups on the food guide pyramid and include the recommended number of servings.

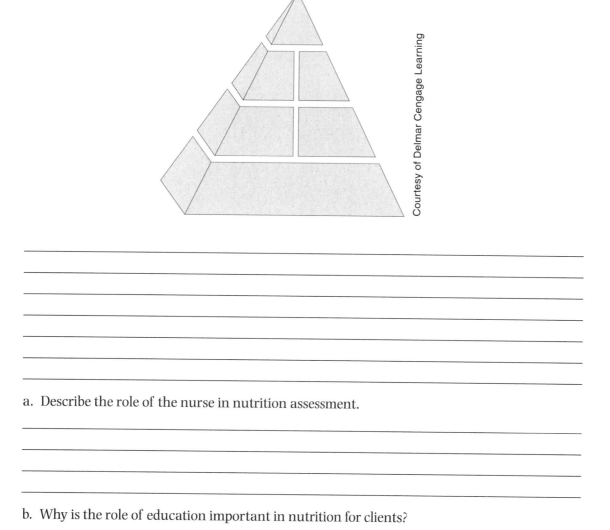

_____
_____
_____
_____
_____
_____

a. Describe the role of the nurse in nutrition assessment.

_____
_____
_____

b. Why is the role of education important in nutrition for clients?

_____
_____
_____
_____

2. Label the parts of the digestive system. Write a major function for each.

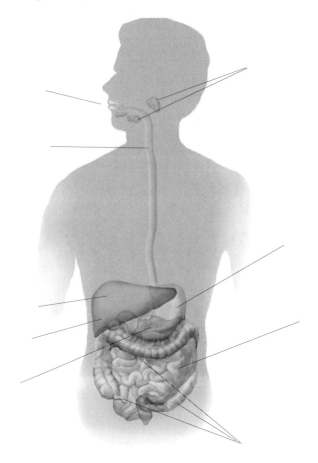

Courtesy of Delmar Cengage Learning

   a. What is the function for each of these nutrients?

   Water _____

   Carbohydrates _____

   Fats _____

   Proteins _____

   Vitamins _____

   Minerals _____

3. Calculate the desired weight and caloric needs for each of the following clients.

   a. The first client is a male who is 5 ft. 11 in. tall, with a large build.

   Desired weight _____

   Basal energy needs _____

   This client's actual weight is 215 lb. What would be his actual basal energy needs?

   Actual weight: 210 ÷ 2.2 = _____ kg

   _____ kg × 1 × 24 = _____ basal kcal (basal energy needs)

   He maintains a moderately active lifestyle. Determine his total energy requirements:

   _____ (basal kcal) × _____ = _____ total kcal

   Is this client considered obese? _____

b. Your second client is a female who is 5 ft. 2 in. tall, with a small build.

Desired weight _____

Basal energy needs _____

Her actual weight is 97 lb. Determine her actual basal energy needs.

Actual weight: 97 ÷ 2.2 = _____ kg

_____ kg × 1 × 24 = _____ basal kcal (basal energy needs)

She maintains a sedentary lifestyle. What are her total energy requirements?

_____ (basal kcal) × _____ = _____ total kcal

Is this client considered underweight? _____

4. List signs and symptoms of poor nutritional status in each of the following.

Skin: _____

_____

Hair: _____

_____

Nails: _____

_____

Eyes: _____

_____

Weight: _____

_____

Activity: _____

_____

a. What information would you include in a presentation to adolescents about healthy nutrition?

_____

_____

b. How do the physical changes of aging affect nutritional status in the older adult client?

_____

_____

c. List three interventions that can support a healthy nutritional intake for the older client.

(1) _____

(2) _____

(3) _____

d. How can an adequate caloric intake be maintained with the client who is unable to chew food or swallow well?

_____

_____

5. R.W., 29 years old, appears healthy and well nourished on her first prenatal visit. Her weight, at 134 lb., seems appropriate for her height of 5 ft. 4 in. Findings on her physical assessment indicate good nutritional status. She has been a vegetarian for 5 years and would like to know what adjustments she might need to her diet while she is pregnant.

   a. Why is good nutrition important during pregnancy?

   _____

   _____

      How many grams of protein are recommended for this client before pregnancy?

      _____ lb ÷ 2.2 lb/kg = _____ kg

      _____ kg × 0.8 g/kg = _____ gm protein/day

   How does this requirement change for her pregnancy?

   b. Describe one tool that could be used to assess her nutritional intake.

   _____

   _____

   c. What items need to be included for a complete nutritional assessment for this client?

   _____

   _____

   d. Describe any recommendations you would include for her vegetarian diet.

   _____

   _____

   e. What information will you give R.W. about the benefits of lactation for her infant?

   _____

   _____

Self-Assessment Questions

Circle the letter that corresponds to the best answer.

1. Signs of calcium deficiency include osteoporosis, tetany, poor tooth formation, and
   a. rickets.
   b. scurvy.
   c. anemia.
   d. pellagra.

2. Without sufficient carbohydrates, the body converts protein into glucose for energy. This process is called
   a. ketosis.
   b. catabolism.
   c. glycogenolysis.
   d. gluconeogenesis.

3. Which of the following statements is incorrect regarding nutrition needs for the older client?
   a. Calorie needs decrease about 2% to 3% every 10 years.
   b. Water requirements decrease along with fewer total calories.
   c. Canned foods should be avoided if there are cardiac problems.
   d. Protein requirements are stable, about 12% to 14% of total calories.

4. To ensure an adequate nutritional intake of zinc to promote wound healing, your client's diet should include
   a. meat, milk, and whole grains.
   b. bananas, oranges, and prunes.
   c. legumes, raisins, and apricots.
   d. legumes and green leafy vegetables.

5. The client with ulcerative colitis or Crohn's disease may be advised to avoid
   a. eggs, cheese, and milk.
   b. breads, cereal, and rice.
   c. raw fruits and whole grains.
   d. animal fats and milk products.

6. While caring for your client, you note decreased skin turgor, sunken eyes, and weight loss. Which of the following findings would the nurse anticipate?
   a. Increased venous filling times
   b. Decreased body temperature
   c. Increased protein intake
   d. Decreased urine output

7. The constructive process of metabolism is called
   a. catabolism.
   b. anabolism.
   c. oxidation.
   d. basal metabolism.

8. Inorganic nutrients include
   a. carbohydrates.
   b. fats.
   c. vitamins.
   d. minerals.

9. Which is *not* a source for sensible water loss?
   a. Urine
   b. Diarrhea
   c. Respiration
   d. Vomit

10. What type of carbohydrate requires no digestion and is quickly absorbed?
    a. Monosaccharides
    b. Disaccharides
    c. Polysaccharides
    d. Glycogen

Rest and Sleep

Key Terms

Match the following terms with their correct definitions.

___ 1. Biological clock

___ 2. Bruxism

___ 3. Cataplexy

___ 4. Chronobiology

___ 5. Circadian rhythm

___ 6. Hypersomnia

___ 7. Insomnia

___ 8. Narcolepsy

___ 9. Parasomnia

___ 10. REM disorder

___ 11. Rest

___ 12. Restless leg syndrome

___ 13. Sleep

___ 14. Sleep apnea

a. Alteration in sleep pattern characterized by excessive sleep, especially in the daytime.

b. Condition characterized by profoundly disturbed sleep due to behavioral or physiological events.

c. State of altered consciousness during which an individual experiences fluctuations in level of consciousness, minimal physical activity, and general slowing of the body's physiologic processes.

d. Grinding of teeth during sleep.

e. Syndrome wherein breathing periodically ceases during sleep for a period of 30 to 60 seconds; often associated with heavy snoring.

f. State of relaxation and calmness, both mental and physical.

g. Science of studying biorhythms.

h. Difficulty in falling asleep initially or in returning to sleep once awakened.

i. Sleep alteration manifested as sudden uncontrollable urges to fall asleep during the daytime.

j. Condition wherein the paralysis normally occurring during REM sleep is absent or incomplete and the sleeper acts out the dream that is occurring.

k. Condition characterized by uncomfortable sensations of tingling or crawling in the muscles, and twitching, burning, prickling, or deep aching in the foot, calf, or upper leg when at rest (lying or sitting).

l. Biorhythm that cycles on a daily basis.

m. Sudden loss of muscle control.

n. Internal mechanism capable of measuring time in a living organism.

___15. Sleep cycle

___16. Sleep deprivation

o. Sleepwalking.

p. Sequence of sleep that begins with the four stages of non–rapid eye movement sleep in order, with a return to stage 3 and then stage 2, followed by passage into the first rapid eye movement stage.

___17. Sleep hygiene

___18. Somnambulism

q. Prolonged inadequate quality and quantity of sleep.

r. Client's habits in preparing for sleep.

Abbreviation Review

Write the meaning or definition of the following abbreviations and acronyms.

1. CPAP _____

2. EEG _____

3. NANDA _____

4. NREM _____

5. NSF _____

6. NSRED _____

7. PLMD _____

8. PMS _____

9. REM _____

10. RLS _____

Exercises and Activities

1. Differentiate the terms *rest* and *sleep.* In what ways is each important to the health/wellness of an individual?

_____

_____

_____

a. What do you do at bedtime to help you sleep?

_____

_____

b. In what ways, if any, has school affected your ability to rest or sleep?

_____

_____

c. If you were hospitalized for a brief period, in what ways do you think it would affect your sleep patterns?

_____

_____

2. What impact might illness or the health care setting have on each of the following factors affecting sleep? List two interventions for each factor that could help promote rest/sleep for clients.

Factor	Impact of Illness/Health Care	Interventions
Physical		(1) (2)
Psychological		(1) (2)
Environmental		(1) (2)
Lifestyle		(1) (2)
Diet		(1) (2)

a. What effect does medication have on rest and sleep?

_____

_____

3. Describe REM sleep. How does it differ from NREM sleep?

_____

_____

_____

a. What is the importance of adequate REM sleep for an individual?

_____

_____

b. Describe the sleep pattern for a school-age child. What interventions might help the child to get adequate rest/sleep in a health care setting?

_____

_____

c. Describe the sleep pattern for an older adult. What interventions might encourage rest and sleep in these clients?

_____

_____

4. L.P., a 68-year-old client, is scheduled for surgery in the morning. When you assessed him earlier, he seemed comfortable. You are making rounds again at 1 A.M. and you find him still awake. When you ask if he needs anything, L.P. assures you that he is fine, but he "just can't seem to get to sleep." You ask if he is having any pain, and he says he is fairly comfortable right now. After a little more discussion, you decide that he might be anxious about his surgery. You also note that his room seems a little warm, and his roommate, who is sleeping soundly, is also snoring loudly.

a. What nursing diagnosis might be appropriate for L.P.?

_____

_____

b. What factors could be interfering with his ability to sleep?

_____

_____

c. Describe interventions that you could use to encourage this client to sleep.

_____

_____

d. L.P. is being discharged home. When his wife arrives, she says, "At least I was able to get a little more sleep while he was in the hospital. He usually wakes me up several times a night at home." What questions might you want to ask his wife?

_____

_____

_____

Self-Assessment Questions

Circle the letter that corresponds to the best answer.

1. Your client has a history of loud snoring, breathing pauses of 30 to 60 seconds, and daytime sleepiness. Based on this sleep assessment, your client may be experiencing
   a. narcolepsy.
   b. parasomnia.
   c. sleep apnea.
   d. hypersomnia.

2. A somnambulist is an individual who
   a. has difficulty falling asleep.
   b. has daytime sleepiness.
   c. treats sleep disorders.
   d. sleepwalks.

3. All but which of the following are treatments used for sleep apnea?
   a. Dental appliances
   b. Medication
   c. Surgery
   d. CPAP

4. The nurse is conducting a sleep assessment on an elderly client. The nurse understands that the client is at increased risk for
   a. restless leg syndrome.
   b. somnambulism.
   c. hypersomnia.
   d. sleep terrors.

5. The client with sleep apnea is at a greater risk for hypertension and
   a. narcolepsy.
   b. headache.
   c. bruxism.
   d. stroke.

6. A nurse who works on the night shift is at greater risk of sleep deprivation due to an alteration in
   a. environment.
   b. lifestyle.
   c. aging.
   d. diet.

7. Nearly half of normal adult NREM sleep is spent in
   a. stage 1.
   b. stage 2.
   c. stage 3.
   d. stage 4.

8. What food items frequently disrupt sleep?
   a. Alcohol and tea
   b. Spicy foods and chips
   c. Cola and snacks
   d. Chocolate and coffee

9. A medication that may cause insomnia is
   a. hydroxyzine.
   b. diphenhydramine.
   c. captopril.
   d. amitriptyline.

10. The hallmark symptom of narcolepsy is
    a. cataplexy.
    b. snoring.
    c. leg movements.
    d. bruxism.

Safety/Hygiene

Key Terms

Match the following terms with their correct definitions.

d 1. Body image
j 2. Chemical restraint
c 3. Dental caries
e 4. Gingivitis
h 5. Halitosis
b 6. Hygiene
k 7. Perineal care

n 8. Physical restraint
g 9. Poison

a 10. Pyorrhea
l 11. Restraint

i 12. Self-care deficit

f 13. Sensory overload
m 14. Stomatitis

a. Periodontal disease.
b. Science of health.
c. Cavities.
d. Individual's perception of physical self, including appearance, function, and ability.
e. Inflammation of the gums.
f. Increased perception of the intensity of auditory and visual stimuli.
g. Any substance that when taken into the body interferes with normal physiologic functioning; may be inhaled, injected, ingested, or absorbed by the body.
h. Bad breath.
i. State wherein an individual is not able to perform one or more activities of daily living.
j. Medication used to control client behavior.
k. Cleansing of the external genitalia and perineum and the surrounding area.
l. Protective device used to limit the physical activity of a client or to immobilize a client or extremity.
m. Inflammation of the oral mucosa.
n. Equipment that reduces the client's movement.

Abbreviation Review

Write the meaning or definition of the following abbreviations and acronyms.

1. ADL activities of daily living
2. CDC _____
3. CHD _____
4. CMS _____

5. CPR _____

6. FDA _____

7. GCS _____

8. HDL _____

9. ID _____

10. JCAHO _____

11. MSDS _____

12. NANDA _____

13. OBRA _____

14. OSHA _____

15. PCA _____

Exercises and Activities

1. Why is safety an important issue for clients?

   nurses are responsible for providing professional, quality care to the client in a safe environment.

   a. Why is safety important for health care workers?

   #1 priority. A safe environment reduces the risk of accidents and subsequent alterations in health and life style. Also cost of health care services.

   b. In what ways does OSHA assist health care workers?

   "Right to know laws.

   pg. 417

   c. Explain right-to-know laws.

   employee right to know laws state that employees are legally entitled to info. regarding hazardous substance!

   d. What is contained on a material safety data sheet?

   _____

   _____

2. You have been asked to help with orientation for new nursing students at your facility. What would you include in a safety presentation to them? Include safety measures for clients and for the nursing students.

   _____

   _____

   _____

   _____

   _____

   _____

a. What safety instructions would you give to a client who has recently been admitted to your facility?

_____

_____

3. Why is fire such a serious risk in a health care facility?

because of immobilized and incapacitated clients... softy is our # one concern.

_____

a. List five interventions that can prevent or reduce the risk of fire in the health care setting.

(1) five exits are marked clearly

(7) know where fire extiguishers are and how to use them

(2) practice fire evacuation procedures

(3) keep halls clear of obstacles

(4) post emergency phone # near phone

(5) check electrical cords for damage

(6) teach clients about fire hazards

b. What would you do if a fire were discovered?

R.A.C.E. = rescue individuals, activate 911, confine the fire, evacuate/extinguish fire

4. Describe risk factors and list three interventions for each developmental age to facilitate safety.

Developmental Age	Risk Factors	Interventions
Infant/toddler	-explore enviorment	(1) Careful adult supervision (2) (3)
School-age child	-explore enviorment outside the home	(1) Stranger awareness (2) trafic safty (3) protective equipment
Adolescent/ young adult	-death- car accident -STD -substance abuse -violence -pregnancy	(1) Educational efforts of parents, schools and community health (2) care providers must focus on (3) environmental safty.
Adult	-anxiety -sleep -fatigue -altered health -strain maintenance	(1) exercise, nutritions (2) Occupational safty (3)

a. How does the aging process affect a client's safety?

- falls cause injury -loss of muscle stregth
- poor vision   - loss of balance
- effects of medication - disease

b. In what ways does proper hygiene promote health or healing for the client?

provides comfort/relaxation, self image, promotes cleanliness/ healthy skin. Its part of client safty

5. S.J. is an 83-year-old client with a history of congestive heart failure and pneumonia that has resolved. She is also healing from a right hip fracture that resulted from a fall at home. Medications include a diuretic and occasional mild analgesic for pain. S.J. responds slowly when you try to get her attention and is often confused about where she is. Her appetite is usually poor, but she will take about half her food with some encouragement. Caregivers refer to her as "frail" and have noted reddened areas over her back and left ankle. Although she is in a wheelchair for part of the day, she has lost strength and mobility in her legs and spends most of her time in bed. She is usually incontinent.

a. Evaluate S.J.'s risk status for skin integrity using Table 20-1 in your text.

_____

_____

b. What fall risk factors are present for this client?

_____

_____

c. List several interventions that could protect S.J. from injury.

(1) _____

(2) _____

(3) _____

(4) _____

(5) _____

(6) _____

(7) _____

(8) _____

d. Restraints have been ordered for S.J. to be used during the night. What special precautions must be taken?

_____

_____

e. You are prepared to medicate S.J. and discover that she has no identification band. How would you proceed?

_____

_____

f. If S.J. were to be transferred to home care with portable oxygen, what safety advice would you give to her family?

_____

_____

Self-Assessment Questions

Circle the letter that corresponds to the best answer.

1. The nurse discovers a fire in a client's room. The first priority for the nurse is
   a. ensuring the client's safety. ①
   b. calling the fire department. ②
   c. trying to extinguish the fire. ④
   d. closing doors to other rooms. ③

2. A client with wrist restraints in place must be assessed at least every 2 hours for
   a. vital signs.
   b. range of motion.
   c. proper body mechanics.
   d. circulation and sensation.

3. Which of the following statements is correct regarding personal hygiene of the client?
   a. Gloves are not needed for bathing a client. ✗
   b. It is best when performed by nursing staff. ✗
   c. Clients should be encouraged to perform their own perineal care.
   d. Reddened areas on the skin should be massaged during the bath. ✓

4. Assessment of the client's hair during shampoo and combing can provide information about the client's
   a. skin integrity.
   b. medication use.   Pg. 433
   c. fall risk potential.
   d. general health status.

5. Periodontal disease can be prevented through
   a. regular dental care.
   b. good oral hygiene.
   c. using fluoride drops.
   d. massaging the gums.

6. The organization that outlines and enforces regulations that all health facilities must follow with regard to employees and exposure to and handling of potentially infectious materials is
   a. MSDS.
   b. CDC.   Occupational Safty and Health Administration
   c. OSHA.
   d. FDA.   Pg. 417

7. What is it called when a client is not able to perform one or more activities of living?
   a. Risk for injury
   b. Personal preference
   c. Precautionary feedback
   d. Self-care deficit

8. All are safe alternatives to side-rail use except
   a. a low-height bed.
   b. a bed mats.
   c. a bed alarm.
   d. a motion sensor.

9. An alternative to restraint use is
   a. placing the call light in reach.
   b. providing bathroom breaks every 4 hours.
   c. removing extra pillows and blankets.
   d. maintaining the hospital schedule.

10. What type of fire extinguisher would you use for an electrical fire?
    a. Class A - wood, paper, cloth
    b. Class B - liquids → grease, gas, oil   Pg. 429
    c. Class C - electrical
    d. Class D - metals

Infection Control/ Asepsis

Key Terms

Match the following terms with their correct definitions.

d 1. Acquired immunity

oo 2. Agent

x 3. Airborne transmission

ii 4. Antibody

tt 5. Asepsis

rv 6. Aseptic technique

z 7. Bactericide

aaa 8. Biological agent

qa 9. Carrier

k 10. Chain of infection

pp 11. Chemical agent

q 12. Clean object

hh 13. Cleansing

a. Transfer of an agent to a susceptible host by animate means such as mosquitoes, fleas, ticks, lice, and other animals.

b. Practices that reduce the number, growth, and spread of microorganisms.

c. Microorganisms that occur or have adapted to live in a specific environment, such as intestinal, skin, vaginal, or oral flora.

d. Formation of antibodies (memory B cells) to protect against future invasions of an already experienced antigen.

e. Physical transfer of an agent from an infected person to a host through direct contact with that person, indirect contact with an infected person through a fomite, or close contact with contaminated secretions.

f. Process of invasion by and multiplication of pathogenic microorganisms that occurs in body tissue and results in cellular injury.

g. Practices that eliminate all microorganisms and spores from an object or area.

h. Transfer of an agent to a susceptible host by contaminated inanimate objects such as food, milk, drugs, and blood.

i. Route by which an infectious agent enters the host.

j. Object contaminated with an infectious agent.

k. Phenomenon of the development of an infectious process.

l. Infection that was acquired in a hospital or other health care facility and was not present or incubating at the time of the client's admission.

m. Microorganisms that attach to the skin for a brief period of time but do not continuously live on the skin.

_W_ 14. Colonization

_ll_ 15. Communicable agent

_r_ 16. Communicable disease

_y_ 17. Compromised host

_e_ 18. Contact transmission

_ff_ 19. Dirty object

_ss_ 20. Disinfectant

_zz_ 21. Disinfection

_jj_ 22. Edema

_xx_ 23. Erythema

_c_ 24. Flora

_j_ 25. Fomite

_v_ 26. Germicide

_p_ 27. Hand hygiene

bbb 28. Hospital-acquired infection

_aa_ 29. Host

_kk_ 30. Humoral immunity

_gg_ 31. Immunization

ccc 32. Incubation period

_f_ 33. Infection

_mm_ 34. Infectious agent

_vv_ 35. Inflammation

_cc_ 36. Localized infection

_o_ 37. Medical asepsis

_ll_ 38. Mode of transmission

n. Frequency with which a pathogen causes disease.

o. Microorganisms that are always present, usually without altering the client's health.

p. Rubbing together of all surfaces and crevices of the hands using a soap or chemical and water, followed by rinsing in a flowing stream of water.

q. Object on which there are microorganisms that are usually not pathogenic.

r. Disease caused by a communicable agent.

s. Microorganism that causes disease.

t. Person who lacks resistance to an agent and is thus vulnerable to disease.

u. Infectious agent transmitted to a client by direct or indirect contact, via vehicle, vector, or airborne route.

v. Chemical that can be applied to both animate and inanimate objects for the purpose of eliminating pathogens.

w. Multiplication of microorganisms that occurs on or within a host but does not result in cellular injury.

x. Transfer of an agent to a susceptible host through droplet nuclei or dust particles suspended in the air.

y. Person whose normal defense mechanisms are impaired and who is therefore susceptible to infection.

z. Bacteria-killing chemicals found in tears.

aa. Simple or complex organism that can be affected by an agent.

bb. Inoculation with a vaccine to produce immunity against specific diseases.

cc. Infection limited to a defined area or single organ.

dd. Place where the agent can survive.

ee. Total elimination of all microorganisms, including spores.

ff. Object on which there is a high number of microorganisms, some of which are potentially pathogenic.

gg. Process of creating immunity or resistance to infection in an individual.

hh. Removal of soil or organic material from instruments and equipment used in providing client care.

ii. Protein substance that counteracts and neutralizes the effects of antigens and destroys bacteria and other cells.

jj. Detectable accumulation of increased interstitial fluid.

kk. Stimulation of B cells and antibody production.

ll. Process that bridges the gap between the portal of exit of the infectious agent from the reservoir or source and the portal of entry of the susceptible "new" host.

_l_ 39. Nosocomial infection

_s_ 40. Pathogen

_ww_ 41. Pathogenicity

_yy_ 42. Physical agent

_i_ 43. Portal of entry

_nn_ 44. Portal of exit

_dd_ 45. Reservoir

_o_ 46. Resident flora

_ee_ 47. Sterilization

_q_ 48. Surgical asepsis

_t_ 49. Susceptible host

_uu_ 50. Systemic infection

_m_ 51. Transient flora

_bb_ 52. Vaccination

_a_ 53. Vector-borne transmission

_h_ 54. Vehicle transmission

_n_ 55. Virulence

mm. Microorganism that causes infection.

nn. Route by which an infectious agent leaves the reservoir.

oo. Entity capable of causing disease.

pp. Substance that interacts with a host, causing disease.

qq. Person who harbors an infectious agent but has no symptoms of disease.

rr. Infection control practice used to prevent the transmission of pathogens.

ss. Chemical solution used to clean inanimate objects.

tt. Absence of microorganisms.

uu. Infection that affects the entire body with involvement of multiple organs.

vv. Nonspecific cellular response to tissue injury.

ww. Ability of a microorganism to produce disease.

xx. Increased blood flow to an inflamed area.

yy. Factor in the environment capable of causing disease in a host.

zz. Elimination of pathogens, with the exception of spores, from inanimate objects.

aaa. Living organism that invades a host, causing disease.

bbb. Nosocomal infection.

ccc. Time interval between entry of an infectious agent in the host and the onset of symptoms.

Abbreviation Review

Write the meaning or definition of the following abbreviations, acronyms, and symbols.

1. AIDS _____

2. APIC _____

3. CDC _____

4. DNA _____

5. EPA _____

6. ESR _____

7. HBV _____

8. HCV _____

9. HIV _____

10. NANDA _____

11. OR _____

12. OSHA _____

13. pH _____

14. RNA _____

15. TB _____

16. WBC _____

Exercises and Activities

1. Differentiate the terms *infection* and *inflammation*.

   infection is the invasion and multiplication of pathogenic microorganims in body tissue that results in cellular injury. Inflammation is nonspecific cellular response to tissue injury.

   a. Briefly describe the five stages of the inflammatory process.
      (1) inital injury
      (2) Blood flow increases
      (3) Increase capillary permeability leaks out large amount of plasma into damaged tissue
      (4) Leukocytes infiltrate + cleanup bacteria
      (5) Damage tissues are replaced

   b. Describe each of the four stages of the infection process.
      (1) Incubation stage
      (2) Prodromal stage
      (3) illness stage
      (4) Convalescent stage

   c. How would you explain nosocomial infection to another student?
      Infection acquired in the hospital / Rehab

2. Match the essential element on the left with its appropriate location in the diagram.

Source ✓

Biological agent ✓

Susceptible host ✓

Mode of transmission ✓

Portal of entry to host ✓

Portal of exit from source ✓

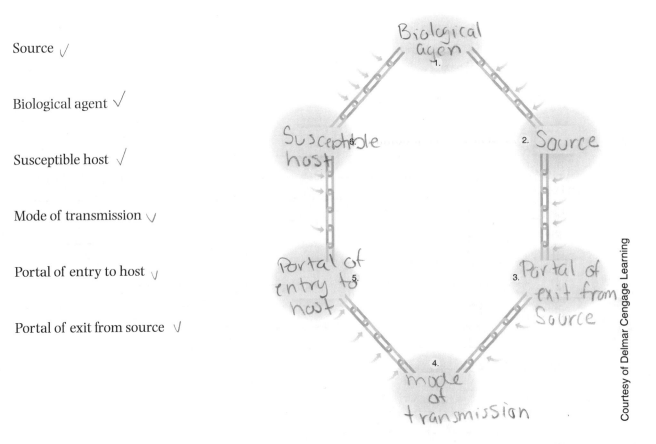

Courtesy of Delmar Cengage Learning

a. Give one specific method to break the chain of infection among the preceding links for the common cold virus.

Modes of transmission: Contact transmission.
Chain broken by wearing gloves, gowns, masks,
Proper disposal of of contaminated objects and Hand
Hygine!

b. What makes hand hygiene the first line of defense for infection control?

to prevent infection control

c. Describe several characteristics that make an individual a more susceptible host for infections.

Age, concurrent diseases, stress,
Immunization/vaccination status, Lifestyle,
nutritional status Heredity

3. In what way is education important for prevention of disease

a. for health care workers?

to break the chain of infection

b. for clients and family members?

to understand why precautions are
taken w/ loved ones

c. You are preparing to talk to the parents of a 5-year-old child who will be attending school. What suggestions can you include about preventing infection and disease (immunizations, staying healthy, avoiding spread of illness, and so on)?

hand washing, good nutrition, sleep,
current immunizations

4. A.W. is a 77-year-old client admitted to a long-term care facility following several small strokes that have affected her ability to speak and swallow. Her nurse notes that A.W.'s nutritional status is poor, and she appears to have difficulty coughing up secretions effectively. Her activity level has greatly diminished, and she spends most of her time in bed. The nurse is concerned because several visitors and staff members have recently become ill with a flu virus.

a. What factors make this client a more susceptible host for disease?

b. List two nursing diagnoses for A.W..

(1) _____

(2) _____

c. How can this client strengthen her immune system?

d. Identify possible fomites in this health care environment.

_____

_____

Self-Assessment Questions

Circle the letter that corresponds to the best answer for each question.

1. Chemical agents that can cause disease include pesticides, food additives, and
   a. spores.
   b. fomites.
   c. radiation.
   d. medications.

2. The most effective way to reduce the incidence of nosocomial infection is for health care workers to
   a. use germicide solutions on all surfaces.
   b. wash hands frequently and thoroughly.
   c. understand the chain of infection transmission.
   d. use aseptic technique with all medical procedures.

3. The nurse notes that the client has a low-grade fever and fatigue following exposure to the measles virus. The nurse understands that the client
   a. will be contagious within 3 days.
   b. is in the incubation period of the disease.
   c. is in the prodromal phase and is contagious.
   d. is in the illness stage, with signs and symptoms of measles.

4. A nurse is preparing to perform a urinary catheterization on a client. For this procedure, the nurse will
   a. maintain a sterile field and surgical asepsis.
   b. use gowning and a closed gloving technique.
   c. dispose of wastes in a sharps-disposal container.
   d. perform the catheterization using medical aseptic technique.

5. A mother is requesting antibiotics to treat a sore throat and cough in her 5-year-old child. The use of antibiotics may be discouraged for which of the following reasons?
   a. The child is too young to benefit from antibiotics.
   b. Antibiotics may impair the child's natural immunity.
   c. The medication may not be covered by health insurance.
   d. Antibiotics destroy normal flora and may not be effective.

6. Microorganisms that are always present are called
   a. resident flora.
   b. pathogens.
   c. bacteria.
   d. viruses.

7. Organisms that can live only inside the cell are called
   a. resident flora.
   b. pathogens.
   c. bacteria.
   d. viruses.

8. All of the following are types of agents capable of causing disease except
   a. bacteria and heat.
   b. pesticides and light.
   c. viruses and fomites.
   d. fungi and medication.

9. Which is *not* an example of a contact mode of transmission?
   a. Secretion from a client
   b. Coughing
   c. Bathing
   d. Specimen containers

10. An example of a specific immune defense is
    a. an antibody
    b. skin
    c. mucous membrane
    d. inflammation

Standard Precautions and Isolation

Key Terms

Match the following terms with their correct definitions.

_C_ 1. Airborne Precautions

_i_ 2. Aseptic Technique

_K_ 3. Barrier Precautions

_d_ 4. Contact Precautions

_f_ 5. Droplet Precautions

_H_ 6. Endemic

_l_ 7. Epidemic

_g_ 8. Hospital-acquired infection

_a_ 9. Isolation

_b_ 10. Reverse isolation

a. Separate from other persons, especially those with infectious diseases.

b. Barrier protection designed to prevent infection in clients who are severely compromised and highly susceptible to infection; also known as protective isolation.

c. Measures taken in addition to Standard Precautions and for clients known to have or suspected of having illnesses spread by airborne droplet nuclei.

d. Measures taken in addition to Standard Precautions and for clients known to have or suspected of having illnesses easily spread by direct client contact or contact with fomites.

e. Practices designed for clients documented as or suspected of being infected with highly transmissible or epidemiologically important pathogens for which additional precautions beyond the Standard Precautions are required to interrupt transmission in hospitals.

f. Measures taken in addition to Standard Precautions and for clients known to have or suspected of having serious illnesses spread by large-particle droplets.

g. Infection that is acquired in the hospital and was not present or incubating at the time of the client's admission.

h. Occurring continuously in a particular population and having low mortality.

i. Infection control practice used to prevent the transmission of pathogens.

j. Preventive practices to be used in the care of all clients in hospitals regardless of diagnosis or presumed infection status.

⟍ 11. Standard Precautions

k. Use of personal protective equipment, such as masks, gowns, and gloves, to create a barrier between the person and the microorganisms and thus prevent transmission of the microorganism.

ℓ 12. Transmission-Based Precautions

l. Infecting many people at the same time and in the same geographic area.

Abbreviation Review

Write the meaning or definition of the following abbreviations and acronyms.

1. AIDS _____

2. BSI _____

3. CDC _____

4. DHHS _____

5. HBV _____

6. HICPAC _____

7. HIV _____

8. MDR _____

9. OSHA _____

10. TB _____

Exercises and Activities

1. In what ways have infection control practices changed since 1985?

_____

_____

_____

a. What is the purpose of the Hospital Infection Control Practices Advisory Committee?

_____

_____

2. What is the role of the nurse in preventing the spread of nosocomial infections?

_____

_____

_____

a. List five actions or techniques to help reduce your occupational exposure to infection and disease.

(1) _____

(2) _____

(3) _____

(4) _____

(5) _____

b. How does reverse isolation protect clients who are highly susceptible to infection?

_____

_____

3. Describe Standard Precautions.

Preventative practices to be used in care of all clients in hospitals regardless of diagnosis or presumed infection status

a. How do Standard Precautions differ from Universal Precautions?

_____

_____

b. Why were Transmission-Based Precautions added to Standard Precautions for infection control procedures?

_____

_____

c. Describe each of the following types of Transmission-Based Precautions:

Airborne Precautions: *Used when clients are suspected to have serious illness spread by airbord droplet*

Contact Precautions: *Used when clients have suspected serious illness. Direct contact w/ client*

Droplet Precautions: *Used when clients are suspected of having illness spread by large particle droplets*

d. Which type of precautions would be appropriate for each of the following diseases?
   (1) Airborne
   (2) Contact
   (3) Droplet
   _3_ Pneumonia
   _2_ Chickenpox
   _3_ Scarlet fever
   _2_ Scabies
   _1_ Measles
   _3_ Rubella
   _2_ Impetigo
   _3_ Meningitis

   _3_ mumps
   _1_ tuberculosis
   _1_ Varicella
   _2_ wound
   _2_ respiratory infection
   _2_ Herps
   _3_ influenza

4. E.Y. is a 74-year-old client who was hospitalized for several days for treatment of dehydration and a gastrointestinal disorder. He is now improving his hydration and nutrition status but has been developing a pressure ulcer on his right buttock. The nurse caring for E.Y. today notes that the wound is open and draining. The drainage from the wound appears purulent and has a foul odor.

a. What types of precautions should be followed in providing this client's care?

_____

_____

b. Describe barrier precautions that will be used by E.Y.'s nurse.

_____

_____

c. If gloves are used while providing care for E.Y., why is hand hygiene still essential?

_____

_____

d. Do family members need to follow any special precautions while visiting E.Y.?

_____

_____

e. How would you address family members' concerns about why this client is now being "isolated."

_____

_____

Self-Assessment Questions

Circle the letter that corresponds to the best answer.

1. The primary impact of the CDC guidelines in 1970 and 1975 was to
    a. introduce Body Substance Isolation.
    b. determine seven categories of isolation.
    c. establish Blood and Body Fluid Precautions.
    d. allow users to decide which guideline was appropriate for a given situation.

2. The most important and basic aspect of Standard Precautions is to
    a. know the medical diagnosis.
    b. limit contact with the client.
    c. wash hands frequently.
    d. use gown and gloves.

3. A nurse is caring for a client who is suspected of having pulmonary tuberculosis. The nurse will use personal protective equipment that includes
    a. goggles.
    b. sterile gloves.
    c. a surgical mask.
    d. an N95 respirator.

4. The nurse caring for a client diagnosed with varicella zoster (shingles) will use
    a. Contact Precautions.
    b. Universal Precautions.
    c. barrier nursing procedures.
    d. a negative air pressure room.

5. The nurse is most likely to use reverse isolation with a client who
   a. has a latex allergy.
   b. is immunocompromised because of chemotherapy.
   c. requires multiple medical procedures.
   d. may have a serious undiagnosed disease.

6. A client is noted to have purulent drainage from a wound. The nurse caring for this client will first
   a. tell the client about precautions to take at home.
   b. encourage all personnel to use good hand hygiene.
   c. institute appropriate precautions and obtain a culture.
   d. speak with the physician the next day about precautions.

7. According to OSHA regulations, all health care facilities must provide
   a. hepatitis B vaccine at a minimal charge.
   b. protective equipment.
   c. training about occupational exposure every 2 years.
   d. containers for sharps disposal every 6 feet.

8. Used needles can only be:
   a. capped using the one-handed "scoop" technique.
   b. recapped using both hands.
   c. broken for disposal.
   d. thrown away.

9. What is the appropriate type of precaution for a client with diphtheria?
   a. Airborne
   b. Contact
   c. Droplet
   d. Precautions are not needed for this client.

10. Which is *not* a psychological intervention for the client in isolation?
    a. Encouraging verbalization of feelings
    b. Encouraging visitors with appropriate barrier precautions
    c. Supporting existing coping mechanisms
    d. Discussing with team members the isolation process

Bioterrorism

Key Terms

Match the following terms with their correct definitions.

___ 1. Anthrax

___ 2. Bioterrorism

___ 3. Centers for Disease Control and Prevention

___ 4. Chemical, Biological, Radiological, Nuclear, and Explosive Enhanced Response Force Packages

___ 5. Chemical warfare agent

___ 6. Expeditionary medical support

___ 7. First responders

___ 8. Nerve agents

___ 9. Plague

___10. Radiation sickness

___11. Ricin

___12. Sarin

___13. Smallpox

___14. Terrorism

___15. Zoonotic disease

a. A highly contagious and frequently fatal viral disease.

b. Using any product, weapon, or threat of using a harmful act or substance to kill or injure others.

c. Disease caused by *Bacillus anthracis* bacteria.

d. A total package that includes everything necessary to screen and treat clients.

e. Poison made from castor beans.

f. Result of exposure to ionizing radiation.

g. EMEDS package plus a surgical suite.

h. Fast-acting clear, colorless, tasteless gas.

i. First people who respond to emergency situations.

j. Powerful acetycholinesterase inhibitors.

k. Gases, liquids, or solids that cause injury and death to people, plants, or animals.

l. Federal agency whose goal is to promote health and quality of life.

m. Purposeful use of biological agents for the purpose of harming, killing, and/or instilling fear.

n. Infection caused by the *Yersina pestis* bacteria.

o. Disease of animals that is directly transmissible to humans from the primary animal host.

Abbreviation Review

Write the meaning or definition of the following abbreviations and acronyms.

1. CDC _____

2. CERFPS _____

3. EMEDS _____

4. EOP _____

5. FEMA _____

6. KI _____

7. SNS _____

8. VMI _____

9. VX _____

Exercises and Activities

1. Using Table 23–1 in the text as a reference, describe the three categories of biological agents.

   Category A _____

   Category B _____

   Category C _____

2. Why are biological agents advantageous to use as a weapon?

   _____

   _____

   _____

3. E.C. is a dairy farmer in an area of the Upper Midwest that has naturally occurring anthrax bacteria. What are the three forms of human anthrax?

   _____

   _____

   _____

   a. Explain the most likely cause of E.C.'s anthrax disease.

   _____

   _____

   b. Why is exposure to anthrax spores a particular problem?

   _____

   _____

   c. Why would E.C.'s case not be considered terrorism?

   _____

   _____

   d. If E.C. develops cutaneous anthrax, describe what the lesions look like.

   _____

   _____

   e. What antibiotics would E.C. be most likely to receive if he had no known drug allergies?

   _____

   _____

4. Explain how the smallpox virus causes infection.

_____

_____

_____

   a. Describe the symptoms of smallpox.

_____

_____

   b. If smallpox can be prevented by vaccination, explain why mass vaccinations are no longer recommended.

_____

_____

   c. What precautions would a nurse need to make if a client were diagnosed with smallpox?

_____

_____

5. Plague is considered to be a zoonotic disease. What does this mean?

_____

_____

_____

   a. How is the transmission of bubonic and pneumonic plague different?

_____

_____

   b. How would a terrorist use the plague bacteria as a weapon?

_____

_____

   c. How soon should antibiotics be administered to a plague victim?

_____

_____

6. Identify chemicals that could be used for terrorism.

_____

_____

_____

   a. What was the intended use of chemical agents introduced in World War I?

_____

_____

7. Explain the role of FEMA in a bioterrorism event.

_____

_____

_____

8. How does the Strategic National Stockpile work?

_____

_____

_____

Self-Assessment Questions

Circle the letter that corresponds to the best answer.

1. If a terrorist group uses sarin as a weapon, which actions would a first responder take first?
   a. Move the victims into fresh air.
   b. Remove the contaminated clothing.
   c. Flush the exposed area with copious amounts of water.
   d. Induce vomiting.

2. Following the atomic bomb in Hiroshima, Japan, in World War II, those that were exposed to high doses of radiation developed
   a. skin cancers.
   b. leukemia.
   c. pneumonia.
   d. heart attacks.

3. Potassium iodide (KI) is given in the event of a nuclear explosion. Which of the following is true of KI usage?
   a. It prevents lung cancer.
   b. It prevents radioactive iodine from entering the thyroid gland.
   c. KI protects all the organs of the endocrine system.
   d. It must be taken for two weeks following exposure.

4. JCAHO requires hospitals to have Emergency Operations Plan. What is contained in an Emergency Operations Plan?
   a. Information on how to activate the plan
   b. Who to notify at federal levels
   c. Who to notify at state levels
   d. Which security personnel to call

5. A nurse is caring for a patient who developed anthrax in the respiratory form. What precautions should the nurse take for herself?
   a. Standard precautions when working with bodily fluids.
   b. No precautions necessary, as it is not contagious in the respiratory form
   c. Strict isolation
   d. Respiratory precautions

Fluid, Electrolyte, and Acid–Base Balance

Key Terms

Match the following terms with their correct definitions.

____ 1. Acid

____ 2. Acidosis

____ 3. Alkalosis

____ 4. Anion

____ 5. Arterial blood gases

____ 6. Atom

____ 7. Base

____ 8. Buffer

____ 9. Cation

___10. Compound

___11. Crenation

___12. Decomposition

___13. Dehydration

___14. Dialysis

___15. Diffusion

___16. Edema

a. Decreased oxygen level in the blood.

b. Pressure that a fluid exerts against a membrane; also called filtration force.

c. Solution that has the same molecular concentration as does the cell; also called an isosmolar solution.

d. Substances combined in no specific way.

e. Measurement of levels of oxygen, carbon dioxide, pH, partial pressure of oxygen, partial pressure of carbon dioxide, saturation of oxygen, and bicarbonate in arterial blood.

f. Substance that attempts to maintain pH range, or hydrogen ion concentration, in the presence of added acids or bases.

g. Condition wherein cells decrease in size, shrivel and wrinkle, and are no longer functional when in a hypertonic solution.

h. Condition wherein more water is lost from the body than is replaced.

i. Seepage of fluid into the interstitial tissue as a result of accidental dislodgement of the IV needle from the vein.

j. Pressure exerted against the cell membrane by the water inside a cell.

k. Membrane that allows passage of only certain substances.

l. Normal resiliency of the skin.

m. Equilibrium (balance); consistency of body fluids.

n. Rupture of red blood cells due to osmosis.

o. Administration of fluids, electrolytes, nutrients, or medications by the venous route.

p. Fluid in tissue spaces around each cell.

___17. Electrolyte

q. Measurement of the total concentration of dissolved particles (solutes) per kilogram of water.

___18. Element

r. Diffusion used to separate molecules out of a solution by passing them through a semipermeable membrane.

___19. Extracellular fluid

s. Substance that when dissociated produces ions that will combine with hydrogen ions.

___20. Filtration

t. Condition characterized by an excessive number of hydrogen ions in a solution.

___21. Hemolysis

u. In a solution, liquid, or gas, movement of molecules from an area of high molecular concentration to one of low molecular concentration.

___22. Homeostasis

v. Element or compound that, when dissolved in water or another solvent, dissociates (separates) into ions (electrically charged particles).

___23. Hydrostatic pressure

w. Fluid within the cells.

___24. Hypertonic solution

x. Atoms of the same element that have different atomic weights (i.e., different numbers of neutrons in the nucleus).

___25. Hypotonic solution

y. Product formed when an acid and a base react with each other.

___26. Hypoxemia

z. Concentration of solutes per liter of cellular fluid.

___27. Infiltration

aa. Anything that occupies space and possesses mass.

___28. Interstitial fluid

bb. Ion bearing a positive charge.

___29. Intracellular fluid

cc. Condition characterized by an excessive loss of hydrogen ions from a solution.

___30. Intravascular fluid

dd. Smallest unit of an element that still retains the properties of that element that cannot be altered by any chemical change.

___31. Intravenous therapy

ee. Detectable accumulation of increased interstitial fluid.

___32. Ion

ff. Solution that has a lower molecular concentration than the cell; also called hypo-osmolar solution.

___33. Isotonic solution

gg. Process of fluids and the substances dissolved in them being forced through the cell membrane by hydrostatic pressure.

___34. Isotopes

hh. Diffusion from a region of higher concentration to a region of lower concentration.

___35. Matter

ii. Joined with oxygen.

___36. Mixture

jj. Chemical reaction when two or more atoms, called reactants, bond and form a more complex molecular product.

___37. Molecule

kk. Fluid outside of the cells; includes interstitial, intravascular, synovial, cerebrospinal, and serous fluids; aqueous and vitreous humor; and endolymph and perilymph.

___38. Osmolality

___39. Osmolarity

___40. Osmosis

___41. Osmotic pressure

___42. Oxidized

___43. Permeability

___44. Potential hydrogen (pH)

___45. Salt

___46. Semipermeable membrane

___47. Synthesis

___48. Turgor

ll. Fluid consisting of the plasma in the blood vessels and the lymph in the lymphatic system.

mm. Atoms of the same element that unite with each other.

nn. Ability of a membrane to permit substances to pass through it.

oo. Any substance that in a solution yields hydrogen ions bearing a positive charge.

pp. Ion bearing a negative charge.

qq. Combination of atoms of two or more elements.

rr. Chemical reaction wherein the bonding between atoms in a molecule is broken and simpler products are formed.

ss. Solution that has a higher molecular concentration than the cell; also called a hyperosmolar solution.

tt. Basic substance of matter.

uu. Atom bearing an electrical charge.

vv. The measure of acid and base strength.

Fill in the Blank

Fill in the blanks with information from the key terms used in this chapter.

1. An _____ is an ion bearing a negative charge.

2. A _____ is an ion bearing a positive charge.

3. An _____ is an atom bearing an electrical charge.

4. An _____ is a basic substance of matter.

Abbreviation Review

Write the meaning or definition of the following abbreviations, acronyms, and symbols.

1. ABG _____

2. ADH _____

3. ATP _____

4. BP _____

5. BUN _____

6. Ca^{++} _____

7. CBC _____

8. Cl^- _____

9. CO_2^- _____

10. COOH _____

11. CNS _____

12. D_5W _____

13. dL _____

14. ECF _____

15. GI _____

16. H^+ _____

17. H_2CO_3 _____

18. H_2O _____

19. HCl _____

20. HCO_3^- _____

21. Hct _____

22. Hgb _____

23. I&O _____

24. ICF _____

25. IV _____

26. K^+ _____

27. KCl _____

28. kg _____

29. L _____

30. lb. _____

31. mEq _____

32. mg _____

33. Mg^{++} _____

34. mL _____

35. mm Hg _____

36. MOM _____

37. mOsm/kg _____

38. Na^+ _____

39. NaCl _____

40. NaH_2PO_4 _____

41. $NaHCO_3$ _____

42. $NaHPO_4$ _____

43. NaOH _____

44. NH_2 _____

45. NPO _____

46. O_2 _____

47. OH _____

48. PCO_2 $(PaCO_2)$ _____

49. pH _____

50. PO_2 (PaO_2) _____

51. PO_4^- _____

52. SaO_2 _____

53. TPN _____

54. TPR _____

55. wt _____

Exercises and Activities

1. Complete the following statements:

    a. Understanding fluid and electrolyte balance is important for the nurse because

    _____

    _____

    b. Homeostasis can be described as

    _____

    _____

    c. The body tries to maintain homeostasis by

    _____

    _____

2. Use the following diagrams to describe the processes of osmosis and diffusion.

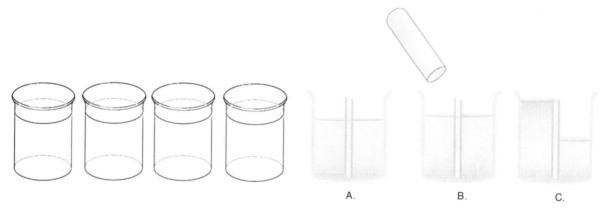

A.   B.   C.

Courtesy of Delmar Cengage Learning

Draw and explain diffusion: Draw and explain osmosis:

a. What is hemolysis and how does it occur?

_____

_____

b. How does dialysis work?

_____

_____

3. Why is it important for the body to maintain the acid–base balance?

_____

_____

_____

a. How does each of the body's three main control systems regulate acid–base balance?

The buffer systems: _____

_____

_____

Respiratory regulation: _____

_____

_____

Renal regulation: _____

_____

_____

b. Which control system is fastest? _____

Which control system is slowest? _____

4. List signs of a fluid imbalance that a nurse might observe on physical examination of a client per age group.

Fluid Volume Excess	Adult	Child
(1)		
(2)		
(3)		
(4)		
Fluid Volume Deficit	Adult	Child
(1)		
(2)		
(3)		
(4)		

a. Why is dehydration a common and serious fluid imbalance in an individual?

_____

_____

b. What are the primary nursing goals in dehydration?

_____

_____

c. Explain why 0.9% NaCl could be used for fluid replacement.

_____

_____

d. What would you tell a client about the role that water plays in health?

_____

_____

5. S.B. is a 29-year-old client who arrived at the hospital with multiple trauma following an automobile accident. Because of injury to his lungs, S.B. is now acutely ill. On assessment, the nurse notes that he is showing signs of hypoxemia, including dyspnea, increased respiratory rate, and an increased heart rate. He has been restless since he was admitted, but now appears to be showing some confusion.

a. The nurse determines that S.B. is exhibiting signs of which acid–base imbalance?

_____

_____

b. What changes in laboratory values would you anticipate?

pH _____

PCO_2 _____

HCO_3 _____

c. Why is a prompt and careful respiratory assessment important for this client?

_____

_____

d. List three actual or risk nursing diagnoses for this client.

(1) _____

(2) _____

(3) _____

e. How does respiratory acidosis differ from metabolic acidosis?

_____

_____

6. Fill in the table.

Acid Base Review

	Respiratory Acidosis	Respiratory Alkalosis
pH		
PCO_2 levels		
HCO_3 levels		
	Metaboic Acidosis	Metabolic Alkalosis
pH		
PCO_2 levels		
HCO_3 levels		

Self-Assessment Questions

Circle the letter that corresponds to the best answer.

1. The human body can tolerate only very slight changes in
   a. fluid volume.
   b. metabolic rate.
   c. respiratory rate.
   d. blood pH value.

2. If blood pH falls below 7.35, acidosis occurs, which may be characterized by a weak and irregular heartbeat, lower blood pressure, and
   a. a decreased level of consciousness (LOC).
   b. a decreased respiratory rate.
   c. spasmodic muscle contractions.
   d. numbness and tingling in the extremities.

3. A client admitted with dehydration may exhibit signs and symptoms that include dry mucous membranes, decreased tearing, decreased urine output, and
   a. decreased pulse rate.
   b. lower blood pressure.
   c. jugular vein distention.
   d. taut, smooth, shiny, pale skin.

4. The hormones ADH, aldosterone, and renin are important to a client's health status because they
   a. maintain the fluid balance by encouraging the kidneys to retain water.
   b. maintain the acid–base balance by causing the excretion of sodium.
   c. stabilize the normal pH level as part of the buffer systems.
   d. bind with excess hydrogen ions in the blood.

5. A client tells the nurse that he has been taking a lot of antacid tablets and milk in an attempt to control heartburn. The nurse should be aware that this client may be at risk for
   a. gastric acidosis.
   b. metabolic acidosis.
   c. metabolic alkalosis.
   d. compensatory alkalosis.

6. The most common indicator in a client who has fluid volume deficit is
   a. thirst.
   b. weakness.
   c. decreased urination.
   d. increased skin turgor.

7. A client has been advised to take a calcium supplement. To increase her absorption of calcium from the gastrointestinal tract, the nurse explains to the client that she should also consume
   a. vitamin C.
   b. vitamin D.
   c. amino acids.
   d. sports drinks.

8. An example of an isotonic solution is
   a. 0.45% NaCl.
   b. 0.9% NaCl.
   c. 3% NaCl.
   d. 5% dextrose in 0.9% NaCl.

9. A _____ solution would cause crenation.
   a. hypotonic
   b. isotonic
   c. hypertonic
   d. osmotic

10. The client received a crushing injury to the leg when a tree fell on it. With a crush injury, the nurse anticipates which of the following electrolytes will be elevated as a result of the intracellular damage?
   a. Sodium
   b. Bicarbonate
   c. Chloride
   d. Potassium

Medication Administration and IV Therapy

Key Terms

Match the following terms with their correct definitions.

n 1. Absorption

v 2. Angiocatheter

g 3. Aspiration

ee 4. Bioavailability

u 5. Butterfly needle

o 6. Chemical name

kk 7. Distribution

a 8. Drug allergy

ff 9. Drug incompatibility

i 10. Drug interaction

jj 11. Drug tolerance

t 12. Enteral instillation

ii 13. Excretion

pp 14. Extravasation

a. Hypersensitivity to a drug.

b. Time it takes the body to eliminate half of the blood concentration level of the original dose.

c. Device made of a radiopaque silicone catheter and a plastic or stainless steel injection port with a self-sealing silicone-rubber septum.

d. Study of the absorption, distribution, metabolism, and excretion of drugs to determine the relationship between the dose of a drug and the drug's concentration in biological fluids.

e. Physical and chemical processing of a drug by the body.

f. Seepage of foreign substances into the interstitial tissue, causing swelling and discomfort at the IV site.

g. Procedure performed to withdraw fluid that has abnormally collected or to obtain a specimen; also, inhalation of regurgitated gastric contents into the pulmonary system.

h. Medications dispensed and labeled in large quantities for storage in the medication room or nursing unit.

i. Effect one drug can have on another drug.

j. Highly unpredictable response that may be manifested by an overresponse, an underresponse, or an atypical response.

k. System of packaging and labeling each dose of medication by the pharmacy, usually for a 24-hour period.

l. Addition of an intravenous solution to infuse concurrently with another infusion.

m. The highest blood concentration of a single dose until the elimination rate equals the rate of absorption.

n. Passage of a drug from the site of administration into the bloodstream.

_oo_ 15. Flashback

_gg_ 16. Flow rate

_bb_ 17. Generic name

_b_ 18. Half-life

_s_ 19. Hypervolemia

_j_ 20. Idiosyncratic reaction

_c_ 21. Implantable port

_f_ 22. Infiltration

_w_ 23. Intracath

_dd_ 24. Intradermal

_ll_ 25. Intramuscular

_mm_ 26. Intravenous

_p_ 27. IV push (bolus)

_e_ 28. Metabolism

_x_ 29. Onset of action

_cc_ 30. Parenteral

_y_ 31. Patency

_m_ 32. Peak plasma level

_d_ 33. Pharmacokinetics

_z_ 34. Phlebitis

_L_ 35. Piggyback

_q_ 36. Plateau

_h_ 37. Stock supply

_aa_ 38. Subcutaneous

_nn_ 39. Toxic effect

_hh_ 40. Trade (brand) name

_k_ 41. Unit dose form

_v_ 42. Vesicant

o. Precise description of the drug's composition (chemical formula).

p. Method of administering a large dose of medication in a relatively short time, usually 1 to 30 minutes.

q. Level at which a drug's blood concentration is maintained.

r. Medication that causes blisters and tissue injury when it escapes into surrounding tissue.

s. Increased circulating fluid volume.

t. Administration of drugs through a gastrointestinal tube.

u. Wing-tipped needle.

v. Intracatheter with a metal stylet.

w. Plastic tube for insertion into a vein.

x. Time it takes the body to respond to a drug after administration.

y. Being freely opened.

z. Inflammation of a vein.

aa. Injection into the subcutaneous tissue.

bb. Name assigned by the U.S. Adopted Names Council to the manufacturer that first develops the drug.

cc. Any route other than the oral–gastrointestinal tract.

dd. Injection into the dermis.

ee. Readiness to produce a drug effect.

ff. Undesired chemical or physical reaction between a drug and a solution, between two drugs, or between a drug and the container or tubing.

gg. Volume of fluid to infuse over a set period of time.

hh. Name assigned a drug by the pharmaceutical company.

ii. Elimination of drugs from the body.

jj. Reaction that occurs when the body becomes accustomed to a specific drug and requires larger doses of the drug to produce the desired therapeutic effects.

kk. Movement of drugs from the blood into various body fluids and tissues.

ll. Injection into the muscle.

mm. Injection into a vein.

nn. Reaction that occurs when the body cannot metabolize a drug, causing the drug to accumulate in the blood.

oo. Rushing of blood back into intravenous tubing when a negative pressure is created on the tubing.

pp. The inadvertent IV administration of a vescicant escaping into the surrounding tissue.

Fill in the Blank

1. The ___U.S. Pharmacopeia___ and the ___National formulary___ are books of drug standards in the United States.

2. The ___generic___, or nonproprietary drug name, is assigned by the U.S. Adopted Names Council. These names are not capitalized.

3. ___U.S. Pharmacopeia___ refers to the routes of medication administration that are *not* the oral-gastrointestinal route.

4. The movement of a drug from the administration site into the bloodstream is known as ___absorption___

Abbreviation Review

Write the meaning or definition of the following abbreviations, acronyms, and symbols.

1. AIDS _____

2. BSA _____

3. c _____

4. cc _____

5. cm _____

6. CVC _____

7. D_5W _____

8. DEA _____

9. dr _____

10. FDA _____

11. fl _____

12. g _____

13. GI _____

14. gr _____

15. gtt _____

16. ID _____

17. IM _____

18. IV _____

19. IVPB _____

20. kg _____

21. KVO _____

22. L _____

23. lb _____

24. ɱ _____

25. MAR _____

26. mcg _____

27. mg _____

28. min _____

29. mL _____

30. NF _____

31. NG _____

32. NPO _____

33. NTG _____

34. oz _____

35. po _____

36. prn _____

37. pt _____

38. PT _____

39. PTT _____

40. qd _____

41. qt _____

42. RBC _____

43. SC/SQ _____

44. tsp _____

45. Tbsp _____

46. USP _____

47. VAD _____

Exercises and Activities

1. Explain the benefits of each of the following methods of medication administration.

    Buccal _____

    Intramuscular _____

    Intravenous _____

    Oral _____

    Respiratory _____

    Subcutaneous _____

    Sublingual _____

    Topical _____

2. What are the nurse's responsibilities related to giving medications?

    _____

    _____

    _____

    a. What was the impact of the Controlled Substance Act of 1970?

    _____

    _____

    b. List and briefly describe the four properties that determine the action of a drug.

    (1) _____

    (2) _____

    (3) _____

    (4) _____

    c. How does the onset of action influence the choice of route for a drug?

_____

_____

    d. Why are most medications given orally?

_____

_____

3. What questions will the nurse ask clients about their medication history?

_____

_____

_____

    a. If a client states she has an allergic reaction to a particular medication, what information is needed?

_____

_____

    b. How can you help prepare a client to take medication at home?

_____

_____

    c. List the seven "rights" of medication administration.

      (1) _____

      (2) _____

      (3) _____

      (4) _____

      (5) _____

      (6) _____

      (7) _____

    d. If you make a medication error, what steps should you take?

_____

_____

    e. What actions should the nurse take if the client refuses to take the prescribed medications?

_____

_____

    f. How is noncompliance different from refusing to take a dose of medication?

_____

_____

4. Give the equivalent (approximate) for each measurement:

1 gr	= _____ mg		1 cup	= _____ oz		1 Tbsp	= _____ mL	
1 g	= _____ mg		1/2 cup	= _____ cc		1 mL	= _____ minim	
1 tsp	= _____ cc		1 kg	= _____ lb		5 ft. 8 in.	= _____ cm	
1 L	= _____ mL		1 lb	= _____ kg		60 kg	= _____ lb	
1 oz	= _____ cc		1 oz	= _____ Tbsp		0.5 mg	= _____ mcg	
0.5 L	= _____ mL		1 tsp	= _____ gtt		gr 1/200	= _____ mg	

a. Determine the correct dosage for the following medication orders.

(1) You need to administer Benadryl 50 mg po every six hours as needed for itching. If each capsule is 25 mg, how many capsules will you give? _____ What is the maximum number of mg of Benadryl your client might receive in 24 hours? _____

(2) You need to administer phenobarbital gr 1/2 po. If each tablet is 60 mg, how many tablets will you give? _____

(3) You are giving ampicillin 325 mg IV to an infant. After the medication is reconstituted, it equals 250 mg/mL. How many cc will you give? _____

(4) You are also administering gentamicin 8 mg IM. The vial contains 40 mg/mL. How many cc will you give?_____ What size syringe will you use? _____ What site will you use for this injection? _____

(5) An IV of 1,000 mL D5W is scheduled to infuse at a rate of 125 mL/hr. If you start it at 1300, when will it finish? _____

(6) On the following diagram of a 3 cc syringe, draw a line at 1.6 cc.

Courtesy of Delmar Cengage Learning

b. What is the body surface area for a newborn, 21 in. in height, weighing 9 lb? _____
What is the body surface area for a child 90 cm in height, weighing 14 kg? _____

c. What information is missing from the following medication orders for Mr. J. Client?

(1) *8/31/xx 1130 Tetracycline 250 mg po x 5 days. Dr. B. Smith*

Missing: _____

(2) *9/1/xx Lanoxin 0.125 mg q AM at 0900 Dr. B. Smith*

Missing: _____

5. Using the computerized medication record (Figure 25-3 in your text), answer the following questions.

What is the client's diagnosis? _____

What does "start date" mean? _____

List the medications that L. White gave at 9 A.M. _____

What does QOD indicate on the Lanoxin order? _____

If the client has chest pain, what will you give? _____

When is Reglan ordered to be given? _____

When was the last time Mr. Patient took pain medication? _____

What were the medication and dose given for pain? _____

Where was the injection given? _____

You are caring for this client from 3 P.M. to 11 P.M. List the drug name, dose, and time of all the medications you will be responsible for giving. _____

6. A new nurse is preparing to give medications to several clients on her unit this morning.

   a. Her first client, J.B., is to have 10 units of regular insulin with breakfast. The nurse remembers from class that insulin is given subcutaneously because _____. J.B. tells the nurse that he usually gives himself injections in his thighs when he is at home and asks the nurse to use a different site. Draw on the following diagram the sites the nurse could use for J.B.

Courtesy of Delmar Cengage Learning

   b. In the next room, the nurse will start one of the two antibiotics due at 8 A.M., IVPB, on A.R. Why will Kim check drug compatibility on the two medications?

   _____

   _____

   Before starting the first antibiotic, the nurse assesses the IV site in A.R.'s right forearm. She recalls that the signs and symptoms of infiltration and phlebitis are

   _____

   _____.

   If the nurse determines that A.R. has phlebitis, she will

   _____

   _____.

   The nurse sets the flow rate for the IV. Because the IV of 1,000 mL is ordered to run for 12 hours, the nurse determines the infusion rate as _____ mL/hr. Because she is not using an infusion pump, she calculates the IV drip rate. The drip factor for this IV tubing is 12 drops/mL. She calculates the IV drip rate as _____ drops per minute. List five actions/interventions that the nurse will include in monitoring this client's IV therapy.

   (1) _____

   (2) _____

   (3) _____

   (4) _____

   (5) _____

c. Her next client, C.W., is on I&O. After C.W. finishes with her clear liquid breakfast tray, the nurse asks what she had to drink. C.W. says, "I had a cup of bouillon, half a cup of juice, and an ounce of water with a pain pill earlier." The nurse writes down _____ mL as C.W.'s fluid intake for breakfast.

d. N.P., a client the nurse remembers from a previous admission, is waiting for her in the next room. He is scheduled to have an IM injection of iron dextran (Imferon) this morning. She will inject this drug deeply into the _____ site using the Z-track method. To use the Z-track method, the nurse will _____
_____.

e. Depending on lab work this morning, S.Z., the nurse's last client, may need to have packed RBCs administered again today. What items will the nurse include in her initial assessment and preparation for S.Z. to receive blood products? _____
_____.

7. Identify the needle gauge, length, and angle of entry that are used in the following types of injections.

Injection Type	Needle Gauge	Needle Length	Angle of Entry
Intradermal			
Subcutaneous			
Insulin			
Intramuscular			

a. Name the muscles that the nurse would give an injection in at the following sites.
   (1) Upper arm _____
   (2) Thigh _____
   (3) Buttocks _____
   (4) Hip _____

b. The client is receiving a transfusion of packed red blood cells for anemia. The nurse needs to observe for signs of a trasnsfusion reaction. List the symptoms.

_____
_____

Self-Assessment Questions

Circle the letter that corresponds to the best answer for each question.

1. Parenteral drugs are administered by all except which of the following routes?
   a. Intraspinal
   b. Sublingual
   c. Intradermal
   d. Subcutaneous

2. A client is considered to be noncompliant with his medication. The nurse should first determine
   a. whether the client really needs the medicine.
   b. how to get the client to take the medication.
   c. why the client is not taking the drug as prescribed.
   d. whether there is a similar drug the client can take instead.

3. Drug actions are dependent on their absorption, distribution, metabolism, and
   a. excretion.
   b. utilization.
   c. bioavailability.
   d. administration.

4. The nurse caring for a new client notes during the assessment that he has difficulty swallowing. A medication was ordered for this client in tablet form. To avoid aspiration, the nurse will
   a. give the medication by injection.
   b. ask the physician to change the order.
   c. crush the tablet and mix it with water or juice.
   d. find a similar medication that is easier to swallow.

5. The nurse is preparing to give a medication to the client, who states, "This is a new pill. Why are you giving this to me?" The nurse should first
   a. check the medication order again.
   b. tell the client why she needs the medication.
   c. hold the medication until the physician comes in the next morning.
   d. explain why it is important to take the medications prescribed by the doctor.

6. A nurse is assessing the IV site on a client and notes the presence of swelling and cool, pale skin. The nurse understands that these are signs of
   a. phlebitis.
   b. infiltration.
   c. catheter sepsis.
   d. rapid IV infusion.

7. Anabolic steroids are a schedule ___ drug.
   a. I
   b. II
   c. III
   d. IV

8. Diazepam is a schedule ___ drug.
   a. I
   b. II
   c. III
   d. IV

9. A severe life-threatening reaction to a drug is called
   a. urticaria.
   b. anaphylaxis.
   c. tolerance.
   d. a toxic effect.

10. A nurse on your unit has an emergency situation occurring and asks you to administer medications already prepared. You should
   a. give the medications.
   b. help with the emergency.
   c. prepare and administer the medications yourself.
   d. refuse and leave the medications in the medication room.

Assessment

Key Terms

Match the following terms with their correct definitions.

i 1. Adventitious breath sound
  abnormal ↑

u 2. Affect
  expression of mood or emotions

l 3. Auscultation

a 4. Borborygmi – *can hear w/o stethoscope*

m 5. Bradycardia
  * brady = slow

v 6. Bradypnea ↓ 10

dd 7. Bronchial sound – *normal sounds*

s 8. Bronchovesicular sound

j 9. Crackles

d 10. Cyanosis

cc 11. Dyspnea
  * pnea = breathing

t 12. Eupnea – *normal breathing*

k 13. Health history

ff 14. Hyperventilation ↑ 20

a. High-pitched, loud, rushing sounds produced by the movement of gas in the liquid contents of the intestine.

b. Physical examination technique that uses the sense of touch to assess texture, temperature, moisture, organ location and size, vibrations and pulsations, swelling, masses, and tenderness.

c. High-pitched, harsh sound heard on inspiration when the trachea or larynx is obstructed.

d. Bluish or dark purple discoloration of the lips, skin, or nail beds.

e. Indirect measurement of cardiac output obtained by counting the number of peripheral pulse waves over a pulse point.

f. Low-pitched grating sound on inhalation and exhalation.

g. Respiratory rate greater than 24 beats per minute.

h. Abnormal, low-pitched breath sound, louder on exhalation.

i. Abnormal breath sound.

j. Abnormal breath sound that resembles a popping sound, heard in inhalation and exhalation, not cleared by coughing.

k. Review of the client's functional health patterns prior to the current contact with a health care agency.

l. Physical examination technique that involves listening to sounds in the body that are created by movement of air or fluid.

m. Heart rate less than 60 beats per minute in an adult.

n. Physical examination technique that uses short, tapping strokes on the surface of the skin to create vibrations of underlying organs.

_Z_ 15. Hypoventilation ↓12

_W_ 16. Inspection

_ee_ 17. Orthostatic hypotension

_b_ 18. Palpation

_n_ 19. Percussion

_f_ 20. Pleural friction rub

_bb_ 21. Pulse amplitude

_o_ 22. Pulse deficit

_e_ 23. Pulse rate

_p_ 24. Pulse rhythm

_r_ 25. Review of systems

_y_ 26. Sibilant wheeze — whistlelike

_q_ 27. Snellen chart ✳

_h_ 28. Sonorous wheeze — loud

_c_ 29. Stridor

_x_ 30. Tachycardia   ✳ Tachy=fast

_g_ 31. Tachypnea

_aa_ 32. Vesicular sound

o. Condition in which the apical pulse rate is greater than the radial pulse rate.

p. Regularity of the heartbeat.

q. Chart containing various-sized letters with standardized numbers at the end of each line of letters. (Eye test)

r. Brief account of any recent signs or symptoms related to any body system.

s. Medium-pitched and blowing sounds heard equally on inspiration and expiration from air moving through the large airways.

t. Easy respirations with a rate of breaths per minute that is age appropriate.

u. Outward expression of mood or emotions.

v. Respiratory rate of 10 or fewer breaths per minute.

w. Physical examination technique that involves thorough visual observation.

x. Heart rate in excess of 100 beats per minute in an adult.

y. Abnormal breath sound, high pitched and whistlelike in nature, during inhalation and exhalation.

z. Breathing characterized by shallow respirations.

aa. Soft, breezy, low-pitched sound heard longer on inspiration than expiration that results from air moving through the smaller airways over the lung periphery, with the exception of the scapular area.

bb. Measurement of the strength or force exerted by the ejected blood against the arterial wall with each contraction.

cc. Difficulty breathing as observed by labored or forced respirations through the use of accessory muscles in the chest and neck.

dd. Loud, tubular, hollow-sounding breath sound normally heard over the sternum.

ee. Significant decrease in blood pressure that results with dizziness or lightheadedness when a person moves from a lying or sitting (supine) position to a standing position.

ff. Breathing characterized by deep, rapid respirations.

Abbreviation Review

Write the meaning or definition of the following abbreviations, acronyms, and symbols.

1. BP _____

2. cm _____

3. LLQ _____

4. LOC _____

5. LUQ _____

6. P _____

7. PERRLA _____

8. R _____

9. RLQ _____

10. ROS _____

11. RUQ _____

12. T _____

Exercises and Activities

Pg. 553

1. Personal data including name, address, birth date, and gender are known as _demographic_ information.

2. In addition to physical assessment, identify four other sources of objective data.
   a. _inspection - look_
   b. _palpation - touch_
   c. _Percussion - tapping_
   d. _ausculation - listening_

3. What does *light accommodation* stand for in assessing for PERRLA?
   Pupils, equal, Round, reactive to, Light, accomodation

4. What is the frequency of bowel sounds if they are normally active?
   5-20 per min or 1 every 5-15 seconds

5. What are the purposes of the health history and physical assessment?
   Health history - functional health patterns before contact with health agency, physical assessment are observations, while assessing (objective).

   a. What findings might indicate that a client has been abused?
   pg 559 _Refusal to be touched, not able to maintain eye contact, unwillingness to talk about bruises/burns/injuries._

6. In which section of the health history would each of the following items be found?
   a. Completed hepatitis immunization _____
   b. Smokes one pack of cigarettes a day _____
   c. Last Pap test 6 months ago _____
   d. Experiencing stress from a new job _____
   e. Client rates his health as an 8 on a scale of 1 to 10 _____
   f. Sister and maternal grandmother have high blood pressure _family history._
   g. Develops a rash with penicillin _allergy_

h. Began having severe stomach pain 1 hour ago _____

i. Sleeps 7 hours a night, feels rested _____

j. Thyroidectomy at age 24 _____

k. Takes acetaminophen 650 mg every 4 hours PRN for headache _____

l. Chickenpox at age 5, no sequelae _____

7. Write at least two interventions that might be helpful for assessing each of the following:

An elderly client: _____
_____

A client who is hearing impaired: _____
_____

A client who is dyspneic: _____
_____

A client who does not speak English: _____
_____

A client who is in pain: _____
_____

8. What items are included in the assessment of vital signs?

NORMS: →
pg. 500

a. Give normal findings for T-P-R and BP.
Tempature: axillary 97.6°f, tympanic 98.6°f, oral 98.6°f,
rectal 99.6°f. Pulse: 60-100 beats/min. Respirations:
12-20 resp./min. B/P: Hypotension 90/60, Hypertension 140/90

b. Why are vital signs an important part of an assessment?
"signs of life", connect external inspection w/ internal
inspection.

c. What factors can affect an individual's temperature, pulse, respirations, and blood pressure?
temp: hot/cold drinks, smoking

d. Convert the following temperatures:

97.7°F = _____ °C   38°C = _____ °F
101°F = _____ °C   39°C = _____ °F

e. Explain the following terms:
    (1) Bradycardia   less than 60 beats per min. (adult)
    (2) Bradypnea   respitory rate of 10 of few breath per min.
    (3) Dyspnea   difficulty breathing
    (4) Eupnea   easy respirations, w rate of breaths per minute that is an appropriate
    (5) Hypoventilation   shallow respirations (breathing)

(6) Hyperventilation _deep/rapid respirations (breathing)_
(7) Tachycardia _heart rate ↑ 100 beats per minute_
(8) Tachypnea _respitory rate ↑ 24 beats per minute_

f. Label and draw a line to each of the pulse points on the figure.

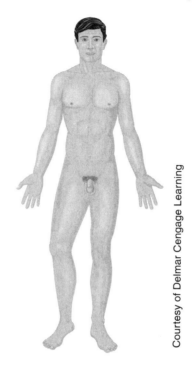

Courtesy of Delmar Cengage Learning

g. Draw an X over each area on this diagram where you would auscultate the lungs. Draw an arrow to show where you would assess the apical pulse.

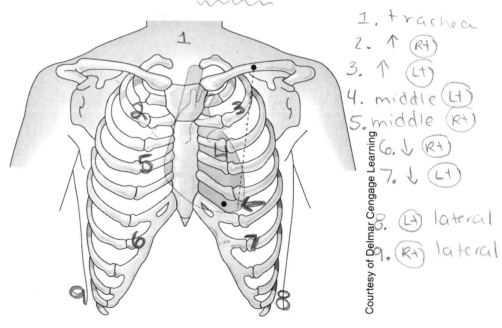

1. trachea
2. ↑ (Rt)
3. ↑ (Lt)
4. middle (Lt)
5. middle (Rt)
6. ↓ (Rt)
7. ↓ (Lt)
8. (Lt) lateral
9. (Rt) lateral

Courtesy of Delmar Cengage Learning

anterior

h. Write a brief description of normal findings for a respiratory assessment on a client.

_____

_____

9. D.M. is a 71-year-old client with a history of cigarette smoking, obesity, hypertension, and diabetes mellitus. Vital signs are temperature 97.9°F, pulse 88, respirations 20, blood pressure 158/92, and a weight today of 213 lb. He is now exhibiting signs and symptoms of peripheral vascular disease, a complication of poorly controlled diabetes. During your assessment of the lower extremities, you note decreased leg hair, skin that is cool to touch, with some loss of sensation.

   a. What information from his health history might be helpful in planning nursing interventions and teaching for D.M.?

   _____

   _____

   _____

   _____

   b. Write three questions you could ask D.M. for the ROS for his legs.

   (1) _____

   (2) _____

   (3) _____

   c. What other information could you obtain during your physical examination of the legs?

   _____

   _____

   d. Where will you palpate the peripheral pulses for D.M.?

   _____

   _____

   e. Write two actual and two risk nursing diagnoses for this client.

   (1) _____

   (2) _____

   (3) _____

   (4) _____

   f. What elements will you include to complete the cardiovascular assessment of this client?

   _____

   _____

   _____

   _____

Self-Assessment Questions

Circle the letter that corresponds to the best answer.

1. The nurse is performing <u>percussion</u> on the client's <u>abdomen</u>, If the assessment findings are nor-mal, the nurse would note
    a. stridor. *-high pitch, loud sound*
    b. tympany.
    c. resonance.
    d. hyperresonance.

2. The nurse is preparing to do a physical assessment on an elderly client with <u>difficulty breathing</u>. Which position will the nurse use for <u>respiratory</u> assessment? *(dyspena)*
    a. Sims
    b. Supine *– to keep pt. comfterable*
    c. Sitting
    d. Dorsal recumbent

3. An abdominal assessment finding that the nurse will report to a supervisor is
    a. positive borborygmi.
    b. audible peristalsis on auscultation.
    c. separation of the rectus abdominis muscle.
    d. finding abdominal organs with light palpation.

4. A nurse is performing a head and neck assessment on the client. To assess for <u>visual acuity</u>, the nurse will use
    a. a Snellen chart.
    b. direct light reflex.
    c. tangential lighting.
    d. an ophthalmoscope.

5. To accurately assess the apical pulse of a client, the nurse will
    a. palpate the brachial artery and count for 30 seconds.
    b. locate the left carotid artery and palpate gently for 1 minute.
    c. locate the fifth intercostal space, midclavicular line, and listen for 60 seconds.
    d. place the stethoscope on the left of the sternum and listen for 30 seconds.

6. The nurse is auscultating the lungs of a client with a respiratory illness. The breath sounds over the periphery of the lungs are <u>normally</u> described as
    a. resonant.
    b. vesicular.
    c. bronchial.
    d. hyperresonant. *when you are a student*

7. A technique requiring significant expertise and instructor supervision is
    a. light palpation.
    b. auscultation.
    c. visual observation.
    d. deep palpation.

8. The best position for assessment of the abdomen is
    a. sitting.
    b. dorsal recumbent. – *laying on back, face up – knees bent*
    c. supine. – *laying down, face up*
    d. Sims'. – *hand under pillow, top leg bent, other leg extended (side).*

9. The _____ position is indicated for the assessment of the lungs of a client with cardiopulmonary alterations.
    a. sitting
    b. dorsal recumbent
    c. supine
    d. Sims'

10. All are life-cycle considerations *(true)* for an elderly client except
    a. senses that are less acute. ✓
    b. increased awareness to pain.
    c. decreased height. ✓
    d. slowed respirations. ✓

Pain Management

Key Terms

Match the following terms with their correct definitions.

___ 1. Acupuncture

___ 2. Acute pain

___ 3. Adjuvant medication

___ 4. Afferent pain pathway

___ 5. Analgesia

___ 6. Analgesic

___ 7. Ceiling effect

___ 8. Chronic acute pain

___ 9. Chronic nonmalignant pain

___10. Chronic pain

___11. Colic

___12. Cryotherapy

a. Discomfort identified by sudden onset and relatively short duration, mild to severe intensity, and a steady decrease in intensity over several days or weeks.

b. Discomfort that occurs almost daily, has been present for at least 6 months, and ranges in intensity from mild to severe; also known as chronic benign pain.

c. Descending spinal cord pathway that transmits sensory impulses from the brain.

d. Neuropathic pain that occurs after amputation with pain sensations referred to an area in the missing portion of the limb.

e. Unpleasant sensory and emotional experience associated with actual or potential tissue damage or described in terms of such.

f. Compound that blocks opioid effects on one receptor type while producing opioid effects on a second receptor type.

g. Drug used to enhance the analgesic efficacy of opioids, treat concurrent symptoms that exacerbate pain, and provide independent analgesia for specific types of pain.

h. Use of cold applications to reduce swelling.

i. Analgesics administered via a catheter that terminates in the epidural space.

j. Technique of focusing attention on stimuli other than pain.

k. State of heightened awareness and focused concentration.

l. Discomfort from the internal organs that is felt in another area of the body.

____13. Cutaneous pain

____14. Distraction

____15. Efferent pain pathway

____16. Endorphins

____17. Epidural analgesia

____18. Gate control pain theory

____19. Hypnosis

____20. Intrathecal analgesia

____21. Ischemic pain

____22. Mixed agonist-antagonist

____23. Modulation

____24. Myofascial pain syndromes

____25. Neuralgia

____26. Nociceptor

____27. Noxious stimulus

____28. Pain

____29. Pain threshold

____30. Pain tolerance

____31. Patient-controlled analgesia

____32. Perception

m. Stress management strategy in which muscles are alternately tensed and relaxed.

n. Underlying pathology that causes pain.

o. Central nervous system pathway that selectively inhibits pain transmission by sending signals back down to the dorsal horn of the spinal cord.

p. Paroxysmal pain that extends along the course of one or more nerves.

q. Noxious stimulus that triggers electrical activity in the endings of afferent nerve fibers (nociceptors).

r. Process of applying a low-voltage electrical current to the skin through cutaneous electrodes.

s. Phenomenon of requiring larger and larger doses of an analgesic to achieve the same level of pain relief.

t. Discomfort resulting when the blood supply of an area is restricted or cut off completely.

u. Level of intensity at which pain becomes appreciable or perceptible.

v. Device that allows the client to control the delivery of intravenous or subcutaneous pain medication in a safe, effective manner through a programmable pump.

w. Discomfort marked by repetitive painful episodes that may recur over a prolonged period or throughout a client's lifetime.

x. Technique of monitoring negative thoughts and replacing them with positive ones.

y. Discomfort caused by stimulation of the cutaneous nerve endings in the skin.

z. Group of opiate-like substances produced naturally by the brain; these substances raise the pain threshold, produce sedation and euphoria, and promote a sense of well-being.

aa. Pain relief without producing anesthesia.

bb. Ascending spinal cord.

cc. Administration of analgesics into the subarachnoid space.

dd. Receptive neuron for painful sensations.

ee. Nonlocalized discomfort originating in tendons, ligaments, and nerves.

ff. Level of intensity or duration of pain that a person is willing to endure.

____33. Phantom limb pain

gg. Discomfort generally identified as long term (lasting 6 months or longer) that is persistent, nearly constant, or recurrent and that produces significant negative changes in a person's life.

____34. Progressive muscle relaxation

hh. Insertion of small needles into the skin at selected (hoku) sites.

____35. Recurrent acute pain

ii. Substance that relieves pain.

____36. Referred pain

jj. Condition of acute abdominal pain.

____37. Reframing

kk. Discomfort that occurs almost daily over a long period, has the potential for lasting months or years, and has a high probability of ending; also known as progressive pain.

____38. Relaxation technique

ll. Theory that proposes that the cognitive, sensory, emotional, and physiological components of the body can act together to block an individual's perception of pain.

____39. Somatic pain

mm. Group of muscle disorders characterized by pain, muscle spasm, tenderness, stiffness, and limited motion.

____40. Tolerance

nn. Process whereby the pain impulse travels from the receiving nociceptors to the spinal cord.

____41. Transcutaneous electrical nerve stimulation

oo. Method used to decrease anxiety and muscle tension.

____42. Transduction

pp. Discomfort felt in the internal organs.

____43. Transmission

qq. Ability to experience, recognize, organize, and interpret sensory stimuli.

____44. Visceral pain

rr. Medication dosage beyond which no further analgesia occurs.

Abbreviation Review

Write the meaning or definition of the following abbreviations, acronyms, and symbols.

1. APS _____

2. AHCPR _____

3. ATC _____

4. EMLA _____

5. IASP _____

6. MRI _____

7. NPO _____

8. NSAID _____

9. PCA _____

10. PRN _____

11. TAC _____

12. TENS _____

13. TMJ _____

14. VAS _____

15. WHO _____

Exercises and Activities

1. In what ways is the role of the nurse important in pain relief?

_____

_____

_____

_____

a. What is the importance of pain control to an individual's health?

_____

_____

_____

_____

b. When is pain deemed chronic?

_____

_____

_____

_____

c. How can pain be a diagnostic tool?

_____

_____

_____

_____

2. Draw and label the pain pathway from the stimulus to the muscle response.

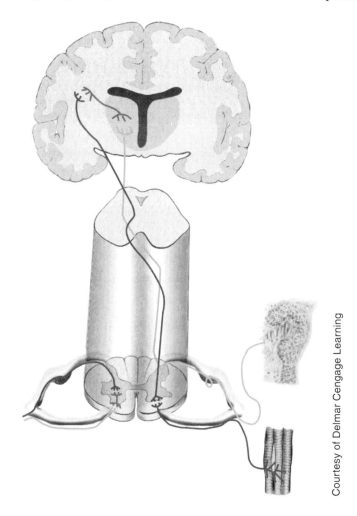

Courtesy of Delmar Cengage Learning

a. How does each of the following factors affect how an individual experiences pain?

Age: _____

_____

Previous experiences with pain: _____

_____

Cultural norms: _____

_____

b. Briefly describe the three general principles of pain management.

_____

_____

3. How does the nurse determine the amount of pain a client is experiencing?

    _____

    _____

    _____

    a. Compare and give examples for the three categories of pain control interventions.

	Examples	Advantages	Disadvantages
Pharmacological			
Noninvasive			
Invasive			

    b. How do nonopioid analgesics differ from opioid analgesics?

    _____

    _____

    c. What are the nurse's responsibilities in administration of analgesics?

    _____

    _____

4. A client gives the following description of a headache:

    "About 2 hours ago I started getting this awful headache right in the back of my head, just above my neck. I've had plenty of headaches before, but this one just came on with no warning, and now it feels like someone is pounding a hammer inside my head. I started feeling sick to my stomach and even vomited a couple of times, but it didn't help. All I had at home to take for the headache was some mild pain medicine, but it didn't even touch the pain. Since my mother died a couple of years ago from a stroke, every headache I get really worries me."

    a. What subjective and objective information would be helpful to assess this client's level of pain?

    _____

    _____

    b. For a complete description of the pain, list at least five specific questions you will ask this client.

    (1) _____

    (2) _____

    (3) _____

    (4) _____

    (5) _____

    c. What terms might clients use to describe the quality of their pain?

    _____

    _____

  d. Give an example of a nursing diagnosis for this client.

  _____

  _____

  e. State the goal for the client using the above nursing diagnosis.

  _____

  _____

5. F.L. is a 34-year-old client who had an amputation of her right leg below the knee as a result of extensive trauma 3 years ago. Since then, she has experienced chronic neuropathic pain ranging from mild to moderate. With a prosthesis, she is able to care for her family and do housework, but she has difficulty sitting for extended periods of time or walking long distances. F.L. has tried several types of pain medication over the past year but states that the ones that give enough relief make her feel too sleepy.

  a. What type of pain is F.L. experiencing?

  _____

  _____

  b. List five ways in which the pain F.L. is experiencing differs from acute pain.

  (1) _____

  (2) _____

  (3) _____

  (4) _____

  (5) _____

  c. Does this client's pain serve as a protective mechanism?

  _____

  _____

  d. F.L. says that she would like to try something to help ease her pain besides just medication. Suggest two interventions and explain your rationale.

  (1) _____

  _____

  _____

  (2) _____

  _____

  _____

  e. Why will she need ongoing pain assessments?

  _____

  _____

  _____

  _____

Self-Assessment Questions

Circle the letter that corresponds to the best answer.

1. To reverse respiratory depression in a client receiving Duramorph, the nurse would administer
   a. naloxone.
   b. an amphetamine.
   c. an opioid agonist.
   d. a neurolytic agent.

2. The nurse is assessing a client's level and intensity of pain 2 days postsurgery. The most effective way for the nurse to determine the client's pain level is to
   a. evaluate the amount of pain medication taken.
   b. ask the client to describe her perception of the pain.
   c. note the facial expressions and the presence of guarding.
   d. assess the client's mobility and level of self-care activities.

3. As part of a comprehensive pain management plan, noninvasive interventions may include relaxation techniques, guided imagery, distraction, and
   a. radiation.
   b. cryotherapy.
   c. nerve blocks.
   d. nonopioid analgesia.

4. The primary advantage of using PCA is that it
   a. has fewer systemic side effects.
   b. can be used in the home setting.
   c. gives clients greater control over their pain.
   d. uses lower doses of medication to achieve pain relief.

5. A nurse is caring for a client who continues to experience neck and back pain following an automobile accident 1 year ago. Because of the chronic pain, this client is most likely to
   a. use analgesic medication effectively.
   b. display signs that resemble those of anxiety.
   c. exhibit the same behaviors as a client in acute pain.
   d. benefit from nonpharmacological pain relief methods.

6. Twisting an ankle results in
   a. cutaneous pain.
   b. somatic pain.
   c. visceral pain.
   d. referred pain.

7. Signs of chronic pain include
   a. loss of libido and weight.
   b. localized pain and normal vital signs.
   c. guarding and normal pupils.
   d. diaphoresis and fatigue.

8. Myocardial infarction may cause
   a. hormone changes.
   b. colic.
   c. ischemic pain.
   d. myofascial pain.

9. Which side effect of opioid analgesics requires immediate intervention?
   a. Nausea
   b. Constipation
   c. Pruritis
   d. Respiratory depression

10. A noninvasive intervention for pain that uses features of both relaxation and distraction is called
    a. guided imagery.
    b. biofeedback.
    c. reframing.
    d. cognitive-behavioral.

Diagnostic Tests

Key Terms

Match the following terms with their correct definitions.

___ 1. Agglutination

    a. Visualization of the vascular structures through the use of fluoroscopy with a contrast medium.

___ 2. Agglutinin

    b. Globular protein that is produced in the body and catalyzes chemical reactions within the cells by promoting the oxidative reactions and synthesis of various chemicals.

___ 3. Agglutinogen

    c. Blood in the urine.

___ 4. Analyte

    d. Chalky-white contrast medium.

___ 5. Aneurysm

    e. Venous catheter inserted into the superior vena cava through the subclavian or internal or external jugular vein.

___ 6. Angiography

    f. Use of high-frequency sound waves to visualize deep body structures; also called an echogram.

___ 7. Antibody

    g. Study of x-rays or gamma ray–exposed film through the action of ionizing radiation.

___ 8. Antigen

    h. Diminished production of urine.

___ 9. Arteriography

    i. Minimally depressed level of consciousness during which the client retains the ability to maintain a continuously patent airway and to respond appropriately to physical stimulation or verbal commands.

___10. Ascites

    j. Graphic recording of the heart's electrical activity.

___11. Aspiration

    k. Any antigenic substance that causes agglutination by the production of agglutinin.

___12. Bacteremia

    l. Clumping together of red blood cells.

___13. Barium

    m. Immunoglobulin produced by the body in response to bacteria, viruses, or other antigenic substances.

___14. Biopsy

    n. Substance, usually a protein, that causes the formation of an antibody and reacts specifically with that antibody.

___15. Central line

    o. Excision of a small amount of tissue.

___16. Computed tomography

    p. Product of incomplete fat metabolism.

___17. Conscious sedation

___18. Contrast medium

___19. Culture

___20. Cytology

___21. Electrocardiogram

___22. Electroencephalogram

___23. Electrolyte

___24. Endoscopy

___25. Enzyme

___26. Fluoroscopy

___27. Hematuria

___28. Invasive

___29. Ketone

___30. Lipoprotein

___31. Lumbar puncture

___32. Magnetic resonance imaging

___33. Necrosis

___34. Noninvasive

___35. Occult blood

___36. Oliguria

___37. Papanicolaou test

___38. Paracentesis

___39. Phlebotomist

q. Aspiration of cerebrospinal fluid from the subarachnoid space.

r. Process of urine elimination.

s. Instrument that converts electrical energy to sound waves.

t. Susceptibility of a pathogen to an antibiotic.

u. Smear method of examining stained exfoliative cells.

v. Individual who performs venipuncture.

w. Radiopaque substance that facilitates roentgen (x-ray) imaging of the body's internal structures.

x. Specific kind of antibody whose interaction with antigens manifests as agglutination.

y. Procedure performed to withdraw fluid that has abnormally collected or to obtain a specimen.

z. Tissue death as the result of disease or injury.

aa. Accessing body tissues, organs, or cavities through some type of instrumentation procedure.

bb. Colorless derivative of bilirubin formed by the normal bacterial action of intestinal flora on bilirubin.

cc. Alert and with vital signs within the client's normal range.

dd. Aspiration of fluid from the abdominal cavity.

ee. Blood in the stool that can be detected only via a microscope or chemical means.

ff. Radiologic scanning of the body with x-ray beams and radiation detectors that transmit data to a computer, which in turn transcribes the data into quantitative measurement and multidimensional images of the internal structures.

gg. Descriptor for procedure wherein the body is not entered with any type of instrument.

hh. Port that has been implanted under the skin with a catheter inserted into the superior vena cava or right atrium through the subclavian or internal jugular veins.

ii. Immediate, serial images of the body's structure or function.

jj. Abnormal accumulation of fluid in the abdomen.

kk. Weakness in the wall of a blood vessel.

ll. Growing of microorganisms to identify a pathogen.

mm. Graphic recording of the brain's electrical activity.

___40. Pneumothorax

nn. Sharply pointed surgical instrument contained in a cannula.

___41. Port-a-Cath

oo. Visualization of a body organ or cavity through a scope.

___42. Radiography

pp. Puncturing of a vein with a needle to aspirate blood.

___43. Sensitivity

qq. Study of cells.

___44. Stable

rr. Blood lipid bound to protein.

___45. Stress test

ss. Condition of bacteria in the blood.

___46. Thoracentesis

tt. Substance that is measured.

___47. Transducer

uu. Substance that, when in solution, separates into ions and conducts electricity.

___48. Trocar

vv. Radiographic study of the vascular system following the injection of a radiopaque dye through a catheter.

___49. Type and cross-match

ww. Condition wherein air or gas accumulates in the pleural space, causing the lungs to collapse.

___50. Ultrasound

xx. Measure of a client's cardiovascular response to exercise tolerance.

___51. Urobilinogen

yy. Laboratory test that identifies the client's blood type (e.g., A or B) and determines the compatibility of the blood between potential donor and recipient.

___52. Venipuncture

zz. Aspiration of fluids from the pleural cavity.

___53. Void

aaa. Imaging technique that uses radio waves and a strong magnetic field to make continuous cross-sectional images of the body.

Abbreviation Review

Write the meaning or definition of the following abbreviations and symbols.

1. ABG _____

2. C&S _____

3. CSF _____

4. CT _____

5. ECG (EKG) _____

6. EEG _____

7. IVP _____

8. $PaCO_2$ _____

9. PaO_2 _____

10. RBC _____

11. WBC _____

Exercises and Activities

1. Describe the role of the nurse in preparing a client for diagnostic procedures.

   _____

   _____

   _____

   a. What teaching will the nurse do with the client?

   _____

   _____

   b. Explain the importance of informed consent for invasive procedures.

   _____

   _____

2. What is the role of the nurse during invasive diagnostic procedures?

   _____

   _____

   _____

   a. How can the nurse help the client to be more relaxed?

   _____

   _____

   b. List ways to maintain safety for the nurse and the client during the procedure.

   _____

   _____

3. Identify the purpose of each of these common blood tests and list normal values.

	Normal Values	*Purpose*
WBC		
Hemoglobin (Hgb)		
Hematocrit (Hct)		
ABG analysis		
Na^+		
K^+		
Fasting blood sugar (FBS)		
Glucose tolerance test (GTT)		
Blood urea nitrogen (BUN)		
Cholesterol (lipid profile)		

4. What documentation is the nurse responsible for after diagnostic procedures?

_____

_____

_____

5. For each of the following diagnostic procedures, briefly describe the purpose of the test, any special preparation for the client, and nursing assistance or interventions during the procedure.

	Purpose	*Preparation*	*Assistance*
Paracentesis			
Pap smear			
Cardiac catheterization			
Thoracentesis			
Magnetic resonance imaging (MRI)			

6. B.P., a normally active 14-year-old, was brought in by his parents following the sudden onset of a severe headache, nausea, and vomiting. On assessment he appears somewhat irritable and displays stiffness in his neck. His temperature and pulse rate are increased, and he is breathing rapidly. The physician has ordered a lumbar puncture to rule out meningitis. B.P. seems frightened, and the parents are extremely anxious. They insist on staying in the room with their son during the procedure.

a. How does the nurse explain this procedure to B.P.?

_____

_____

b. What preparation is necessary?

_____

_____

c. What position should B.P. assume?

_____

_____

d. How does the nurse assist the physician and B.P. during the procedure?

_____

_____

e. How can the nurse help B.P.'s parents during the procedure?

_____

_____

_____

_____

7. The physician suspects that K.T. has colon cancer. The physician has ordered the following diagnostic tests: Hgb, Hct, CEA, FOBT, abdominal ultrasound, and abdominal CT.

   a. K.T. wants to know why blood is being drawn and what is the doctor hoping to find. How should the nurse respond?

   _____

   _____

   _____

   b. List the normal laboratory values for:
      (1) Hgb _____
      (2) Hct _____
      (3) CEA _____

   c. The nurse instructs K.T. regarding the guiaic test ordered.
      (1) What drugs could affect the results of this test?

      _____

      (2) Why should red meat be avoided in the diet for at least three days prior to this test?

      _____

   d. K.T. asks if his bladder needs to be full for the abdominal ultrasound. What should the nurse tell K.T. about an ultrasound exam?

   _____

   _____

   e. The abdominal CT requires the use of contrast media. What safety measures should the nurse take regarding K.T.?

   _____

   _____

   f. K.T. has **K**nowledge *Deficit* related to diagnostic testing listed as one of his problems on the nursing care plan. What interventions can the nurse take to help K.T.?

   _____

   _____

Self-Assessment Questions

Circle the letter that corresponds to the best answer.

1. A nurse is caring for a client who is having an IVP. To monitor the client, the nurse should be aware that the most serious hazard of an allergic reaction to the dye is
   a. oliguria.
   b. urticaria.
   c. respiratory distress.
   d. low blood pressure.

2. A practitioner has ordered a urine sample for a creatinine clearance test. The most appropriate method to collect this is from a
   a. timed sample.
   b. sterile specimen.
   c. random collection.
   d. clean-voided specimen.

3. A nurse is caring for a client who has experienced a bronchoscopy. Following this procedure, it is important for the nurse to
   a. observe the client for signs of tachycardia.
   b. withhold fluids until the gag reflex returns.
   c. advise the client that he may experience dysphagia.
   d. place the client in a high Fowler's position to minimize coughing.

4. The nurse is aware that the most serious complication of thoracentesis is
   a. dyspnea.
   b. infection.
   c. dysrhythmia.
   d. pneumothorax.

5. A client is recovering after having a cardiac catheterization. Following this procedure, it is important for the client to
   a. maintain a side-lying position with the knees bent.
   b. limit fluid intake for several hours until the medication has worn off.
   c. keep the extremity in which the catheter was placed straight and immobile.
   d. collect urine for 24 hours for proper disposal related to the use of radiographic dyes.

6. The nurse correctly describes conscious sedation to the client as
   a. a state of relaxation using biofeedback techniques.
   b. anesthesia delivered by a nurse working in an "expanded role."
   c. a state in which the client is awake and aware but unable to move.
   d. a depressed level of consciousness in which the client can breathe on his own.

7. Immunoglobulins produced by the body in response to bacteria are called
   a. antigens.
   b. antibodies.
   c. agglutinogens.
   d. agglutinins.

8. In an allergic reaction, you would expect to find an increase in _____ when checking the differential count.
   a. neutrophils
   b. eosinophils
   c. lymphocytes
   d. monocytes

9. Which urine test does *not* measure adrenal cortex function?
   a. 17-Hydroxycorticosteroids
   b. Vanillylmandelic acid
   c. Aldosterone assay
   d. Bence Jones protein

10. Which radiologic study can be performed on a client who has an allergy to shellfish?
    a. Cardiac catheterization
    b. Adrenal angiography
    c. Barium enema
    d. Intravenous pyelogram

Basic Procedures

Key Terms

Match the following terms with their correct definitions.

___ 1. Antipyretic

___ 2. Antiseptic handwash

___ 3. Antiseptic hand rub

___ 4. Apnea

___ 5. Caries

___ 6. Doppler

___ 7. Gingivitis

___ 8. Halitosis

___ 9. Hand hygiene

___10. Logrolling

___11. Pyrexia

___12. Stomatitis

___13. Surgical hand antisepsis

a. A device used when the pulse cannot be detected by palpation.

b. Bad breath.

c. Cessation of breathing for several seconds.

d. Dental cavities.

e. Fever-reducing medication.

f. Inflammation of the gums.

g. Inflammation of the oral mucosa.

h. Temperature above the normal range.

i. The rubbing together of all surfaces and crevices of the hands using plain soap and water.

j. Turning the client as one unit, keeping the head, neck, hip, and back in alignment.

k. Using an alcohol-based rub to cleanse hands.

l. Using antiseptic handwash or antiseptic hand rub preoperatively by surgical personnel to eliminate transient and reduce resident hand flora.

m. Using antimicrobial substances and water to cleanse hands.

Abbreviation Review

Write the meaning or definition of the following abbreviations and acronyms.

1. ABCD _____

2. AED _____

3. CDC _____

4. CPR _____

5. EMS _____

6. I&O _____

7. PMI _____

8. PROM _____

9. ROM _____

10. VRE _____

Exercises and Activities

1. What are the three essential elements to hand hygiene?

   (1) _____

   (2) _____

   (3) _____

2. List the conditions or times in which hand hygiene should be completed.

   _____

   _____

   _____

   _____

   _____

3. Explain why the hospitalized client is at increased risk for a health care acquired infection.

   _____

   _____

   _____

4. Identify five items used by health care workers to protect themselves from exposure to potentially hazardous body fluids. Include an explanation of when these items are used.

   (1) _____

   (2) _____

   (3) _____

   (4) _____

   (5) _____

5. Describe the correct position/location for each pulse point.

   a. Temporal _____

   b. Carotid _____

   c. Apical _____

   d. Brachial _____

   e. Radial _____

   f. Ulnar _____

   g. Femorai _____

   h. Popliteal _____

   i. Posterior tibial _____

   j. Pedal/dorsal pedal _____

6. What is a nosocomial infection? What are its prevention measures?

_____

_____

_____

_____

7. Describe the anatomical landmarks used when assessing an apical pulse.

_____

_____

_____

8. Explain the five phases of Karotkoff sounds when taking a blood pressure.
   (1) _____
   (2) _____
   (3) _____
   (4) _____
   (5) _____

9. The client is short of breath. The nurse obtains a pulse oximeter reading. The client asks how an oximeter works. How would the nurse explain this to the client?

_____

_____

_____

10. Correct body mechanics are essential in order to avoid _____

_____

_____

11. What is PROM? What is the benefit of PROM? Describe the technique.

_____

_____

_____

_____

12. Place a check mark in the correct action per joint on the table below when performing PROM for the client.

	Neck	_Shoulder_	_Elbow_	_Hip_	_Knee_
Flexion					
Extension					
Hyperextention					
Abduction					
Adduction					
Internal rotation					
External rotation					

Self-Assessment Questions

Circle the letter that corresponds to the best answer.

1. Clients at high risk for falls include all of the following except
   a. those with prolonged hospitalization.
   b. those taking sedatives.
   c. confused clients.
   d. those without history of physical-restraint use.

2. What is *not* a key concept to remember when positioning a client?
   a. Pressure
   b. Friction
   c. Skin color
   d. Nutrition

3. What is *not* considered a common complication of immobility?
   a. Skin breakdown
   b. Incontinence
   c. Muscle wasting
   d. Clot formation

4. Activity is important because it
   a. improves muscle tone and increases venous return.
   b. stimulates peristalsis and decreases muscle tone.
   c. is an important part of the healing process and decreases peristalsis.
   d. decreases venous return and stimulates peristalsis.

5. Of the following, the best descriptor of massage is that it
   a. cannot help rid the body of metabolic wastes.
   b. does not stimulate circulation.
   c. can open lines of communication.
   d. may detract from the therapeutic relationship.

6. M.W., a frail 80-year-old woman, is hospitalized with a stroke. She cannot move her left side. Which of the following is an indication that she should be repositioned more frequently than every two hours?
   a. Areas of redness on the right heel that resolve within 5 minutes
   b. Areas of redness on the occiput that resolve in 45 minutes
   c. When M.W. complains of constipation
   d. M.W. should only be positioned on her immobile side

7. M.W. requires a bed bath. Which of the following statements is correct when providing daily hygiene?
   a. Wash the chin and mouth area first.
   b. Cleanse the eyes from outer canthus to inner canthus.
   c. Cleanse the eyes from inner to outer canthus first.
   d. Start from the top down, so begin with her forehead.

8. The client broke his left leg in a skiing accident. The doctor ordered the client to be non–weight bearing for six-weeks. Therefore, the client needs to use crutches. Which gait should the nurse teach the client?
   a. Swing-through gait
   b. Two point gait
   c. Three-point gait
   d. Four-point gait

Intermediate Procedures

Key Terms

Match the following terms with their correct definitions.

___ 1. Ampule

___ 2. Catheterization

___ 3. Colostomy

___ 4. Dorsogluteal muscle

___ 5. Intramuscular injection

___ 6. Nebulizer

___ 7. Sterile technique

___ 8. Subcutaneous injection

___ 9. Vastus lateralis muscle

___ 10. Vial

a. Consists of those practices that eliminate all micro-organisms and spores from an object or area.

b. Passing a rubber or plastic tube into the bladder via the urethra.

c. An opening surgically created from the ascending, transverse, or descending colon to the abdominal wall.

d. Containers that hold a single dose of medication.

e. A small glass bottle with a rubber seal at the top.

f. Method used to administer medications into the loose connective tissues just below the dermis of the skin.

g. Method used to administer medications into the deep muscle tissue.

h. Muscle located on the anterior lateral aspect of the thigh.

i. Muscle located in the upper outer quadrant of the buttock.

j. Device that is used to aerosolize medications into a mist for delivery directly into the lungs.

Abbreviation Review

Write the meaning or definition of the following abbreviations, acronyms, and symbols.

1. ABG _____

2. COPD _____

3. FlO2 _____

4. Gl _____

5. IV _____

6. MAR _____

7. NG _____

8. OD _____

9. OR _____

10. OS _____

11. OSHA _____

12. OTC _____

13. OU _____

14. PEG _____

15. SaO2 _____

16. SMI _____

Exercises and Activities

1. Why is open intermittent irrigation of a urinary catheter usually done?

    _____

    _____

2. What assessment findings would indicate a need for irrigation?

    _____

    _____

    _____

3. Why are heat and/or cold therapies used?

    _____

    _____

    _____

    _____

    a. What safety measures does the nurse use to protect the client during each therapy?

    Heat _____

    Cold _____

    b. What are contraindications to heat therapy?

    _____

    _____

    c. When should the nurse end the individual treatment for a client receiving heat therapy?

    _____

    _____

    d. When should the nurse end the treatment session for a client receiving cold therapy?

    _____

    _____

4. What are the seven "rights" of medication administration?

    a. _____

    b. _____

    c. _____

    d. _____

    e. _____

    f. _____

    g. _____

5. What actions should the nurse take if a client refuses a medication?

   _____

   _____

   _____

6. What actions should the nurse take if a medication error occurs?

   _____

   _____

   _____

7. What is the Z-track method? What medications are administered using this method?

   _____

   _____

   _____

8. Preparations for applying a transdermal patch include:

   _____

   _____

   _____

9. The nurse is preparing to insert an indwelling catheter before the client goes to surgery. What should the nurse say to the client about this procedure?

   _____

   _____

   _____

   a. What position does the client need to be placed in before inserting the catheter?

      _____

      _____

   b. The nurse removes the outer wrapper and sets the catheter tray on a clean dry surface. Describe how the tray should be opened.

      _____

      _____

   c. The nurse dropped the packet of sterile betadine solution onto the floor. Describe how the nurse might handle this breach of sterile technique.

      _____

      _____

   d. If the client was female, describe how the nurse cleanses around the urinary meatus.

      _____

      _____

   e. If the client was male, describe how the nurse cleanses around the urinary meatus.

      _____

      _____

f. What should be documented regarding the catheter insertion?

_____

_____

10. The nurse needs to administer the following medications to the client. Explain the steps of each medication:

Lanoxin 0.25 mg orally every day _____

_____

Robitussin 5 mL every 4 hours _____

_____

Fentanyl 25 mg patch every 72 hours _____

_____

11. Identify the anatomical landmarks the nurse uses to administer the following intramuscular injections:

a. Deltoid muscle _____

b. Vastus lateralis muscle _____

c. Dorsogluteal muscle _____

d. Ventrogluteal muscle _____

12. Explain the needle size (gauge) and angle of entry for the following types of injections.

Site	Needle Gauge	Angle of Entry
Intradermal		
Subcutaneous		
Intramuscular		

13. The client has a dressing following abdominal surgery. The nurse inspects the dressing frequently. Describe what the nurse assesses the dressing for.

_____

_____

_____

a. The wound is draining foul-smelling fluid and the physician orders a wound culture. Explain how the nurse obtains a wound culture.

_____

_____

b. The physician decides the wound should be irrigated twice a day. What equipment should the nurse assemble for this procedure?

_____

_____

    c. The nurse explains to the client the procedure of wound irrigation. How would you explain it in terms a client might understand?

_____

_____

14. The client needs to have oxygen therapy. Identify the volume of oxygen that the nurse should set each piece of equipment at.

    a. Nasal cannula _____

    b. Simple mask _____

    c. Partial rebreather mask _____

    d. Non-rebreather mask _____

    e. Venturi mask _____

15. The client has a tracheostomy and requires suctioning occasionally. As the nurse prepares the equipment, what amount of suction should the wall suction unit be set at for each of the following?

    For an adult: _____

    For a child: _____

    For an infant: _____

16. The client receives medication through a gastrostomy tube. Explain how the nurse prevents medication from clogging the tube.

_____

_____

_____

Self-Assessment Questions

Circle the letter that corresponds to the best answer.

1. When catheterizing a client, in which hand do you hold the catheter?
   a. Right hand
   b. Left hand
   c. Either hand
   d. Dominant hand

2. What type of bladder irrigation is preferred for surgical procedures such as prostate resections?
   a. Open bladder irrigation
   b. Closed bladder irrigation
   c. Intermittent open bladder irrigation
   d. None are recommended.

3. Cold therapy can
   a. decrease blood flow to an area.
   b. increase systemic temperature.
   c. increase tissue metabolism.
   d. promote vasodilation.

4. What is the maximum amount of time a client should sit in a sitz bath?
   a. 10 minutes
   b. 15 minutes
   c. 20 minutes
   d. 25 minutes

5. When administering a douche or irrigation, the temperature should be at
   a. 90° to 95°F.
   b. 95° to 100°F.
   c. 100° to 105°F.
   d. 105° to 110°F.

Advanced Procedures

Key Terms

Match the following terms with their correct definitions.

___ 1. Hemophilia

___ 2. Macrodrip tubing

___ 3. Microdrip tubing

___ 4. Piggyback

___ 5. Sutures

a. Delivers 10 to 15 gtt/mL.

b. A surgical means of closing a wound, generally removed 7 to 10 days after surgery.

c. An inherited bleeding disorder.

d. Delivers 60 gtt/mL.

e. A drug that is mixed and joined to the primary IV bag.

Abbreviation Review

Write the meaning or definition of the following abbreviations and acronyms.

1. CDC _____

2. IV _____

3. MAR _____

4. NG _____

5. NPO _____

6. ONC _____

7. OSHA _____

Exercises and Activities

1. What are the three primary methods of obtaining blood specimens? Which is the most common?

   _____

   _____

   _____

2. Why would a client be receiving IV fluids?

   _____

   _____

   _____

3. What assessment signs and symptoms of an IV site would indicate infection or phlebitis?

_____

_____

_____

4. The client has a nasogastric tube. What are the reasons a client may have a nasogastric tube?

_____

_____

_____

   a. What are the two most common forms of NG tubes?

   _____

   _____

   b. Why is NG insertion a clean technique instead of a sterile one?

   _____

   _____

   c. What equipment should the nurse assemble when preparing for NG tube insertion?

   _____

   _____

   d. Describe how the nurse knows that the NG tube is correctly situated in the stomach.

   _____

   _____

5. The physician ordered an IV for the client. Why are IV fluids used instead of oral fluids?

_____

_____

_____

   a. Describe the uses for the following gauges of IV needles.
       (1) 18–19-gauge needles _____
       (2) 20–22-gauge needles _____
       (3) 22–24-gauge needles _____

   b. The nurse prepares the IV solution and the tubing but accidentally overfills the drip chamber. How should the nurse correct this?

   _____

   _____

   c. After the IV is inserted and the fluid is running freely, the client reaches to pick up a piece of paper that has fallen to the floor. The client becomes anxious when seeing blood in the IV tubing. How should the nurse respond?

   _____

   _____

   d. Describe the elements of what should be documented following IV insertion.

   _____

   _____

6. The client has a central venous catheter inserted. The nurse uses sterile technique when changing the insertion site dressing. Why is this a sterile procedure?

_____

_____

_____

7. Explain the difference between continuous and interrupted sutures.

_____

_____

_____

8. If sutures are removed too early, dehiscence may occur. Explain what dehiscence is and what the nurse should do if it occurs.

_____

_____

_____

Self-Assessment Questions

Circle the letter that corresponds to the best answer.

1. The CDC guidelines indicate that IV tubing should be changed every
   a. 24 hours.
   b. 48 hours.
   c. 72 hours.
   d. 48–72 hours.

2. The CDC guidelines indicate that an IV site should be changed every
   a. 24 hours.
   b. 48 hours.
   c. 72 hours.
   d. 48–72 hours.

3. An order reads to administer 2 L of normal saline (NS) IV over 24 hours. The nurse has micro-drip tubing. The IV will be regulated at a rate of
   a. 42 gtt/min.
   b. 83 gtt/min.
   c. 125 gtt/min.
   d. 167 gtt/min.

4. A client is to receive an IV of 5% D/0.45 NS at 2,000 mL for 8 hours. The drip factor is 10 gtt/mL. The nurse will regulate the IV at a rate of
   a. 10 gtt/min.
   b. 21 gtt/min.
   c. 42 gtt/min.
   d. 63 gtt/min.

Anesthesia

Chapter
32

Key Terms

Match the following terms with their correct definitions.

____ 1. Amnesia

____ 2. Analgesia

____ 3. Anesthesia

____ 4. Anesthesiologist

____ 5. Anesthetist

____ 6. Capnography

____ 7. General anesthesia

____ 8. Orthostatic hypotension

____ 9. Regional anesthesia

____10. Sedation

____11. Synergism

a. Method of producing unconsciousness, complete insensibility to pain, amnesia, motionlessness, and muscle relaxation.

b. Inability to remember things.

c. Method of temporarily rendering a region of the body insensible to pain.

d. Significant decrease in blood pressure that results when a person moves from a lying or sitting (supine) position to a standing position.

e. Result of two or more agents working together to achieve a greater effect than either could produce alone.

f. Qualified RN, dentist, or medical doctor who administers anesthetics under the direct supervision of an anesthesiologist or a surgeon.

g. Pain relief without producing anesthesia.

h. Licensed physician educated and skilled in the delivery of anesthesia who also adds to the knowledge of anesthesia through research or other scholarly pursuits.

i. Absence of normal sensation.

j. Reduction of stress, excitement, or irritability via some degree of central nervous system depression.

k. Monitoring the exhaled carbon dioxide in anesthetized patients.

Abbreviation Review

Write the meaning or definition of the following abbreviations, acronyms, and symbols.

1. BP _____

2. CNS _____

3. CRNA _____

4. CSF _____

5. EKG _____

6. ETT _____

7. HR _____

8. PCA _____

9. PDPH _____

10. RR _____

Exercises and Activities

1. Describe the role of the nurse in providing care to a client before surgery.

   _____

   _____

   _____

   a. Medications that may be administered prior to surgery include:

   _____

   _____

   b. List at least five items that must be documented in the client's chart before surgery.

   (1) _____

   (2) _____

   (3) _____

   (4) _____

   (5) _____

   c. Why are oral fluids and food normally withheld before surgery?

   _____

   _____

   d. When in the preoperative preparation, should the informed consent be obtained?

   _____

   _____

2. What is the difference between sedation and general anesthesia?

   _____

   _____

   _____

   a. What client monitoring is needed during sedation?

   _____

   _____

b. In what ways might a client's anxiety and pain affect the medication required before and during surgery?

_____

_____

c. Describe the recovery phase from general anesthesia related to the following factors: Oxygenation/ventilation:

_____

_____

Heart rate and blood pressure:

_____

_____

d. List five factors that can contribute to a client's hypothermia or shivering.

(1) _____

(2) _____

(3) _____

(4) _____

(5) _____

3. Briefly describe the following methods of postoperative pain management and give at least one advantage and disadvantage or risk for each.

	Description	_Advantage(s)_	_Disadvantage(s)/Risk(s)_
PCA			
Regional analgesia			
Opioids			

4. S.L. is a 22-year-old client who has been admitted in active labor with her first pregnancy. S.L.'s mother and husband have stayed by her side since she arrived, giving her support and reassurance with each contraction. She is anticipating a vaginal birth using breathing and relaxation techniques they have been practicing. However, after 2 hours, her obstetrician feels that the baby is showing changes in its heart rate that indicate a Cesarean delivery would be necessary. To prepare for the surgery, S.L. is to receive epidural anesthesia.

a. S.L.'s mother asks you what an epidural is. How could you explain it to her?

_____

_____

b. What preparation will be needed before the epidural is administered?

_____

_____

c. In what ways might an epidural block be safer than general anesthesia for S.L. and the baby?

_____

_____

d. What types of residual effects might be noted as the anesthetic wears off following surgery?

_____

_____

e. List three factors that could contribute to a fluid imbalance during surgery.

   (1) _____

   (2) _____

   (3) _____

5. M.C. had right shoulder surgery following an injury sustained in a football game. He had a general anesthetic (halothane). Preoperatively his vital signs were as follows: T 98.6, P 60, R 20, and BP 110/70. He had an estimated blood loss of 200 cc during surgery. His dressing has a small amount of bloody drainage present. He is also complaining of a sore throat.

   a. The nurses assess M.C.'s vital signs upon return to his room. His postoperative vital signs are as follows: T 98.4, P 100, R 22, and BP 90/58. What may be the cause in the change of vital signs?

   _____

   _____

   b. Who should the nurse contact about the vital signs and why?

   _____

   _____

   c. Describe common side effects from the anesthetic halothane.

   _____

   _____

   d. The nurse reviews the chart and notes that M.C. was given succinolcholine chloride as an adjunct to the anesthesia. Explain why this drug was used during the surgery.

   _____

   _____

   e. M.C. complains of a sore throat. He is worried that he may have contracted the common cold during the surgery, as that is the only time he ever has a sore throat. What should the nurse tell M.C. about his sore throat?

   _____

   _____

   f. M.C. also complains of nausea after the surgery. What position should the nurse assist M.C. into in case he begins to vomit?

   _____

   _____

Self-Assessment Questions

Circle the letter that corresponds to the best answer.

1. Following general anesthesia, the ability of the client to respond to verbal commands and maintain his own airway are indicators of
   a. complete recovery.
   b. residual sensory block.
   c. skeletal muscle contraction.
   d. the initial phase of emergence.

2. A client in labor is receiving regional analgesia for labor pain. Because of the effects of this method of pain control, the nurse tells the client that she must remain on
   a. bed rest.
   b. EKG monitoring.
   c. intake and output.
   d. Foley catheterization.

3. The anesthetic most commonly used for epidural blocks is
   a. Epicaine.
   b. Marcaine.
   c. Xylocaine.
   d. Sublimaze.

4. A client has received regional anesthesia for a surgical procedure. Because the sympathetic nerves are the last type of nerve to recover, the client may experience
   a. an abnormal heart rate.
   b. orthostatic hypotension.
   c. increased pain sensation.
   d. blood pressure elevation.

5. Which of the following drugs may be used for surgical procedures that require the client to have complete skeletal muscle relaxation?
   a. Pavulon
   b. Xylocaine
   c. Prostigmin
   d. Carbocaine

6. The nurse is caring for a client who is experiencing a postdural puncture headache. Interventions will include **all** except which of the following?
   a. Analgesics
   b. Increased IV fluids
   c. Epidural blood patch
   d. Ambulation with assistance

7. The client is recovering from an epidural block anesthesia that included a long-acting opioid. During assessment, the nurse notes that the client has a respiratory rate of 10 breaths/minute. The best action for the nurse is to
   a. initiate cardiopulmonary resuscitation.
   b. notify the anesthesia provider.
   c. record normal emergence from anesthesia.
   d. continue monitoring respiratory rate and blood pressure.

8. The anesthetic most commonly used for local anesthesia is
    a. Epicaine.
    b. Marcaine.
    c. Xylocaine.
    d. Sublimaze.

9. Joint Commission on Accreditation of Healthcare Organizations standards for monitoring a client undergoing procedural sedation require that
    a. HR and oxygenation be continuously monitored.
    b. capnography be used.
    c. RR and pulmonary ventilation adequacy be monitored.
    d. Both a and c are required.

10. Nerve blocks last
    a. 30 minutes to 4 hours.
    b. 1 to 6 hours.
    c. 1 to 12 hours.
    d. up to 24 hours.

Surgery

Key Terms

Match the following terms with their correct definitions.

___ 1. Aldrete score

___ 2. Ambulatory surgery

___ 3. Asepsis

___ 4. Aseptic technique

___ 5. Circulating nurse

___ 6. Dehiscence

___ 7. Evisceration

___ 8. First assistant

___ 9. Informed consent

a. Associate of the surgeon, referring physician, or surgical resident who assists the surgeon to retract tissue, aids in the removal of blood and fluids at the operative site, and assists with hemostasis and wound closure.

b. Time during the surgical experience that begins when the client is transferred to the operating room table and ends when the client is admitted to the postanesthesia care unit.

c. Time during the surgical experience that begins at the end of the surgical procedure and ends when the client is discharged from medical care by the surgeon in addition to being discharged from the hospital or institution.

d. RN responsible and accountable for management of personnel, equipment, supplies, the environment, and communication throughout a surgical procedure.

e. Area surrounding the client and the surgical site that is free from all microorganisms; created by draping of the work area and the client with sterile drapes.

f. RN, LP/VN, or surgical technologist who provides services under the direction of the circulating nurse and who is qualified by training or experience to prepare and maintain the integrity, safety, and efficiency of the sterile field throughout an operation.

g. Surgical operation performed under general, regional, or local anesthesia and involving fewer than 24 hours of hospitalization.

h. Treatment of injury, disease, or deformity through invasive operative methods.

i. Complication of wound healing wherein the wound edges and layers separate below the skin.

___10. Intraoperative phase

j. Legal form signed by a competent client and witnessed by another person that grants permission to the client's physician to perform the procedure described by the physician and that demonstrates the client's understanding of the benefits, risks, and possible complications of the procedure, as well as alternate treatment options.

___11. Perioperative

k. Without microorganisms.

___12. Postoperative phase

l. Scoring system for objectively assessing the physical status of clients recovering from anesthesia; serves as a basis for dismissal from the postanesthesia care unit and ambulatory surgery; also known as the postanesthetic recovery score.

___13. Preoperative phase

m. Period of time comprising the preoperative, intraoperative, and postoperative phases of surgery.

___14. Scrub nurse

n. Complication of wound healing characterized by a complete separation of wound edges accompanied by visceral protrusion.

___15. Sterile

o. Collection of principles used to control and/or prevent the transfer of pathogenic microorganisms from sources within (endogenous) and outside (exogenous) the client.

___16. Sterile conscience

p. Time during the surgical experience that begins when the client decides to have surgery and ends when the client is transferred to the operating table.

___17. Sterile field

q. Individual's personal sense of honesty and integrity with regard to adherence to the principles of aseptic technique, including prompt admission and correction of any errors and omissions.

___18. Surgery

r. Absence of microorganisms.

Abbreviation Review

Write the meaning or definition of the following abbreviations, acronyms, and symbols.

1. AORN _____
2. EENT _____
3. NPO _____
4. OR _____
5. PACU _____
6. PCA _____

Exercises and Activities

1. Why is a thorough preoperative nursing assessment essential for the surgical client?

   _____

   _____

   _____

   a. Identify the sources of data for a nursing preoperative assessment.

      _____

      _____

   b. List three of the most common fears of clients who are facing surgery.

      (1) _____

      (2) _____

      (3) _____

   c. What signs and symptoms can indicate anxiety in the client?

      _____

      _____

   d. List the four purposes of preoperative teaching.

      (1) _____

      (2) _____

      (3) _____

      (4) _____

2. What items and preparation need to be documented before a surgical procedure?

   _____

   _____

   _____

   a. Why are renal and hepatic status in the client important?

      _____

      _____

   b. What factors in a client's medical history increase the risk for infection?

      _____

      _____

   c. List specific preoperative activities that prepare the client the morning of surgery.

      _____

      _____

      _____

3. Identify items and procedures that promote asepsis in the surgical suite.

_____

_____

_____

   a. Describe the concept of a "sterile conscience."

   _____

   _____

   b. Identify each of the following figures:

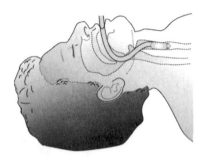

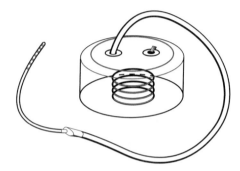

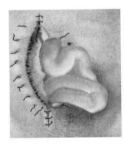

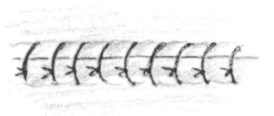

Courtesy of Delmar Cengage Learning

4. How will the nurse in the postanesthesia care unit monitor a client's respiratory and cardiovascular status?

   _____

   _____

   _____

   a. List five signs of respiratory distress.

      (1) _____

      (2) _____

      (3) _____

      (4) _____

      (5) _____

   b. Why is the postoperative client at risk for aspiration?

   _____

   _____

c. What observations and care are required for surgical wound dressing and any drains?

_____

_____

_____

_____

d. How often does the PACU nurse monitor vital signs?

_____

_____

5. O.Q., a 70-year-old client, has been admitted from a long-term care facility where he has been a resident for the past 3 weeks. He is now scheduled for a lower extremity amputation related to long-term peripheral vascular disease, a result of his diabetes. At first, O.Q. refused surgery, saying he was "just going to die anyway," but he recently decided to have the procedure done, after strong encouragement from his family. During the preoperative assessment, the nurse notes that O.Q. is moderately anxious and shows signs of poor nutrition and skin breakdown from his lack of mobility. His wife mentions that he has a hearing aid with him but does not like to use it.

a. What items will the nurse include in O.Q.'s preoperative teaching? How might his anxiety affect his ability to learn?

_____

_____

_____

b. What complications do elderly clients have associated with surgical procedures?

_____

_____

_____

c. Because O.Q. is diabetic and insulin dependent, what complications is he at risk for developing?

_____

_____

_____

d. Identify nursing interventions that will help prevent skin breakdown during and after surgery.

_____

_____

e. What factors are present for O.Q. that could delay wound healing?

_____

_____

_____

_____

6. S.C. was in a motor vehicle accident and sustained internal injuries. The surgeon performed a splenectomy and a partial bowel resection on S.C.

a. How would the nurse explain this set of procedures to the client's spouse?

_____

_____

b. S.C. weighed 257 pounds before surgery. How will her weight affect her postoperative recovery?

_____

_____

c. List three factors that increase the risk of surgical complications as the result of obesity and anesthesia use.

(1) _____

(2) _____

(3) _____

d. As the nurse assists S.C. with her cares, S.C. suddenly sneezes. She complains of severe burning at the incision. As the nurse inspects the wound, the nurse notes loops of bowel protruding from the wound. What activities should the nurse immediately do?

_____

_____

_____

e. Provide an example of how the nurse documents the evisceration and the care provided.

_____

_____

7. The nurse prepares to enter the operating room. Before donning gown and gloves, the nurse performs handwashing.

a. What is the rationale for handwashing before gowning and gloving?

_____

_____

b. How is this type of handwashing different from handwashing used in other areas of the hospital?

_____

_____

c. What is the rationale for the nurse removing jewelry when gloves will be worn?

_____

_____

8. S.S., age 6, had a tonsillectomy and adenoidectomy after repeated bouts of strep throat.

a. Explain the surgical procedure in terms that S.S.'s parents can understand.

_____

_____

b. What is the rationale for placing S.S. in a side-lying position postoperatively?

_____

c. The nurse prepared the room with suction equipment before S.S. returned from surgery. Why would suction be necessary?

_____

_____

Self-Assessment Questions

Circle the letter that corresponds to the best answer.

1. The nurse is caring for ambulatory (same-day) surgery clients. Which of the following actions by the nurse will be most important in preventing nosocomial infection?
   a. Using aseptic technique
   b. Administering antibiotics prophylactically
   c. Having the client cough and deep-breathe
   d. Teaching the client about ways to prevent infection

2. The postoperative phase of recovery for the client begins when the surgical procedure is completed and lasts until the client is
   a. well enough to be discharged home.
   b. fully recovered from the effects of anesthesia.
   c. discharged from medical care by the surgeon.
   d. returned to the general medical–surgical unit from PACU.

3. To assess renal function in the preoperative client, the physician orders a
   a. urine C&S.
   b. PTT and APTT.
   c. 24-hour urine collection.
   d. BUN and serum creatinine assessment.

4. The nurse is caring for a postoperative client who now has an Aldrete score of 10. Based on this information, the nurse will
   a. administer pain medication.
   b. likely transfer the client from PACU.
   c. notify the physician about the client's respiratory depression.
   d. continue monitoring the client every 15 minutes until a score of 20 is achieved.

5. Because of the effects of medication, a neurological assessment for the postoperative client does not include the client's
   a. level of consciousness.
   b. ability to answer questions.
   c. responsiveness to verbal stimulation.
   d. orientation to person, place, and time.

6. A nurse is preparing to instruct the client on postoperative care to be done at home. The best time for the nurse to begin teaching is
   a. at the time of the client's admission.
   b. immediately after the surgical procedure.
   c. when family members arrive to take the client home.
   d. after the client has received medication for pain and nausea.

7. The nurse is caring for an elderly client 1 day after surgery. Because this client is at risk for atelectasis, the nurse will
   a. maintain the client on supplemental oxygen.
   b. limit fluid intake to decrease fluid in the lungs.
   c. limit pain medication to prevent respiratory depression.
   d. instruct the client to cough, deep-breathe, and move often.

8. The nurse is performing an assessment on a client who is recovering from abdominal surgery. Which of these findings by the nurse may indicate an impending wound dehiscence?
   a. Abdominal distension
   b. Sudden increase in drainage
   c. The client's statement of pain
   d. Low-grade fever and tachycardia

9. A cholecystectomy is an example of a _____ type of surgery.
   a. diagnostic
   b. curative
   c. palliative
   d. restorative

10. Recovery time from anesthesia is _____ in the overweight client compared to the client of average weight.
    a. slower
    b. faster
    c. more critical
    d. unchanged

Oncology

Key Terms

Match the following terms with their correct definitions.

___ 1. Alopecia

    a. A treatment that involves aspirating and storing a fraction of bone marrow, exposing the client to high-dose drug therapy or total-body irradiation, and then reinfusing the bone marrow after treatment is complete.

___ 2. Anorexia

    b. Cancers occurring in blood-forming organs.

___ 3. Antineoplastic

    c. Inflammation of the oral mucosa.

___ 4. Benign

    d. Loss of appetite.

___ 5. Biologic response modifier

    e. Use of drugs to treat illness, especially cancer.

___ 6. Bone marrow transplant

    f. Escape of fluid into the surrounding tissue.

___ 7. Cachexia

    g. Not progressive; favorable for recovery.

___ 8. Cancer

    h. Partial or complete baldness or loss of hair.

___ 9. Carcinogen

    i. State of malnutrition and protein wasting

___10. Carcinoma

    j. To heal or restore health

___11. Chemotherapy

    k. Becoming progressively worse and often resulting in death.

___12. Curative

    l. A treatment for esophageal and early-stage lung cancer where light-activated drugs target cancer cells, leaving surrounding healthy tissue unharmed.

___13. Differentiation

    m. Spread of cancer cells to distant areas of the body by way of the lymph system or bloodstream.

___14. Extravasation

    n. Acquisition of characteristics or functions different from those of the original.

___15. Leukemia

    o. Cancer occurring in epithelial tissue.

___16. Lymphoma

    p. Agent that destroys malignant cells by stimulating the body's immune system.

___17. Malignant

    q. Agent that inhibits the growth and reproduction of malignant cells.

___18. Metastasis

    r. Substance that initiates or promotes the development of cancer.

___19. Neoplasm

    s. Tumor of the lymphatic system.

___20. Oncology

___21. Palliative surgery

___22. Photodynamic therapy

___23. Radiotherapy

___24. Reconstructive surgery

___25. Sarcoma

___26. Stomatitis

___27. Tumor marker

___28. Vesicant

t. Study of tumors.

u. Cancer occurring in connective tissue.

v. Any abnormal growth of new tissue.

w. Disease resulting from the uncontrolled growth of cells, which causes malignant cellular tumors.

x. Surgery to relieve symptoms in more advanced stages of cancer that does not alter the course of the disease.

y. Treatment of cancer with high-energy radiation.

z. Surgery to reestablish function or rebuild for a better cosmetic effect.

aa. Substance found in the serum that indicates the possible presence of malignancy.

bb. Agent that may produce blisters and tissue necrosis.

Abbreviation Review

Write the meaning or definition of the following abbreviations and acronyms.

1. ACS _____

2. AHCPR _____

3. BCG _____

4. BMT _____

5. CCNS _____

6. CCS _____

7. CNS _____

8. CT _____

9. DNA _____

10. EPA _____

11. TENS _____

12. TNM _____

Types of Cancers: Fill in the Blank

Fill in the blanks with information from the key terms used in this chapter.

1. Cancers occurring in infection-fighting tissues such as lymphatic tissue are known as

   _____ .

2. Cancers occurring in blood-forming organs such as bone marrow are known as

   _____ .

3. Cancers occurring in connective tissues such as bone are known as

   _____ .

4. Cancers occurring in epithelial tissues like the colon are known as

   _____ .

Exercises and Activities

1. How do cancer cells differ from normal cells?

   _____

   _____

   _____

   a. Describe how tumor markers help in cancer detection.

   _____

   _____

   b. How does staging of tumors differ from grading of tumors?

   _____

   _____

   c. What is a stage I tumor?

   _____

   _____

2. The seven warning signs of cancer are remembered with the acronym CAUTION. Identify what each of the letters represents.

   C _____

   A _____

   U _____

   T _____

   I _____

   O _____

   N _____

3. List three lifestyle factors that can increase an individual's risk for cancer.

   _____

   _____

   _____

   a. According to Table 34-1, cigarette smoking is a risk factor for which types of cancer?

   _____

   _____

   b. You are asked to present a class on healthy behaviors to women. What would you include in your teaching to help them lower their risk for cancer? What recommendations would you make for health screening for early detection?

   _____

   _____

   _____

   _____

4. How are palliative and reconstructive surgery used in the treatment of cancer?

_____

_____

_____

a. Describe how each of these treatments destroys cancer cells.

Radiation: _____

_____

Chemotherapy: _____

_____

Biotherapy: _____

_____

Bone marrow transplantation: _____

_____

b. What precautions are important for nurses to consider when administering chemotherapy?

_____

_____

c. What precautions are important for health care workers when a client is treated with radiation?

_____

_____

d. Identify the cause of and three nursing interventions for the following complications.

	Cause	Interventions
Bone marrow dysfunction		1. 2. 3.
Poor nutrition		1. 2. 3.
Fatigue		1. 2. 3.
Dyspnea		1. 2. 3.
Ascites		1. 2. 3.

    d. List four medical emergencies that can develop with advanced cancer.

       (1) _____

       (2) _____

       (3) _____

       (4) _____

5. C.R., a 72-year-old client, has been admitted to your unit following a collapse in her apartment. Although usually in good health, she had noticed increasing fatigue and leg pain, with a lesion developing on the right lower leg. After feeling ill all morning, she attempted to stand up, but sudden, severe pain in her leg and general weakness caused her to fall and hit her head. A neighbor found her the next day, and she was admitted to the hospital. C.R. has now been diagnosed with multiple myeloma, a malignancy affecting the bone marrow and soft tissue. She has refused surgery but is undergoing radiation. C.R. has very limited mobility and weight-bearing on her right side. During your morning care, you note two large, draining, purplish red lesions on her right leg, two new discolored areas on her left leg, and one on her back. Pressure on her right leg causes a great deal of pain, and she now has very little appetite.

    a. List four actual nursing diagnoses for this client.

       (1) _____

       (2) _____

       (3) _____

       (4) _____

    b. Draw a line under the nursing diagnosis in the preceding list that you believe is most important, and identify at least three nursing interventions.

       (1) _____

       (2) _____

       (3) _____

    c. What side effects of radiation do you need to monitor for?

    _____

    _____

    d. What impact can pain have on the client with cancer?

    _____

    _____

    _____

    _____

    e. Because C.R. is most likely in an advanced stage of cancer, what are your goals for her?

    _____

    _____

    _____

    _____

Self-Assessment Questions

Circle the letter that corresponds to the best answer.

1. A nurse is caring for a client with breast cancer. Because the cancer has metastasized to the bone, the nurse will monitor for signs and symptoms of which serious complication?
   a. Hypokalemia
   b. Osteomyelitis
   c. Hypercalcemia
   d. Spinal cord compression

2. Your client is exposed to vinyl chloride, a carcinogen, at his job. Because of his occupational exposure, you will include in your health teaching that it is especially important for him to
   a. lose weight.
   b. stop smoking.
   c. avoid drinking alcohol.
   d. take vitamin supplements.

3. For clients with cancer that has metastasized, palliative surgery may be used to
   a. restore health.
   b. relieve symptoms.
   c. minimize deformity.
   d. improve the survival rate.

4. You are caring for a client with pancreatic cancer. Because he is showing signs of cachexia, you determine that your client would benefit most from
   a. antibiotics.
   b. pain control.
   c. oxygen therapy.
   d. nutritional guidance.

5. A nursing student is assigned to care for a client with a grade IV tumor. Based on this information, the instructor explains to the student that this client's tumor
   a. involves at least four lymph nodes.
   b. is most responsive to chemotherapy.
   c. is undifferentiated with a poor prognosis.
   d. involves metastasis to another organ or bone.

6. Food substances that may reduce cancer risk are
   a. cabbage and broccoli.
   b. cauliflower and brussels sprouts.
   c. kohlrabi and legumes.
   d. all of the above.

7. When grading tumors, the higher the grade, the
   a. more cells are differentiated.
   b. better the prognosis.
   c. worse the prognosis.
   d. less cells are aggressive.

8. When caring for a client with internal radiation
   a. several nurses should be assigned to the client so that exposure time is minimized.
   b. the nurse should prepare items for client care in the room.
   c. the nurse should not remain in the room for longer than an hour.
   d. special precautions should be taken with body secretions as a sealed source.

9. Hallmarks of malnutrition are
   a. weight loss of 5% and serum albumin of 3.8 g/dL.
   b. weight loss of 10% and serum albumin of 3.5 g/dL.
   c. weight loss of 20% and serum albumin of 3.3 g/dL.
   d. none of the above.

10. A major problem that can occur when cancer metastasizes to bone is
    a. paralytic ileus.
    b. electrolyte imbalance.
    c. infertility.
    d. pathological fracture.

Respiratory System

Key Terms

Match the following terms with their correct definitions.

___ 1. Adventitious breath sound

___ 2. Asthma

___ 3. Atelectasis

___ 4. Audible wheeze

___ 5. Bronchial sound

___ 6. Bronchiectasis

___ 7. Bronchitis

___ 8. Bronchovesicular sound

___ 9. Caseation

___ 10. Cavitation

___ 11. Chemoreceptor

___ 12. Coarse crackle

___ 13. Diffusion

___ 14. Emphysema

___ 15. Epistaxis

a. Lung disease wherein air accumulates in the tissues of the lungs.

b. Condition wherein blood accumulates in the pleural space of the lungs.

c. Persistent, intractable asthma attack.

d. Condition wherein air or gas accumulates in the pleural space of the lungs, causing the lungs to collapse.

e. Condition characterized by intermittent airway obstruction due to antigen antibody reaction.

f. Receptor that monitors the levels of carbon dioxide, oxygen, and pH in the blood.

g. Abnormal sound, including sibilant wheezes (formerly wheezes), sonorous wheezes (formerly rhonchi), fine and coarse crackles (formerly rales), and pleural friction rubs.

h. Inflammation of the bronchioles and alveoli accompanied by consolidation, or solidification of exudate, in the lungs.

i. Collection of pleural fluid within the pleural cavity.

j. Process of exchanging oxygen and carbon dioxide.

k. Phospholipid that is present in the lungs and lowers surface tension to prevent collapse of the airways.

l. Breath sound normally heard in the area of the scapula and near the sternum; medium in pitch and intensity, with inspiratory and expiratory phases of equal length.

m. Lung disorder characterized by chronic dilation of the bronchi.

n. Exchange of gases between the atmosphere and the lungs.

o. Exchange of oxygen and carbon dioxide at the cellular level.

___16. External respiration

___17. Fine crackle

___18. Hemopneumothorax

___19. Hemothorax

___20. Internal respiration

___21. Liquefaction necrosis

___22. Lung stretch receptor

___23. Perfusion

___24. Pleural effusion

___25. Pleural friction rub

___26. Pleurisy

___27. Pneumonia

___28. Pneumothorax

___29. Primary tubercle

___30. Respiration

___31. Sibilant wheeze

___32. Sonorous wheeze

___33. Status asthmaticus

___34. Stridor

p. Movement of air into and out of the lungs.

q. Death and subsequent change of tissue to a liquid or semi-liquid state; often descriptive of a primary tubercle.

r. Abnormal breath sound that is low pitched and snoring in nature and is louder on expiration.

s. Nodule that contains tubercle bacilli and forms within lung tissue.

t. Condition arising from inflammation of the pleura, or sac, that encases the lung.

u. Abnormal breath sound that is creaky and grating in nature and is heard on inspiration and expiration.

v. Receptor that monitors the patterns of breathing and prevents overexpansion of the lungs.

w. Collapse of a lung or a portion of a lung.

x. Wheeze that can be heard without the aid of a stethoscope.

y. Inflammation of the bronchial tree accompanied by hypersecretion of mucus.

z. Process whereby the center of the primary tubercle formed in the lungs as a result of tuberculosis becomes soft and cheeselike due to decreased perfusion.

aa. Process whereby a cavity is created in the lung tissue through the liquefaction and rupture of a primary tubercle.

bb. Moist, low-pitched crackling and gurgling lung sound of long duration.

cc. Hemorrhage of the nares or nostrils; also known as nosebleed.

dd. Dry, high-pitched crackling and popping lung sound of short duration.

ee. Abnormal breath sound that is high pitched and musical in nature and is heard on inhalation and exhalation.

ff. Blood flow through an organ or body part.

gg. Loud, tubular, hollow-sounding breath sound normally heard over the sternum.

hh. Process whereby a substance moves from an area of higher concentration to an area of lower concentration.

___35. Surfactant

ii. Soft, low breath sound heard over the majority of lung tissue.

___36. Ventilation

jj. Collection of air and blood in the pleural cavity.

___37. Vesicular breath sound

kk. Abnormal, high-pitched, musical breathing sound caused by a blockage in the throat or larynx.

Abbreviation Review

Write the meaning or definition of the following abbreviations, acronyms, and symbols.

1. ABG _____
2. ACS _____
3. AFB _____
4. APTT _____
5. ARDS _____
6. ASO _____
7. BCG _____
8. CAT _____
9. CHF _____
10. CO_2 _____
11. COLD _____
12. COPD _____
13. HIV _____
14. MDRTB _____
15. min _____
16. PE _____
17. PFT _____
18. PPD _____
19. PT _____
20. SaO_2 _____
21. SARS _____
22. TB _____
23. URI _____

Exercises and Activities

1. Describe the normal pathway of oxygen through the respiratory system to the bloodstream.

   _____

   _____

   _____

a. Identify the structures of the respiratory system on the diagram.

Alveoli

Diaphragm

Epiglottis

Larynx

Left lower lobe

Left upper lobe

Mainstem bronchus

Nasopharynx

Respiratory bronchiole

Right lower lobe

Right middle lobe

Right upper lobe

Trachea

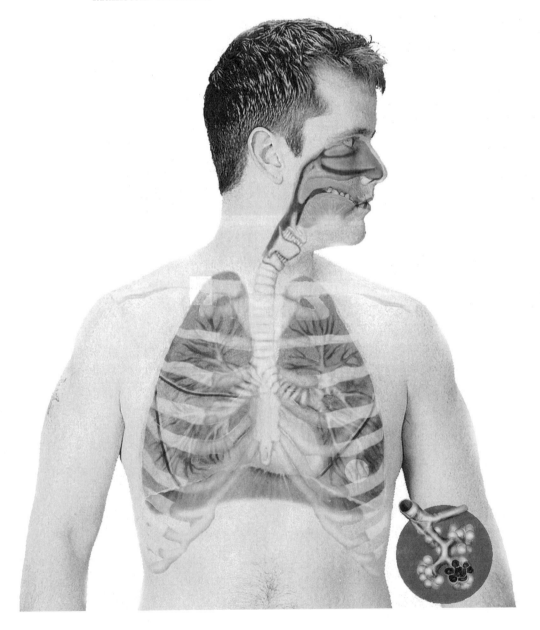

Courtesy of Delmar Cengage Learning

b. Differentiate external respiration and internal respiration.

_____

_____

c. What is the role of surfactant?

_____

_____

d. Differentiate the terms *ventilation* and *perfusion.*

_____

_____

e. What makes us breathe?

_____

_____

f. How is the ability to breathe affected in COPD/COLD?

_____

_____

2. Describe the items that the nurse would include in a respiratory assessment.

_____

_____

_____

a. Write four questions that the nurse might ask clients about their health history.

(1) _____

(2) _____

(3) _____

(4) _____

b. Match the correct term to the definition and then place the assigned number on the diagram where each type of sound would be best heard.

____ (1) Adventitious breath sound

____ (2) Audible wheeze

____ (3) Bronchial wheeze

____ (4) Bronchovesicular sound

____ (5) Coarse crackle

____ (6) Fine crackle

a. Abnormal, high-pitched musical breathing sound caused by a blockage in the throat or larynx.

b. Soft, low breath sound heard over the majority of lung tissue.

c. Loud, tubular, hollow breath sound normally heard over the sternum.

d. Abnormal breath sound that is high-pitched and musical in nature and is heard on inhalation and exhalation.

e. Dry, high-pitched crackling and popping lung sound of short duration.

f. Moist, low-pitched crackling and gurgling lung sound of long duration.

___ (7) Pleural friction rub

___ (8) Sibilant wheeze

___ (9) Sonorous wheeze

___(10) Stridor

___(11) Vesicular breath sound

g. Wheeze that can be heard without the aid of a stethoscope.

h. Abnormal breath sound that is creaky and grating in nature and is heard on inspiration and expiration.

i. Abnormal breath sound that is low-pitched and snoring in nature and is louder on expiration.

j. Breath sounds normally heard in the area of the scapula and near the sternum; medium in pitch and with inspiratory and expiratory phases of equal duration.

k. Abnormal sound including sibilant wheezes, sonorous wheezes, fine and coarse crackles, and pleural friction rubs.

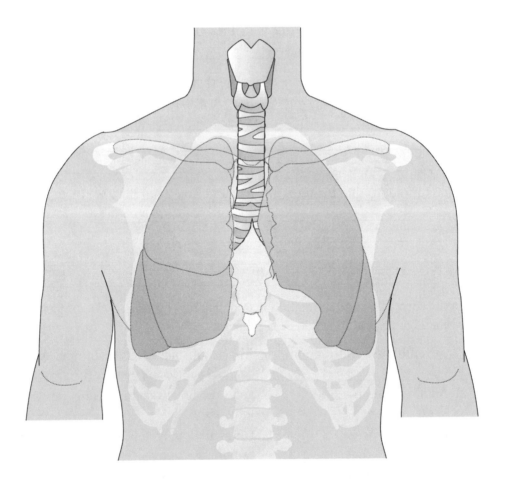

Courtesy of Delmar Cengage Learning

c. Outline on the diagram the areas where you will hear each of the normal breath sounds.

3. G.N., a 63-year-old grain farmer, smokes 2 packs of cigarettes a day and is now hospitalized with pneumonia. The nurse notes he is dyspneic when walking or talking. He also has circumoral cyanosis. Which of the following nursing interventions should the nurse do first?

a. Elevate the head of the bed.
b. Obtain an oximetry reading.
c. Apply oxygen via mask.
d. Obtain a sputum culture.

_____

_____

4. What factors increase the risk of tuberculosis?

_____

_____

_____

a. What are the common signs and symptoms of tuberculosis?

_____

_____

b. How is tuberculosis diagnosed?

_____

_____

c. Describe the medication and treatment for tuberculosis today.

_____

_____

d. What factors can contribute to the safety of health care workers exposed to tuberculosis?

_____

_____

e. Why is the hospitalized client with tuberculosis placed in a negative pressure room?

_____

_____

5. Compare the following disorders of the respiratory system.

	Risk Factors	Signs and Symptoms	Nursing Interventions
Pneumonia			
Pulmonary edema			
Pulmonary embolus			
Pneumothorax			

6. S.W. is a typically active 8-year-old who was first diagnosed with asthma when he began having episodes of congestion and breathing difficulties around the age of 2. Although he had several trips to the emergency room by the time he was 6 years old, he has been healthy since then, with occasional URIs. This week, however, S.W. developed a particularly bad cold that has now started another round of asthma symptoms. Although he did not seem to have much trouble at first, S.W.'s mother brought him in to start treatment. S.W.'s nurse hears wheezing even before using the stethoscope. His mother says, "S.W.'s older brother has asthma, too, but we keep him on his medicine and bring him in if he gets too sick."

   a. List the predisposing factors for asthma.

   _____

   _____

   b. Describe the changes that take place in the airways with asthma.

   _____

   _____

   c. Why is a detailed history important in treating S.W.'s asthma?

   _____

   _____

   d. What subjective symptoms might S.W. be experiencing?

   _____

   _____

   e. List five objective findings that S.W.'s nurse might detect on assessment.

   (1) _____

   (2) _____

   (3) _____

   (4) _____

   (5) _____

   f. Describe several nursing interventions that are appropriate for S.W.'s care.

   _____

   _____

   g. What should the nurse include in patient teaching regarding asthma for the client and family?

   _____

   _____

7. The physician decides to have a chest tube inserted in the client who has a left pleural effusion as the result of cancer. Number the following items according to the order in which they will occur.

   _____ a. Assess lung sounds.
   _____ b. Gather supplies: chest tube tray, betadine prep solution, and tape.
   _____ c. Obtain consent.
   _____ d. Position client.

_____ e. Document where the tube was placed, and the amount and type of drainage.
_____ f. Apply dressing.
_____ g. Obtain vital signs.
_____ h. Assess for pain and discomfort.
_____ i. Assess for the presence of crepitus.

Self-Assessment Questions

Circle the letter that corresponds to the best answer.

1. While assessing a client's respiratory system, the nurse remembers that a normal finding of the respiratory assessment is
   a. asymmetry of the chest wall and occasional use of the accessory muscles.
   b. bronchial breath sounds over the anterior chest of high pitch and long duration.
   c. vesicular breath sounds over the majority of the lung fields with occasional fine crackles.
   d. bronchovesicular breath sounds by the scapulae posteriorly and near the sternum anteriorly.

2. A client has an increased risk for a pulmonary embolism if she is
   a. on Coumadin therapy.
   b. diabetic or uses oral contraceptive pills.
   c. between the ages of 20 and 35.
   d. anemic and has episodes of dyspnea.

3. During a physical assessment of the client, the nurse notes Cheyne-Stokes respirations. The description of this respiratory pattern is
   a. irregular periods of increased rate and depth of respiration.
   b. apnea alternating with short periods of shallow respirations.
   c. abnormally slow breathing of increased depth and associated cyanosis.
   d. slow, shallow respirations increasing in rate and depth, alternating with apnea.

4. A nurse is caring for a client with a chest tube in place. If the chest tube is dislodged, the first action of the nurse will be to
   a. evaluate respiratory effort and notify the physician.
   b. replace the tube using sterile gloves and aseptic technique.
   c. cover the opening with petrolatum gauze and apply pressure.
   d. assess the opening on the chest wall for lacerations and drainage.

5. The nurse is examining a client with pneumonia. What abnormal assessment findings are likely to be noted?
   a. Friction rub and stridor
   b. Fine and coarse crackles
   c. Hyperresonance and fever
   e. Bronchovesicular breath sounds

6. The nurse suspects pulmonary edema in a client who has
   a. a chronic cough with purulent sputum.
   b. noticeable wheezing and pain on inspiration.
   c. a cough that produces a large amount of pink, frothy sputum.
   d. absent breath sounds with a mediastinum shift toward the affected side.

7. Chemoreceptors normally initiate respiration in response to a(n) _____ of carbon dioxide in the blood.
   a. change
   b. decrease
   c. increase
   d. low level

8. A client with _____ is more likely to exhibit wheezing.
   a. congestive heart failure or atelectasis
   b. a lung abscess or pleurisy
   c. pneumonia or atelectasis
   d. bronchitis or asthma

9. Group A beta-hemolytic streptococci infections of the upper respiratory system are associated with serious sequelae such as
   a. laryngitis.
   b. rheumatic fever.
   c. sinusitis.
   d. pharyngitis.

10. Which of the following states a change that does *not* occur in an elderly client's respiratory status?
    a. The cough reflex increases.
    b. The aspiration risk increases.
    c. Ciliary activity diminishes.
    d. The medulla becomes less sensitive to changes in carbon dioxide levels.

Cardiovascular System

Key Terms

Match the following terms with their correct definitions.

___ 1. Aneurysm

___ 2. Angina pectoris

___ 3. Annulus

___ 4. Arteriosclerosis

___ 5. Ascites

___ 6. Atherosclerosis

___ 7. Baseline level

___ 8. Bradycardia

___ 9. Cardiac tamponade

___10. Dyspnea

___11. Dysrhythmia

___12. Embolus

___13. Hemolysis

___14. Homan's sign

___15. Hypertrophy

___16. Implantable cardioverter-defibrillator

___17. Myocardial infarction

___18. Myocarditis

___19. Necrosis

a. Irregularity in the rate, rhythm, or conduction of the electrical system of the heart.

b. Test to check for the presence of clots in the leg.

c. Inflammation of the myocardium of the heart.

d. Short, high-pitched squeak heard as two inflamed pericardial surfaces rub together.

e. Inflammation in the wall of a vein without clot formation.

f. Treatment that involves injecting a chemical into the vein, causing the vein to become sclerosed (hardened) so blood no longer flows through it.

g. Heart rate in excess of 100 beats per minute in an adult.

h. Formed clot that remains at the site where it formed.

i. Removal of fluid from the pericardial sac.

j. Condition of suddenly awakening, sweating, and having difficulty breathing.

k. Weakness in the wall of a blood vessel.

l. Abnormal accumulation of fluid in the peritoneal cavity.

m. Lab value that serves as a reference point for future value levels.

n. Increase in muscle mass.

o. Formation of a clot because of blood pooling in the vessel, trauma to the vessel's endothelial lining, or a coagulation problem with little or no inflammation in the vessel.

p. Inflammation of the membrane sac surrounding the heart.

q. Fluttering or pounding sensation in the chest.

r. Formation of a clot due to an inflammation in the wall of the vessel.

s. Tissue death as the result of disease or injury.

___20. Orthopnea

___21. Palpitation

___22. Paroxysmal nocturnal dyspnea

___23. Percutaneous balloon valvuloplasty

___24. Pericardial friction rub

___25. Pericardiocentesis

___26. Pericarditis

___27. Peripheral resistance

___28. Phlebitis

___29. Phlebothrombosis

___30. Primary hypertension

___31. Sclerotherapy

___32. Secondary hypertension

___33. Stasis dermatitis

___34. Stent

___35. Tachycardia

___36. Thrombectomy

___37. Thrombophlebitis

___38. Thrombosis

___39. Thrombus

___40. Transesophageal echocardiography

___41. Varicosities

___42. Vein ligation

___43. Vein stripping

___44. Virchow's triad

t. Breakdown of red blood cells.

u. Difficulty breathing.

v. Heart rate less than 60 beats per minute in an adult.

w. Valvular ring in the heart.

x. Insertion of a balloon in a stenosed valve to expand the narrowed valvular space.

y. Pressure within a vessel that resists the flow of blood.

z. Inflammation of the skin due to decreased circulation.

aa. Surgical removal of a clot.

bb. Formation of a clot in a vessel.

cc. Tiny metal tube with holes in it that prevents a vessel from collapsing and keeps the atherosclerotic plaque pressed against the vessel wall; any material used to hold tissue in place or provide support.

dd. Necrosis (death) of the myocardium caused by an obstruction in a coronary artery.

ee. Difficulty breathing while lying down.

ff. Mass, such as a blood clot or an air bubble, that circulates in the bloodstream.

gg. Implantable device that senses a dysrythmia and automatically sends an electrical shock directly to the heart to defibrillate it.

hh. Cardiovascular disease of fatty deposits on the inner lining, the tunica intima, of vessel walls.

ii. Narrowing and hardening of arteries.

jj. Chest pain caused by a narrowing of the coronary arteries.

kk. Diagnostic ultrasonic imaging of the cardiac structures through the esophagus.

ll. Tying off an involved section of a vein with suture.

mm. Three factors (pooling of blood, vessel trauma, and a coagulation problem) that lead to the formation of a clot.

nn. Visibly prominent, dilated, and twisted veins.

oo. Collection of fluid in the pericardial sac hindering the functioning of the heart.

pp. Introducing a wire into a vein to strip the walls of the vein.

qq. Elevated blood pressure greater than 140/90 mm Hg with cause unknown.

rr. Elevated blood pressure greater than 140/90 mm Hg due to another condition within the body.

Anatomy and Physiology Key Terms

Match the following terms with their correct definitions.

___ 1. Afterload

___ 2. Cardiac cycle

___ 3. Cardiac output

___ 4. Contractility

___ 5. Depolarization

___ 6. Heart sounds

___ 7. Preload

___ 8. Repolarization

___ 9. Stroke volume

___10. Vasoconstriction

___11. Vasodilation

a. Contraction of the heart.

b. Recovery phase of the heart.

c. Volume of blood pumped per minute by the left ventricle.

d. Impulse has gone through the conduction system of the heart and the ventricles contracted.

e. Volume of blood pumped per contraction.

f. Amount of pressure within the ventricles.

g. Force needed to open the semilunar valves.

h. Increase in the diameter of the vessel.

i. Sound heard by auscultation of the heart.

j. Strength of cardiac contraction.

k. Decrease in the diameter of the vessel.

Abbreviation Review

Write the meaning or definition of the following abbreviations, acronyms, and symbols.

1. ABG _____

2. ACE _____

3. ALG _____

4. APPT _____

5. AST _____

6. ATG _____

7. AV _____

8. CABG _____

9. CAD _____

10. CBC _____

11. CHF _____

12. CK or CPK _____

13. CPR _____

14. DVT _____

15. EKG _____

16. ESR _____

17. Hct _____

18. HDL _____

19. Hgb _____

20. HTN _____

21. IABP _____

22. ICD _____

23. ICU _____

24. INR _____

25. LAD _____

26. LDH _____

27. LDL _____

28. MI _____

29. MRI _____

30. MUGA _____

31. PAC _____

32. PAT _____

33. PSVT _____

34. PT _____

35. PTCA _____

36. PTT _____

37. PVC _____

38. SA _____

39. TEE _____

40. VF _____

41. VLDL _____

42. VT _____

Exercises and Activities

1. Write in the correct terms on the diagram of the heart.

   Aorta

   Aortic valve

   Inferior vena cava

   Left atrium

   Left pulmonary artery

   Left ventricle

   Mitral valve

   Pulmonary valve

   Pulmonary veins

   Right atrium

   Right pulmonary artery

   Right ventricle

   Septum

   Superior vena cava

   Tricuspid valve

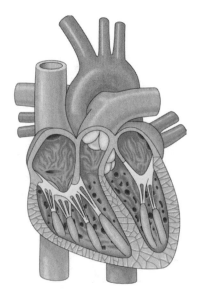

Courtesy of Delmar Cengage Learning

a. Describe the pathway of blood flow through the heart, including the valves (starting with the vena cava).

_____

_____

b. Fill in the blanks with the following terms to describe the electrical pathway of the heart.

atria

AV node

bundle branches

bundle of His

myocardial cells

P wave

Purkinje fibers

QRS complex

right atrium

SA node

ventricles

What makes the heart beat? The heart has a conduction system that starts with its own pacemaker. This pacemaker, or the _____ , is a small amount of nervous tissue in the _____ . From this spot, an electrical impulse spreads across both _____ like ripples in a pond and causes them to contract. You can see this on an EKG strip as a _____ . The electrical impulse then travels to the _____ , where it pauses briefly. This short pause (a tenth of a second) gives the ventricles time to fill with blood. The impulse then proceeds down the AV bundle, which is also called the _____ , and continues to the right and left _____ . From there, the impulse travels to the _____ . These fibers transmit the electrical impulse into the _____ , which make the right and left _____ of the heart contract (systole). On an EKG strip, this is seen as the _____ .

c. Why are ventricular dysrhythmias more serious than atrial dysrhythmias?

_____

_____

2. What information does the nurse need to obtain from clients about their health history?

_____

_____

_____

a. List five unalterable risk factors for heart disease.

(1) _____

(2) _____

(3) _____

(4) _____

(5) _____

b. How can diet and lifestyle choices modify an individual's risk for heart disease?

_____

_____

   c. Why do clients often fail to seek health care for signs and symptoms of cardiac problems?

   _____

   _____

3. What elements will the nurse include in a thorough assessment of the cardiovascular system?

   _____

   _____

   _____

   a. Describe typical symptoms that clients often experience with cardiac disorders.

   _____

   _____

   b. How can clients be assessed for increased fluid volume?

   _____

   _____

   c. Why are breath sounds monitored in clients with cardiac problems?

   _____

   _____

   d. Differentiate findings for arterial occlusion versus venous occlusion in the legs.

   _____

   _____

4. Compare the following dysrhythmias, including their cause and treatment:

	Description	Cause	Treatment
Atrial tachycardia			
Premature ventricular contractions			
Ventricular tachycardia			
Third-degree AV block			

   a. List the cause, assessment findings, and treatment for the following inflammatory disorders:

	Cause	Signs/Symptoms	Treatment
Infective endocarditis			
Myocarditis			
Mitral valve prolapse			

5. List typical symptoms of a myocardial infarction. How might the symptoms be different for a female client than a male?

_____

_____

_____

a. What is a silent myocardial infarct?

_____

_____

b. How does an MI damage the heart?

_____

_____

c. List nursing interventions that will promote recovery for the client following an MI.

_____

_____

d. What client teaching would be needed before discharge?

_____

_____

e. Why does congestive heart failure occur after a myocardial infarction?

_____

_____

f. What diagnostic tests are done when diagnosing CHF?

_____

_____

g. What is the rational for teaching the client to weigh himself or herself daily?

_____

_____

6. J.W., a 59-year-old plumber, was diagnosed several years ago with primary hypertension. At the time, he was motivated to lose 20 lb, cut back on his smoking, and modify his diet. However, J.W. eventually became noncompliant when medications that his physician incorporated into his stepped-care treatment plan seemed to cause uncomfortable side effects. J.W. is now admitted to the hospital with heart failure, the result of continued damage from his hypertension.

a. Briefly describe the stepped-care approach for management of hypertension.

_____

_____

b. Why can hypertension lead to heart failure?

_____

_____

c. Name several other conditions that can result in heart failure.

_____

_____

d. If J.W. is diagnosed with left-sided heart failure, what signs and symptoms might be noted on his assessment?

_____

_____

e. List at least five observations that would indicate that the right side of his heart is also failing.

(1) _____

(2) _____

(3) _____

(4) _____

(5) _____

f. What medical and nursing interventions will improve J.W.'s heart function?

_____

_____

g. What blood pressure reading indicates hypertension?

_____

_____

h. What dietary modifications could the client undertake?

_____

_____

i. List three categories of antihypertensive medication.

(1) _____

(2) _____

(3) _____

7. N.A., age 77, has atrial fibrillation. He takes Lanoxin and Coumadin daily. What is the rationale for taking an aminoglycoside and anticoagulant for this condition?

_____

_____

_____

a. When the nurse assesses vital signs, at which pulse rate should the physician be notified when the client is on Lanoxin?

_____

_____

b. Identify the symptoms of digitoxicity.

_____

_____

c. What is a normal serum digoxin level?

_____

_____

d. What is the antidote for digoxin overdose?

_____

_____

e. What laboratory test is done for clients taking anticoagulants? And what is the expected range for clients taking Coumadin?

_____

_____

f. What is the antidote for Coumadin overdose?

_____

_____

g. What dietary considerations should be taught to the client taking anticoagulants?

_____

_____

Self-Assessment Questions

Circle the letter that corresponds to the best answer.

1. The cardiac output is equal to the
    a. resting pulse rate for 1 minute.
    b. pulse rate multiplied by the stroke volume.
    c. volume of blood pumped by the left ventricle with each contraction.
    d. volume of blood circulated by the heart in relation to the blood pressure.

2. According to Virchow's triad, the clients most at risk for developing a clot are those with
    a. decreased clotting ability, leg trauma, and obesity.
    b. hypertension, phlebitis, and a positive Homan's sign.
    c. pooling of blood, vessel trauma, and a coagulation problem.
    d. venous stasis, a family history of heart disease, and inactivity.

3. Following a myocardial infarction, your client has started thrombolytic therapy with streptokinase. Which of the following would indicate a serious side effect of this therapy?
    a. Tarry stools
    b. Hypertension
    c. Enlarged lymph nodes
    d. Decreased urine output

4. The first heart sound (S_1) is the sound of the
    a. beginning of diastole.
    b. closing of the mitral and tricuspid valves.
    c. opening of the aortic and pulmonic valves.
    d. closing of the valves on the right side of the heart.

5. Premature ventricular contractions are usually caused by
   a. anxiety.
   b. hypertension.
   c. myocardial ischemia.
   d. coronary artery disease.

6. The nurse is caring for a client who had been on bed rest following surgery. During the assessment, the nurse notes a hardened area in the right calf with warmth and tenderness. The best action for the nurse is to
   a. notify the physician.
   b. gently massage the area to relieve pain.
   c. encourage the client to increase ambulation.
   d. apply an ice pack.

7. A nurse is caring for a client who has been admitted with CHF. The nurse will administer a vasodilator such as nitroglycerine to this client to
   a. relieve angina.
   b. decrease fluid retention.
   c. improve myocardial contractility.
   d. decrease the amount of blood returning to the heart.

8. The volume of blood pumped by the ventricle with each contraction is called the
   a. cardiac output.
   b. stroke volume.
   c. minute volume.
   d. stroke index.

9. Clients with congestive heart failure may have this heart sound.
   a. S_1
   b. S_2
   c. S_3
   d. S_4

10. The T wave represents the
    a. repolarization of the atria.
    b. repolarization of the ventricles.
    c. contraction of the atria.
    d. contraction of the ventricles.

Hematologic and Lymphatic Systems

Key Terms

Match the following terms with their correct definitions.

____ 1. Agranulocytosis

____ 2. Apheresis

____ 3. Autologous

____ 4. Bands

____ 5. Blastic phase

____ 6. Erythrocytapheresis

____ 7. Fibrinolysis

____ 8. Hemarthrosis

____ 9. Hematocrit

____10. Hematopoiesis

____11. Hemolysis

____12. Hyperuricemia

____13. Idiopathic

____14. Leukocytosis

____15. Leukopenia

____16. Lymphoma

____17. Phlebotomy

____18. Purpura

____19. Reticulocyte

____20. Secondary malignancy

____21. Sickle

____22. Thrombocytopenia

a. Process of breaking fibrin apart.

b. Intensified phase of leukemia that resembles an acute phase in which there is an increased production of white blood cells.

c. Acute condition causing a severe reduction in the number of granulocytes (basophils, eosinophils, and neutrophils).

d. Decrease in the number of platelets in the blood.

e. Removal of blood from a vein.

f. Increased number of white blood cells.

g. Increased uric acid blood level.

h. Removal of unwanted blood components.

i. Percentage of blood cells in a given volume of blood.

j. Procedure that removes abnormal red blood cells and replaces them with healthy ones.

k. Decreased number of white blood cells.

l. Second malignant condition that develops after successful treatment of an initial malignancy.

m. Bleeding into the joints.

n. Increased circulation of immature neutrophils.

o. Process of blood cell production and development.

p. Occurring without a known cause.

q. Immature red blood cell.

r. Condition in which red blood cells become crescent shaped and elongated.

s. Reddish purple patches on the skin indicative of hemorrhage.

t. Tumor of the lymphatic system.

u. Breakdown of red blood cells.

v. Collected "from self."

Abbreviation Review

Write the meaning or definition of the following abbreviations, acronyms, and symbols.

1. ABVD _____
2. ALL _____
3. AML _____
4. APTT _____
5. ATG _____
6. CHOP _____
7. CLL _____
8. CML _____
9. COPP _____
10. CVP _____
11. DIC _____
12. ESR _____
13. Hct _____
14. Hgb _____
15. HLA _____
16. ITP _____
17. LDH _____
18. MOPP _____
19. NHL _____
20. PCA _____
21. PMN _____
22. PT _____
23. PTT _____
24. RBC _____
25. TIBC _____
26. WBC _____

Exercises and Activities

1. What does plasma contain?

_____

_____

a. Identify the following components of blood, giving their purpose and normal laboratory values.

	Purpose	Normal Values
RBCs		
WBCs		
Platelets		

b. How do RBCs contribute to oxygenation?

_____

_____

c. How does having anemia affect oxygenation?

_____

_____

d. What is the average life span of RBCs?

_____

_____

e. Why can reticulocyte counts be used as a diagnostic tool?

_____

_____

2. Label the following diagram of the lymph system.

Axillary node

Cervical node

Inguinal node

Iliac node

Intestinal node

Lymphatic vessel (2)

Palatine tonsil

Peyer's patch

Spleen

Submandibular node

Thymus gland

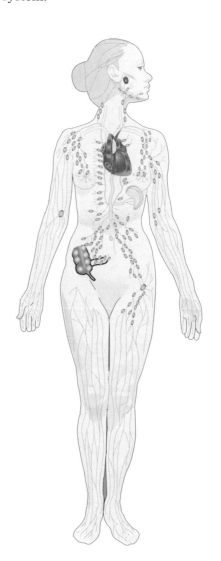

Courtesy of Delmar Cengage Learning

a. Identify the purpose of each of the following:

Lymph nodes: _____

_____

Spleen: _____

_____

Thymus: _____

_____

b. How does the lymphatic system prevent edema?

_____

_____

c. How is lymph different from plasma?

_____

_____

d. Identify the two main functions of the lymphatic system.

_____

_____

3. Identify the nursing procedures for administering a blood transfusion.

_____

_____

_____

a. Why can a person with type O negative blood be a universal blood donor?

_____

_____

b. Why is a person with type AB blood considered a universal receiver?

_____

_____

c. What is the nurse's responsibility if a blood reaction occurs?

_____

_____

d. Identify the signs and syptoms of a transfusion reaction that the nurse needs to be observant for.

_____

_____

4. Write several questions that you would ask clients about their health history.

(1) _____

(2) _____

(3) _____

(4) _____

(5) _____

(6) _____

a. What physical findings would be important in assessment of the client?

_____

_____

b. Briefly describe symptoms and diagnostic tests for the following disorders.

	Symptoms	Diagnostic Tests
Iron deficiency anemia		
Polycythemia		
Acute lymphocytic leukemia		
Thrombocytopenia		
Hodgkin's lymphoma		

c. How would you explain a bone marrow transplant to a client?

_____

_____

d. What types of clients are at risk for developing DIC?

_____

_____

5. You are caring for 3-year-old B., who was brought in because of persistent bleeding from his lip after falling from a chair at home. While talking with B.'s mother, you discover that B. would sometimes get a bruise where he was given his immunizations. He also seemed to get a lot of bruises after he started walking. She mentions that last week B. had a nosebleed that seemed to last a lot longer than it should have. Physical assessment findings and laboratory tests indicate that B. has hemophilia A, an inherited bleeding disorder.

a. Briefly describe the normal clotting mechanism of the blood. How does hemophilia A interfere with this normal clotting process?

_____

_____

_____

_____

b. B.'s mother asks you how B. could have gotten this disease. How would you answer her?

_____

_____

c. What other signs and symptoms might be noted with hemophilia?

_____

_____

d. List three risk nursing diagnoses for B.

(1) _____

(2) _____

(3) _____

e. What treatment is used for hemophilia A?

_____

_____

f. What teaching will B.'s family need for home care?

_____

_____

_____

_____

6. C.P., a 22-year-old college student, saw the physician because she feels so tired. She is pale, with tachycardia and dyspnea on exertion. She admits to finishing a heavy menstrual cycle a week ago. The pysician ordered a serum hemoglobin with her results being 8.5 g/dl. The doctor concluded C.P. has iron deficiency anemia. What other lab tests are used to confirm this diagnosis?

_____

_____

_____

a. The physician ordered Feosol, an iron preparation, for C.P. What dietary considerations should the nurse discuss with C.P. regarding Feosol?

_____

_____

b. Why is an increased intake of vitamin C also recommended for clients with iron deficiency anemia?

_____

_____

c. Identify food sources that are high in iron content.

_____

_____

d. Why should the nurse include information about constipation when teaching the client about Feosol?

_____

_____

e. What additional information should the nurse give the client regarding activity and excerise while she is anemic?

_____

_____

Self-Assessment Questions

Circle the letter that corresponds to the best answer.

1. A client has been diagnosed with thrombocytopenia. The nurse understands that this is a coagulation disorder that includes
   a. a lack of clotting factors in the blood.
   b. microthrombi in arterioles and venules.
   c. a decrease in the number of platelets in the blood.
   d. a syndrome alternating between clotting and hemorrhaging.

2. The nurse is caring for a client with leukemia. The nurse recalls that with this diagnosis, the most likely cause of death would be
   a. DIC.
   b. pneumonia.
   c. heart failure.
   d. hemorrhage.

3. The first sign of Hodgkin's lymphoma in a client is usually
   a. unexplained weight loss.
   b. easy bleeding and bruising.
   c. painless swelling of a lymph node.
   d. tender, enlarged lymph nodes and fever.

4. A nurse is performing an admission assessment on a client with a diagnosis of polycythemia. Which of the following findings would the nurse anticipate when reviewing his laboratory results?
   a. High hematocrit
   b. Low hemoglobin
   c. Low WBC count
   d. Increased polymorphs

5. A client has been diagnosed with bacterial sepsis. Because this is a predisposing condition for DIC, the nurse will monitor the client for
   a. chills and fever.
   b. general fatigue and malaise.
   c. swollen and tender lymph nodes.
   d. reddish patches on the skin and oozing.

6. Your client is newly diagnosed with Hodgkin's disease. She asks you to tell her about it. You begin by saying that Hodgkin's disease is
   a. a rare lymphoma with an unknown cause.
   b. a malignancy of the blood-forming tissues.
   c. a type of anemia resulting in an increased RBC supply.
   d. an inherited hemolytic anemia caused by a recessive gene.

7. Erythropoietin stimulates the bone marrow to produce more
   a. reticulocytes.
   b. platelets.
   c. granulocytes.
   d. lymphocytes.

8. Agranulocytes are classified into two groups, monocytes and
   a. neutrophils.
   b. lymphocytes.
   c. eosinophils.
   d. basophils.

9. The only intravenous solution given during a blood transfusion is
   a. 5% dextrose in 0.9% sodium chloride.
   b. 5% dextrose in 0.45% sodium chloride.
   c. 0.9% sodium chloride.
   d. 0.45% sodium chloride.

10. A complication not likely to occur in polycythemia is
    a. cerebral vascular accident.
    b. myocardial infarction.
    c. emphysema.
    d. hemorrhage.

Gastrointestinal System

Key Terms

Match the following terms with their correct definitions.

_____ 1. Adhesion

_____ 2. Ascites

_____ 3. Calculus

_____ 4. Cholelithiasis

_____ 5. Cirrhosis

_____ 6. Colostomy

_____ 7. Constipation

_____ 8. Diverticula

_____ 9. Diverticulosis

_____10. Effluent

_____11. Gastric ulcer

_____12. Glycogenesis

_____13. Glycogenolysis

_____14. Hematemesis

_____15. Hemorrhoid

_____16. Ileostomy

_____17. Intussusception

_____18. Jaundice

_____19. Ligation

_____20. Melena

a. Saclike protrusion of the intestinal wall that results when the mucosa herniates through the bowel wall.

b. Yellow discoloration of the skin, sclera, mucous membranes, and body fluids that occurs when the liver is unable to fully remove bilirubin from the blood.

c. Stool containing partially broken down blood; usually black, sticky, and tarlike.

d. Erosion formed in the esophagus, stomach, or duodenum resulting from acid/pepsin imbalance.

e. Distal end of the gastrointestinal (GI) or urinary system brought to the outside of the body and sutured into place.

f. Scar tissue from previous surgeries or disease processes.

g. Abnormal accumulation of fluid in the peritoneal cavity.

h. Liquid output from an ileostomy.

i. Test for microscopic blood done on stool.

j. Conversion of glycogen into glucose.

k. Erosion in the stomach.

l. Concentration of mineral salts in the body leading to the formation of stone.

m. Presence of gallstones or calculi in the gallbladder.

n. Opening created in the small intestine at the ileum.

o. Vomiting of blood.

p. Abnormal growth of tissue.

q. Condition characterized by hard, infrequent stools that are difficult or painful to pass.

r. Condition in which multiple diverticula are present in the colon.

s. Conversion of glucose into glycogen.

t. Application of a band or tie around a structure.

___21. Occult blood test (guaiac)

___22. Peptic ulcer

___23. Polyp

___24. Postprandial

___25. Steatorrhea

___26. Stoma

___27. Volvulus

u. Fatty stool.

v. Swollen vascular tissue in the rectal area.

w. After eating.

x. Twisting of a bowel on itself.

y. Opening created anywhere along the large intestine.

z. Chronic degenerative changes in the liver cells and thickening of surrounding tissue.

aa. Telescoping of one part of the intestine into another.

Key Terms: Inflammatory Conditions of the Gastrointestinal System

Match the following terms with their correct definitions.

___ 1. Appendicitis

___ 2. Cholecystitis

___ 3. Diverticulitis

___ 4. Gastritis

___ 5. Hepatitis

___ 6. Pancreatitis

___ 7. Peritonitis

___ 8. Stomatitis

a. Inflammation of the stomach mucosa.

b. Inflammation of a diverticula.

c. Inflammation of the peritoneum.

d. Inflammation of the oral mucosa.

e. Inflammation of the vermiform appendix.

f. Inflammation of the gallbladder.

g. Acute or chronic inflammation of the pancreas.

h. Acute or chronic inflammation of the liver.

Abbreviation Review

Write the meaning or definition of the following abbreviations, acronyms, and symbols.

1. ALT _____

2. AST _____

3. CBD _____

4. CEA _____

5. EGD _____

6. ERCP _____

7. ET _____

8. GERD _____

9. GGT _____

10. HAV _____

11. HBIG _____

12. HC1 _____

13. HCV _____

14. HDV _____

15. IBD _____

16. LDH _____

17. LES _____

18. NG _____

19. NPO _____

20. NSAID _____

21. PT _____

22. PTT _____

23. RLQ _____

24. TIPS _____

25. UC _____

26. UGI _____

Exercises and Activities

1. Label this diagram of the digestive system.

> Appendix
>
> Ascending colon
>
> Descending colon
>
> Duodenum
>
> Esophagus
>
> Gallbladder
>
> Ileum
>
> Jejunum
>
> Liver
>
> Mouth
>
> Pancreas
>
> Rectum
>
> Salivary glands
>
> Sigmoid
>
> Stomach
>
> Transverse colon

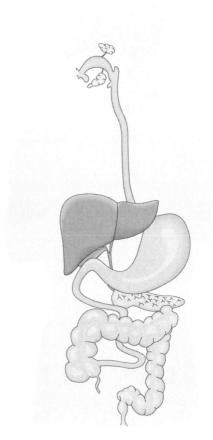

Courtesy of Delmar Cengage Learning

a. Identify two or more functions for each of the following:

Mouth

(1) _____

(2) _____

Gallbladder

(1) _____

(2) _____

Small intestine

(1) _____

(2) _____

Large intestine

(1) _____

(2) _____

Stomach

(1) _____

(2) _____

(3) _____

Pancreas

(1) _____

(2) _____

(3) _____

Liver

(1) _____

(2) _____

(3) _____

(4) _____

(5) _____

b. What changes with aging in the older adult make good nutrition more difficult?

_____

_____

_____

_____

2. If your client has GI symptoms, what types of questions will you ask him or her?

_____

_____

_____

a. What information will be obtained from the physical examination?

_____

_____

b. Describe the order in which the nurse collects data from inspection, palpation, percussion, and auscultation of the abdominal area.

_____

_____

3. Compare symptoms and medical–surgical management for the following GI disorders.

	Signs/Symptoms	Management/Interventions
Gastric ulcer		
Hepatitis		
Cirrhosis		
Oral cancer		

a. What are predisposing factors for developing peritonitis? What objective findings might be present?

_____

_____

b. What laboratory tests would be abnormal in a client with peritonitis?

_____

_____

c. Briefly describe treatment/interventions for the client with peritonitis.

_____

_____

d. What strategies might help a client manage the following GI symptoms?
Constipation: _____

_____

Anorexia: _____

_____

e. How can health care workers protect themselves from acquiring hepatitis?

_____

_____

4. L.O. is a 38-year-old security officer with a small home security company. He is being seen for chronic GI symptoms. Over the past 3 years, he has been experiencing cramping and abdominal pain and a weight loss of several pounds. He sometimes has several loose stools a day and is now having occasional bloody diarrhea. Other than his own food allergies, he is not aware of any particular family history of GI disease. After previously being diagnosed with ulcerative colitis, he was given medication that has been only partially helpful. Now, his increasing bouts of pain and diarrhea are making it very difficult for him to work because he is often away from toilet facilities.

a. How does ulcerative colitis differ from Crohn's disease?

_____

_____

b. What dietary/lifestyle changes might help a client with symptoms of ulcerative colitis?

_____

_____

c. What are the goals for management of this disease?

_____

_____

d. Because medication and dietary management have been unsuccessful in controlling L.O.'s symptoms, what surgical intervention might be indicated?

_____

_____

   e. If untreated, what complications is he at risk for? What complications is a client with Crohn's disease at risk of developing?

_____

_____

   f. How does inflammatory bowel disease have an impact on an individual's life?

_____

_____

5. R.F., a 58-year-old married accountant, was diagnosed with colon cancer. What diagnostic tests are done to confirm this diagnosis?

   a. The treatment for R.F. includes a bowel resection of the descending colon and a subsequent colostomy. R.F. asks the nurse to explain what this means. How does the nurse reply?

_____

_____

   b. When R.F. returns from his surgery, the nurse assesses the new stoma. Describe what a new stoma should look like.

_____

_____

   c. Given the following complications of colon surgery, identify the nursing interventions for each of them.

Hemorrhage _____

_____

Obstruction _____

_____

Prolapse _____

_____

Electrolyte imbalance _____

_____

Skin excoriation _____

_____

   d. When R.F. is preparing for discharge home with his wife, what referrals should the nurse make for him?

_____

_____

Self-Assessment Questions

Circle the letter that corresponds to the best answer.

1. The nurse's assessment findings for the client with GI bleeding may include hematemesis and a black, sticky, tarlike stool called
   a. guaiac.
   b. melena.
   c. steatorrhea.
   d. meconium.

2. The process of converting glycogen to glucose in response to low blood sugar is a function of the
   a. liver.
   b. pancreas.
   c. duodenum.
   d. gallbladder.

3. A client has been diagnosed with infectious hepatitis. As the nurse caring for this client, you understand that to decrease your chance of acquiring this disease, you need to
   a. avoid needlesticks.
   b. use enteric precautions.
   c. use a gown and special respiratory mask.
   d. complete the hepatitis B immunization series.

4. Your client is admitted with a GI disorder. She complains of pain in the upper right quadrant that radiates to the right scapular area 2 hours after eating. She now has nausea and indigestion. The nurse recalls that these are symptoms of
   a. gastritis.
   b. appendicitis.
   c. cholecystitis.
   d. irritable bowel syndrome.

5. A nurse is performing an assessment on a client with a gastric ulcer in the duodenum. The nurse may anticipate symptoms that include pain 2 to 4 hours after eating, pain during the night, and
   a. fatigue.
   b. diarrhea.
   c. weight loss.
   d. weight gain.

6. For the client being treated for ulcers, the physician orders antacids, prostaglandins, and
   a. Indocin.
   b. NSAIDs.
   c. H_2 blockers.
   d. milk products.

7. A common nursing-assessment finding of Crohn's disease is
   a. guaiac.
   b. melena.
   c. steatorrhea.
   d. meconium.

8. Partially digested food and digestive enzymes in the stomach are called
   a. digestion.
   b. haustra.
   c. peristalsis.
   d. chime.

9. Complications that can occur after ostomy surgery are
   a. hemorrhage and rupture.
   b. diverticulitis and infection.
   c. obstruction and prolapse.
   d. hernia and gastric dumping.

10. The output from an ileostomy usually is
    a. thin yellow-green liquid.
    b. thick yellow-green stool.
    c. thin green-brown liquid.
    d. thick green-brown stool.

Urinary System

![black bar]

Key Terms

Match the following terms with their correct definitions.

_____ 1. Anasarca

_____ 2. Azotemia

_____ 3. Cachectic

_____ 4. Calculus

_____ 5. Cystitis

_____ 6. Dialysate

_____ 7. Dialysis

_____ 8. Dysuria

_____ 9. Erythropoiesis

_____10. Fulguration

_____11. Glomerular filtration rate

_____12. Hematuria

_____13. Ileal conduit

_____14. Intravesical

_____15. Litholapaxy

_____16. Lithotripsy

_____17. Micturition

_____18. Nephrotoxic

a. Inability to suppress the sudden urge or need to urinate.

b. Pus in the urine.

c. Within the urinary bladder.

d. Calculus or stone formed in the urinary tract.

e. Difficult or painful urination.

f. Generalized edema.

g. Method of crushing a calculus any place in the urinary system with ultrasonic waves.

h. Production of red blood cells and their release by red bone marrow.

i. Nitrogenous wastes present in the blood.

j. Mechanical means of removing nitrogenous waste from the blood by imitating the function of the nephrons; involves filtration and diffusion of wastes, drugs, and excess electrolytes and/or osmosis of water across a semipermeable membrane into a dialysate solution.

k. Implantation of the ureters into a piece of ileum, which is attached to the abdominal wall as a stoma so urine can be removed from the body.

l. Behind the peritoneum outside the peritoneal cavity.

m. Severe pain in the kidney that radiates to the groin.

n. Concentration of mineral salts, known as stones.

o. Process of expelling the urine from the urinary bladder; also called urination or voiding.

p. Crushing of a bladder stone and immediate washing out of the fragments through a catheter.

q. Bacterial infection of the renal pelvis, tubules, and interstitial tissue of one or both kidneys.

r. Being in a state of malnutrition and wasting.

___19. Nocturia

___20. Nocturnal enuresis

___21. Oliguria

___22. Overflow incontinence

___23. Polyuria

___24. Pyelonephritis

___25. Pyuria

___26. Renal colic

___27. Residual urine

___28. Retroperitoneal

___29. Stress incontinence

___30. Urge incontinence

___31. Urgency

___32. Urinary incontinence

___33. Urinary retention

___34. Urolithiasis

s. Incontinence that occurs during sleep.

t. Solution used in dialysis, designed to approximate the normal electrolyte structure of plasma and extracellular fluid.

u. Leakage of urine when a person does anything that strains the abdomen, such as coughing, laughing, jogging, dancing, sneezing, lifting, making a quick movement, or even walking.

v. Leaking of urine when the bladder becomes very full and distended.

w. Urine remaining in the bladder after the individual has urinated.

x. Involuntary loss of urine from the bladder.

y. Procedure to destroy tissue with long high-frequency electric sparks.

z. Inability to void when there is an urge to void.

aa. Inflammation of the urinary bladder.

bb. Quality of a substance that causes kidney tissue damage.

cc. Amount of fluid filtered from the blood into the capsule per minute.

dd. Presence of red blood cells in the urine.

ee. Excessive urination at night.

ff. Excreting abnormally large volumes of urine.

gg. Feeling the need to urinate immediately.

hh. Diminished output of urine.

Abbreviation Review

Write the meaning or definition of the following abbreviations and acronyms.

1. ACKD _____

2. ACS _____

3. AML _____

4. ARF _____

5. ATN _____

6. A-V _____

7. BPH _____

8. BUN _____

9. C&S _____

10. CAPD _____

11. EABV _____

12. ESR _____

13. ESRD _____

14. ESWL _____

15. GFR _____

16. IVP _____

17. KUB _____

18. NIDDK _____

19. NSAID _____

20. PKD _____

21. UTI _____

Exercises and Activities

1. What are the four functions of the kidneys?

(1) _____

(2) _____

(3) _____

(4) _____

a. Draw the kidneys, ureters, and bladder in the correct location on the diagram.

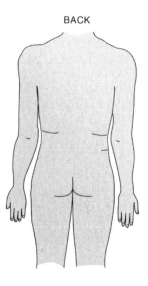

BACK

b. List six warning signs for kidney disease.

(1) _____

(2) _____

(3) _____

(4) _____

(5) _____

(6) _____

Courtesy of Delmar Cengage Learning

c. List the changes in older adults that make them more prone to having problems with:

Urination _____

_____

Infection _____

_____

Kidney failure _____

_____

2. Which clients need a more thorough than usual assessment of the urinary system?

_____

_____

_____

a. Identify several subjective and objective assessment findings for clients with kidney disorders.

_____

_____

_____

b. What terms would be used to document these findings?

Pus in the urine _____

Painful urination _____

Blood in the urine _____

c. A client on your rehabilitation unit tells you one morning, "It hurts when I urinate." Write five questions that you might ask to get more information.

(1) _____

(2) _____

(3) _____

(4) _____

(5) _____

3. List medical, surgical, or lifestyle interventions for the following symptoms.

	Interventions
Stress incontinence	
Nocturnal enuresis	
Urge incontinence	

a. Which clients are predisposed for developing renal calculi? What signs and symptoms might they experience?

_____

_____

b. Briefly describe two forms of medical–surgical treatment for calculi.

_____

_____

_____

_____

c. What dietary changes may be recommended for clients who have renal calculi?

_____

_____

d. Describe how the nurse would explain the procedure of straining the urine to the client with renal calculi.

_____

_____

4. Your client, who is 29 years old, has developed chronic renal failure because of an inherited poly-cystic kidney disease. As she waits for a transplant, what information will she need about her diet and activity?

_____

_____

_____

a. How would you explain the differences between peritoneal dialysis and hemodialysis?

_____

_____

b. What special precautions are needed for a client who uses hemodialysis?

_____

_____

_____

_____

c. What laboratory tests does the nurse need to monitor with the client who is receiving dialysis?

_____

_____

d. The client has been told to avoid foods that are high in potassium. List several sources of foods containing high amounts of potassium.

_____

_____

e. The client has an AV shunt for dialysis in the left forearm. What adaptations for care does the nurse need to consider?

_____

_____

5. K.W., a 22-year-old junior programmer at a local computer firm, missed a couple of days of work 2 weeks ago with a bad sore throat and a fever. He thought he had a mild case of flu because several coworkers had been out sick with it recently. Usually, K.W. is a cheerful, easygoing guy, but now he feels miserable, with a headache, no appetite, and malaise, and he thinks his urine looks a little odd. K.W. says he should be over the flu by now, "so what's wrong with me?"

   a. K.W. is suspected of having acute glomerulonephritis, a disorder frequently caused by which one of the following?

Klebsiella	*Haemophilus influenzae*
Escherichia coli	*Pseudomonas aeruginosa*
Staphylococcus aureus	group A beta-hemolytic streptococcus

   b. Is this an upper UTI or a lower UTI? _____

   c. What other signs and symptoms might K.W. have?

_____

_____

   d. What laboratory results would you anticipate with acute glomerulonephritis?

_____

_____

   e. K.W. says he does not understand how a throat infection could give him a kidney problem. How will you explain this to him?

_____

_____

   f. K.W. wants to know what the treatment is for his disorder. Discuss medical interventions, including medication, diet, and activity.

_____

_____

_____

_____

   g. If K.W.'s kidney disorder becomes chronic, what long-term symptoms and signs would he experience? What would be the treatment?

_____

_____

_____

_____

_____

_____

6. Compare the different types of incontinence and identify causes for the incontinence and nursing interventions for each.

Type of Incontinence	Cause	Nursing Interventions
Stress incontinence		
Urge incontinence		
Overflow incontinence		
Total incontinence		
Nocturnal enuresis		

7. V.L., a 55-year-old white male who smokes and works in a fabric-dying industry, recently saw the physician for hematuria. The physician performed a cystoscopy and found bladder tumors. What risk factors are there for the development of bladder tumors?

_____

_____

_____

   a. The doctor performed fulguration of the tumors. Explain fulguration in terms that V.L. might understand.

_____

_____

   b. How is fulguration different from a TUR?

_____

_____

   c. The doctor decided on BCG therapy for V.L. Explain how this treatment works.

_____

_____

   d. The RN developed the nursing diagnosis of **K**nowledge Deficit related to surgery and treatment regiment. Give an example of a planning goal for this client.

_____

_____

Self-Assessment Questions

Circle the letter that corresponds to the best answer.

1. A nursing student is reviewing the nursing care of a client who is experiencing renal failure. The student recalls that functions of the kidney include helping with acid–base balance, secreting renin to raise blood pressure, and producing a hormone responsible for
    a. sodium excretion.
    b. serum calcium levels.
    c. adrenal gland stimulation.
    d. red blood cell production.

2. During morning report to the student, the nurse states that the client with acute renal failure now has oliguria. The student understands that this indicates that the client is
    a. having pain with urination.
    b. voiding less than 400 mL per day.
    c. voiding more than 1,000 mL per day.
    d. voiding fewer than four times in 24 hours.

3. Fluid restriction will be an appropriate intervention for the client with a diagnosis of
    a. ESRD.
    b. urolithiasis.
    c. pyelonephritis.
    d. urge incontinence.

4. The nurse is providing discharge instructions to a client who has received treatment for urinary calcium calculi. Which of the following statements by the client indicates a need for additional teaching?
    a. "I need to keep track of my intake and output."
    b. "I should drink plenty of water and other fluids every day."
    c. "Too much activity and exercise can make more stones form."
    d. "Milk and other dairy products may cause me to have more stones."

5. The nursing student is assigned to care for a client with kidney failure who receives hemodialysis using an arteriovenous graft. Which of the following will the instructor emphasize to the student?
    a. Weigh the client before and after each dialysis treatment.
    b. Medications should be administered shortly before dialysis.
    c. Absence of a thrill or bruit over the graft site is a normal finding.
    d. Take the blood pressure and pulse on the arm with the graft to assess for circulation.

6. The residual urine left in the bladder should be less than
    a. 25 mL.
    b. 50 mL.
    c. 75 mL.
    d. 100 mL.

7. The majority of urinary tract infections are caused by
   a. *Klebsiella.*
   b. *S. aureus.*
   c. *P. aeruginosa.*
   d. *E. coli.*

8. Elderly clients are more prone to urinary tract infections due to
   a. fecal incontinence.
   b. increased muscle tone.
   c. prostate gland shrinkage.
   d. emptying of the bladder.

9. An example of a lower urinary tract infection is
   a. pyelonephritis.
   b. glomerulonephritis.
   c. cystitis.
   d. urolithiasis.

10. The dietary restriction for a client with uric acid kidney stones is
    a. calcium-rich foods.
    b. purine-rich foods.
    c. foods such as broccoli and chocolate.
    d. oxalate-rich foods.

Musculoskeletal System

Key Terms

Match the following terms with their correct definitions.

b 1. Amphiarthrosis

u 2. Amputation

i 3. Arthroplasty

q 4. Bruxism

a 5. Closed reduction

v 6. Contracture

j 7. Crepitus

o 8. Diarthrosis

c 9. Dislocation

r 10. Fracture

w 11. Heberden's nodes

aa 12. Internal fixation

k 13. Kyphosis

d 14. Locomotor

n 15. Lordosis

h 16. Open reduction

e 17. Orthopedics (orthopaedics)

x 18. Osteoporosis

L 19. Paresthesia

a. Repair of a fracture done without surgical intervention.

b. Condition characterized by slightly movable joints such as the vertebrae.

c. Injury in which the articular surfaces of a joint are no longer in contact.

d. Pertaining to movement or the ability to move.

e. Branch of medicine that deals with the prevention or correction of the disorders and diseases of the musculoskeletal system.

f. Cutting a hole in a plaster cast to relieve pressure on the skin or a bony area and to permit visualization of the underlying body part.

g. Lateral curvature of the spine.

h. Surgical procedure that enables the surgeon to reduce (repair) a fracture under direct visualization.

i. Replacement of both articular surfaces within a joint capsule.

j. Grating or crackling sensation or sound.

k. Increased roundness of the thoracic spinal curve.

l. Abnormal sensation such as numbness or tingling.

m. Immovable joint.

n. Exaggeration of the curvature of the lumbar spine.

o. Freely movable joint.

p. Subcutaneous nodules of sodium urate crystals.

q. Teeth grinding during sleep.

r. Break in the continuity of a bone.

s. Sensation of pain, soreness, and stiffness in an amputated limb.

_o_ 20. Phantom limb pain

_g_ 21. Scoliosis

_t_ 22. Sprain

_y_ 23. Strain

_z_ 24. Subluxation

_m_ 25. Synarthrosis

_p_ 26. Tophi

_f_ 27. Windowing

t. Injury to ligaments surrounding a joint caused by a sudden twist, wrench, or fall.

u. Removal of all or part of an extremity.

v. Permanent shortening of a muscle.

w. Enlargement and characteristic hypertrophic spurs in the terminal interphalangeal finger joints.

x. Increase in the porosity of bone.

y. Injury to a muscle or tendon due to overuse or overstretching.

z. Partial separation of an articular surface.

aa. Repair of fracture using pins, screws, or plates.

Abbreviation Review

Write the meaning or definition of the following abbreviations and acronyms.

1. BMD _____

2. CMS _____

3. CPM _____

4. CRP _____

5. DEXA _____

6. ELISA _____

7. EMG _____

8. NIAMS _____

9. NOF _____

10. OA _____

11. ORIF _____

12. RF _____

13. ROM _____

14. SCD _____

15. SXA _____

16. TMD _____

17. TMJ _____

Exercises and Activities

1. Label each of the bones on this diagram.

Clavicle

Cranium

Femur

Fibula

Humerus

Maleolus

Mandible

Patella

Pelvis

Phalanges

Radius

Rib

Scapula

Sternum

Tibia

Ulna

Vertebral column

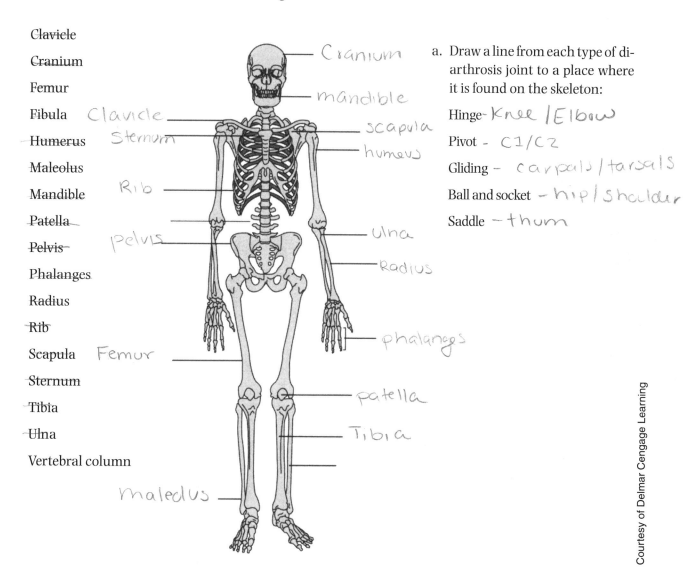

Handwritten labels on skeleton: Cranium, mandible, scapula, humerus, Clavicle, Sternum, Rib, ulna, Radius, Pelvis, phalanges, Femur, patella, Tibia, maleolus

a. Draw a line from each type of di-arthrosis joint to a place where it is found on the skeleton:

Hinge- Knee / Elbow

Pivot - C1/C2

Gliding - carpals / tarsals

Ball and socket - hip / shoulder

Saddle - thum

Courtesy of Delmar Cengage Learning

a. What is the difference between voluntary and involuntary muscle?

Voluntary = have to be told to move
Involuntary = found in organs →organs move the muscles.

b. Identify these spinal curvatures.

- "Hump-back"
- Thoracic Spine
- older person w/ osteoprosis

(Thoracic)

- lateral
- school age

Courtesy of Delmar Cengage Learning

Kyphosis   Scoliosis

The type of curvature seen in pregnancy is ___lordois (lumbar)___
The type of curvature associated with osteoporosis is ___Kyphosis___.
Adolescents are assessed for a curvature called ___Scoliosis___.

2. What is included in an assessment of the musculoskeletal system?
- muscle strength   - gait
- bone intregrity   - ? ADL's
- posture   - Shorten extremities
- Joint function   - pain

pg. 1231

a. List several findings that would be abnormal for a joint.

_____

_____

b. How could you assess for ROM
for the neck? ___70° (Lt) and (Rt) rotation___

for the hip? ___45° abduction___

for the shoulder? ___180° abduction, 180° forward flexion,___
___50° hyperextension, 90° External rotation___

c. Why is an assessment made of the client's ability to perform activities of daily living (ADL)?

_____

_____

3. Name and describe the types of fractures pictured here.

a. _Comminuted_

b. _Open / compound_

Courtesy of Delmar Cengage Learning

c. Your client had a long arm cast applied 1 hour ago. How will you assess the cast?

List the six P's for the neurovascular assessment of this client.

Pg 1239

(1) _Paresthesia (numbness - tingling)_
(2) _pain_
(3) _Pallor (capillary refill check - 2-4 seconds)_
(4) _Paralysis_
(5) _puffiness (edema)_
(6) _pulselessness._

How often will you assess the client?

15 - 30 minutes for seveal hours and then every 3-4 hours.

d. Describe the signs and symptoms of three complications of a fracture.

Infection: _Reslt of an open fx. Also from sx (if needed). Slows healing._

Fat embolism: _(normally associated w/long bone fx., multiplue fx, or crushing Injury. Occurs w/in 24-72 hours. Involves pain in lungs._

Compartment syndrome: _____

e. List three types of traction. Describe nursing care for a client in traction.

1. Skeletal traction, 2. Skin traction, 3. Manual traction.

4. Identify ten risk factors for osteoporosis.

(1) Female

(2) history of fx.

(3) thin (sm) bones

(4) family history

(5) w/o estrogen replacment

(6) amenorrhea

(7) eating disorders

(8) low calcium

(9) inactive

(10) smoking/drinking

P.y.
124 2

a. What will you include in teaching for a client who is newly diagnosed with osteoporosis?

Diet: diet high in calcium + Vitamin D no smoking/alcohol.

Safety: Fx. risk, take medication

Activity: practice good body mechanics, encorage movement to prevent more bone loss.

b. Why are individuals with osteoporosis more likely to suffer fractures?

because both mineral and protien matrix deminish → bones become soft.

5. K.C., a 61-year-old client, has been diagnosed with osteoarthritis. Although she used to be quite active with her family and gardening, she is having increasing problems with stiffness and pain in her knees, especially the right knee. An old injury to the right knee many years ago is probably contributing to the additional pain and loss of mobility on that side now. K.C. acknowledges that she needs to lose some of her extra weight and at first attributed her knee pain to "old age." She asks for more information about this disorder.

a. Describe the signs and symptoms of osteoarthritis.

b. How will you explain the changes that are occurring in OA?

c. What type of lifestyle changes and medication might be suggested for K.C.?

d. Why are NSAID medications effective in the treatment of osteoarthritis?

e. K.C. has lost only a few pounds but has been trying medication and physical therapy and uses a cane for support. Now, however, she can hardly climb the stairs in her house and is in almost constant pain. K.C. is scheduled for arthroplasty on her right knee. Briefly describe this surgery.

_____

_____

f. What nursing care and interventions are needed following total knee replacement?

_____

_____

_____

g. What are your goals for this client?

_____

_____

_____

_____

_____

6. F.P. slipped on a wet floor and fractured the left femoral neck. She was admitted to the hospital and the physician ordered her to be placed in skin traction until her surgery. How is skin traction different from skeletal traction?

_____

_____

_____

a. What are the potential complications for hip arthroplasty surgery?

_____

_____

b. Following surgery, F.P. has an abductor pillow placed between the legs. What is the rationale for this intervention?

_____

_____

c. Clients frequently require a raised toilet seat following this type of surgery. Why is that?

_____

_____

7. B.N. received a traumatic injury below the left knee when he got caught in the power takeoff on a piece of farm equipment. What dietary considerations are there for wound healing in an amputation?

_____

_____

_____

  a. He complains of pain on his missing foot. Describe this type of pain.

  _____

  _____

  b. What are nursing interventions to use if the nursing diagnosis for this client is Disturbed Body Image related to trauma?

  _____

  _____

  c. B.N. asks to have a pillow placed beneath his left knee. The nurse explains that this action is contraindicated. Why?

  _____

  _____

  d. B.N. will be receiving instructions on use of crutches from the physical therapy department. What are some safety considerations for clients who need crutches?

  _____

  _____

7. L.J. works at a factory assembling small machine parts. She complains of numbness in her left hand and is diagnosed with carpal tunnel syndrome. What causes carpal tunnel syndrome?

  _____

  _____

  _____

  a. What are symptoms of carpal tunnel syndrome?

  _____

  _____

  b. What client teaching is important with carpal tunnel syndrome?

  _____

  _____

Self-Assessment Questions

Circle the letter that corresponds to the best answer.

1. The nurse is caring for a client following surgery on the right leg. Because the physician's order is for the client to use a three-point gait, the nurse will instruct the client to move
   a. both crutches with the right leg, then move the left leg.
   b. both crutches, then move both legs by swinging them through.
   c. the right leg with the left crutch, then the left leg with the right crutch.
   d. the right crutch, then the left foot, then the left crutch, then the right foot.

2. A client has recently had a cast applied to the arm. When the nurse assesses this client, which of the following findings would be considered abnormal?
   a. There is a capillary refill of almost 2 seconds in the fingers.
   b. The cast is cool to the touch and sounds dull when percussed.
   c. The client is experiencing pain that is relieved with analgesics.
   d. The client reports a tingling sensation relieved with position change.

3. A client has been recently diagnosed with osteoporosis. When giving discharge instructions to the client, the nurse will include all but which of the following?
   a. Reduce caffeine intake.
   b. Increase protein intake.
   c. Increase calcium intake.
   d. Increase weight-bearing activity.

4. Your client mentions that she used to sew children's clothing several hours a week until she started experiencing burning and numbness in her thumb and fingers, particularly in her right hand. You recall that these are most likely subjective findings for
   a. bursitis.
   b. osteoarthritis.
   c. rheumatoid arthritis.
   d. carpal tunnel syndrome.

5. The nurse is caring for a client who has had a cast applied following a fracture. To complete a neurovascular assessment of the client, the nurse will assess every 15 to 30 minutes for
   a. edema and joint mobility.
   b. drainage and temperature.
   c. pain, edema, and capillary return.
   d. pallor, paresthesia, and level of consciousness.

6. A client is admitted with osteomyelitis in an extremity. When reviewing the care of this client with the nursing assistant, the nurse emphasizes the need to
   a. keep the extremity at complete rest.
   b. elevate the extremity to decrease edema.
   c. begin passive ROM exercises to the extremity.
   d. gently massage the extremity to increase circulation.

7. Nodular formations are *not* produced by
   a. gout.
   b. rheumatoid arthritis.
   c. osteoarthritis.
   d. osteoporosis.

8. The acronym RICE stands for
   a. recovery, ice, compression, and elevation.
   b. rest, intermittent compression, and elevation.
   c. rest, ice, compression, and elevation.
   d. recovery, ice, compression, and enhancement.

9. A fracture that occurs from weakening of the bone is characterized as
   a. pathological.
   b. greenstick.
   c. compound.
   d. telescoped.

Pg 1235

10. A fat embolus usually occurs within:
    a. 6–24 hours.
    b. 12–24 hours.
    c. 24–48 hours.
    d. 24–72 hours.

Pg 1236

Neurological System

Key Terms

Match the following terms with their correct definitions.

___ 1. Affect

___ 2. Agnosia

___ 3. Anosognosia

___ 4. Aphasia

___ 5. Areflexia

___ 6. Ataxia

___ 7. Aura

___ 8. Automatism

___ 9. Autonomic nervous system

___10. Awareness

___11. Bradykinesia

___12. Central nervous system

___13. Cephalalgia

___14. Chorea

___15. Coprolalia

___16. Decerebration

___17. Dysarthria

a. Peculiar sensation preceding a seizure or migraine; may be a taste, smell, sight, sound, dizziness, or just a "funny feeling."

b. Inflammation of the meninges.

c. Paralysis of lower extremities.

d. Difficulty in swallowing.

e. That part of the peripheral nervous system consisting of the sympathetic and parasympathetic nervous systems and controlling unconscious activities.

f. Inability to recognize, either by sight or sound, familiar objects, such as a hand.

g. Cessation of motor, sensory, autonomic, and reflex impulses below the level of injury; characterized by flaccid paralysis of all skeletal muscles, loss of spinal reflexes, loss of sensation, and absence of autonomic function below the level of injury.

h. Specialized area of the brain.

i. Use of uncontrolled, violent, and obscene language.

j. System of the brain and spinal cord.

k. Acute, prolonged episode of seizure activity that lasts at least 30 minutes and may or may not involve loss of consciousness.

l. Lack of awareness regarding deficits.

m. Weakness of one side of the body.

n. Ability to recognize an object by feel.

o. Pain and rigidity in the neck.

p. Nerves that connect the central nervous system to the skin and skeletal muscles and control conscious activities.

q. Headache; also known as cephalgia.

___18. Dysphagia

___19. Emotional lability

___20. Encephalitis

___21. Fasciculation

___22. Functional area

___23. Glasgow Coma Scale

___24. Graphesthesia

___25. Hemiparesis

___26. Hemiplegia

___27. Homonymous hemianopia

___28. Kernig's sign

___29. Meningitis

___30. Mentation

___31. Neuralgia

___32. Neurogenic shock

___33. Neurotransmitter

___34. Nuchal rigidity

___35. Nystagmus

___36. Orientation

___37. Paraplegia

___38. Peripheral nervous system

___39. Postictal

___40. Quadriplegia

___41. Sclerotic

___42. Somatic nervous system

___43. Spinal shock

r. Inability to communicate; often the result of a brain lesion.

s. Slowness of voluntary movement and speech.

t. Dizziness.

u. Hardened tissue.

v. Failure to recognize or care for one side of the body.

w. Objective tool for assessing consciousness in clients with head injuries.

x. Difficult and defective speech due to a dysfunction of the muscles used for speech.

y. Loss of vision in half of the visual field on the same side of both eyes.

z. Constant, involuntary movement of the eye in various directions.

aa. Outward expression of mood or emotion.

bb. Inability to coordinate voluntary muscle action.

cc. Diagnostic test for inflammation in the nerve roots; the inability to extend the leg when the thigh is flexed against the abdomen.

dd. Chemical substance that excites, inhibits, or modifies the response of another neuron.

ee. Mechanical, repetitive motor behavior performed unconsciously.

ff. Loss of emotional control.

gg. Dysfunction or paralysis of both arms, both legs, and bowel and bladder.

hh. Absence of reflexes.

ii. Ability to concentrate, remember, or think abstractly.

jj. Inflammation of the brain.

kk. Awareness of self in relation to person, place, time, and, in some cases, situation.

ll. Hypotensive situation resulting from the loss of sympathetic control of vital functions from the brain.

mm. Involuntary twitching of muscle fibers.

nn. System of cranial nerves, spinal nerves, and the autonomic nervous system.

oo. Ability to identify letters, numbers, or shapes drawn on the skin.

pp. Paralysis of one side of the body.

qq. Paroxysmal pain that extends along the course of one or more nerves.

___44. Status epilepticus

rr. Condition characterized by abnormal, involuntary, purposeless movements of all musculature of the body.

___45. Stereognosis

ss. Extension posturing.

___46. Tetraplegia

tt. The period of time after a seizure has occurred.

___47. Unilateral neglect

uu. Ability to perceive environmental stimuli and body reactions and then respond with thought and action.

___48. Vertigo

vv. A term that is synonymous with quadriplegia.

Abbreviation Review

Write the meaning or definition of the following abbreviations, acronyms, and symbols.

1. ABG _____

2. ACHE _____

3. ACTH _____

4. AD _____

5. ADL _____

6. ALS _____

7. ANS _____

8. CN _____

9. CNS _____

10. CSF _____

11. CT _____

12. CVA _____

13. DAI _____

14. EEG _____

15. EMG _____

16. GABA _____

17. IgG _____

18. LP _____

19. MAO _____

20. MAP _____

21. MRI _____

22. MS _____

23. MSG _____

24. NSA _____

25. NSAID _____

26. $PaCO_2$ _____

27. PERRLA _____

28. PET _____

29. PNS _____

30. PT _____

31. ROM _____

32. SCI _____

33. SPECT _____

34. TIA _____

Exercises and Activities

1. Identify the following landmarks on the diagram below.

   Broca's area

   Cerebellum

   Diencephalon

   Frontal lobe

   Midbrain

   Medulla oblongata

   Occipital lobe

   Parietal lobe

   Pons

   Spinal cord

   Temporal lobe

   Wernicke's area

Courtesy of Delmar Cengage Learning

2. Describe the main function for each of the following.

   Spinal nerves: _____

   _____

   Cranial nerves: _____

   _____

   Somatic nervous system: _____

   _____

   Autonomic nervous system: _____

   _____

3. Give the name and one method of assessing for each cranial nerve.

	Name	Assessment
I		
II		
III		
IV		
V		
VI		
VII		
VIII		
IX, X		
XI		
XII		

4. List the components of a complete nursing assessment of the neurological system.

5. What observations can be used to assess the client for each of the following?
    Communication _____
    Emotional status _____
    Intellectual function _____
    Mental status _____
    Orientation _____

6. How is the Glasgow Coma Scale used to determine the level of consciousness?

    a. What are the components of the Glasgow Coma Scale?

    b. What score indicates the client is in a coma?

    c. Describe questions the nurse might ask when determining if the client is oriented.

7. What signs and symptoms might be noted in a client with increased intracranial pressure?

_____

_____

8. List several factors that can cause an increase in intracranial pressure.

(1) _____

(2) _____

(3) _____

(4) _____

(5) _____

(6) _____

9. Briefly describe the medical–surgical treatment that may be used for a client with a head injury.

_____

_____

10. You are asked to perform frequent assessment on the neurological status of your client. What will you include?

_____

_____

_____

11. List risk factors for stroke. Circle the major risk factor.

(1) _____   (5) _____   (9) _____

(2) _____   (6) _____   (10) _____

(3) _____   (7) _____   (11) _____

(4) _____   (8) _____   (12) _____

12. What intellectual deficits may occur with a stroke?

_____

_____

_____

13. Describe medical–surgical management of the client with a stroke.

_____

_____

_____

a. What is the priority of care in the first 24 to 48 hours?

_____

_____

b. What medications might initially be used with clients who have had a stroke?

_____

_____

14. List 12 factors that can cause seizures.

(1) _____   (5) _____   (9) _____
(2) _____   (6) _____   (10) _____
(3) _____   (7) _____   (11) _____
(4) _____   (8) _____   (12) _____

15. How would you differentiate the three types of generalized seizures?

Tonic-clonic (grand mal): _____

_____

Absence (petit mal): _____

_____

Myoclonic: _____

_____

16. You are helping a client to the bathroom when the client begins to have a tonic-clonic (grand mal) seizure. What actions will you take?

_____

_____

_____

17. What priorities are used when caring for a client in the acute phase of spinal injury?

_____

_____

_____

18. Identify factors that can cause autonomic dysreflexia in the client with spinal injury.

_____

_____

_____

19. Describe immediate care of the client experiencing autonomic dysreflexia.

_____

_____

_____

20. Identify the signs and symptoms and medical treatment for the following neurological disorders.

	Signs/Symptoms	Treatment
Parkinson's disease		
Amyotrophic lateral sclerosis		
Alzheimer's disease		

21. What are the goals of nursing care in the late stage of Alzheimer's disease? Why is respite care important for family caregivers?

_____

_____

_____

22. Until this year, S.A., a 32-year-old high school math teacher, was active as the school's soccer coach, lifted weights at the gym, and enjoyed taking his son for bicycle rides. During the last several months, he had noticed occasional weakness in his legs, which he attributed to long hours coaching and perhaps his age. When S.A. started to walk unsteadily and even fell a couple of times, he became increasingly concerned but hoped it was just fatigue. After an episode of double vision, he agreed to see his physician. Following a thorough health history and physical examination, MS was suspected. Several tests were ordered to try to confirm the diagnosis.

a. What tests can be done to help determine whether S.A. has MS?

_____

_____

b. What other symptoms do clients with MS experience in the early stages of the disease?

_____

_____

c. S.A. asks why his symptoms seem to come and go. How would you describe the disease process to him?

_____

_____

_____

_____

d. If S.A. has the relapsing-remitting type of MS, what will that mean for his symptoms and prognosis?

_____

_____

_____

e. You are reviewing with S.A. lifestyle changes that may be helpful. What measures can he take to limit exacerbations of his disease?

_____

_____

_____

f. Write three nursing diagnoses or goals for S.A.

(1) _____

(2) _____

(3) _____

g. Briefly describe medical management of MS.

_____

_____

h. How can S.A. maintain his mobility as his disease progresses?

_____

_____

    i. What safety measures would you include in teaching S.A. and his wife?

_____

_____

23. The client, D.T., is exhibiting posturing following a severe head injury caused by a motorcycle accident. Explain the differences between flexion and extension posturing.

    a. Describe the three primary mechanisms of brain injury.

_____

_____

    b. D.T. is having trouble maintaining his airway and requires suctioning. Explain why suctioning through the nose is never done with clients with head trauma.

_____

_____

24. M.G., age 22, is the quarterback for the Fighting Panther football team. He shares water bottles with his teammates. He now complains of a severe headache and a fever while denying he received a head injury. The coach recommends that he see a physician who believes M.G. may have meningitis. What other signs and symptoms might M.G. exhibit?

    a. What laboratory and diagnostic tests will be done to confirm the diagnosis?

_____

_____

    b. Explain the rationale for M.G. to receive the following medications.

Antibiotics_____

_____

Anticonvulsants _____

_____

Antipyretics _____

_____

Glucocorticosteroids _____

_____

Osmotic diuretics _____

_____

    c. What precautions should the football team take following the diagnosis of meningitis?

_____

_____

Self-Assessment Questions

Circle the letter that corresponds to the best answer.

1. During a neurological assessment, a nurse asks the client to explain the meaning of a proverb such as "a stitch in time saves nine." The nurse is assessing the client's
   a. language and recall.
   b. intellectual functioning.
   c. orientation and awareness.
   d. understanding of American culture.

2. Several hours following a head injury, the client's score on the Glasgow Coma Scale changes from 13 to 9. The nurse responds appropriately by
   a. notifying the physician.
   b. reassessing after the client has had time to rest.
   c. charting improvement in the client's condition.
   d. continuing to assess at regular intervals, at least every 2 hours.

3. The student nurse is preparing to care for a client with a T-4 spinal injury. The student recalls that this client is at risk of developing autonomic dysreflexia, which can lead to
   a. spinal shock.
   b. cardiac arrest.
   c. a hypertensive crisis.
   d. a loss of respiratory function.

4. The nursing student is caring for a client with a left-sided CVA who is experiencing aphasia. The student anticipates that this client will have difficulty with
   a. coordination.
   b. communication.
   c. chewing and swallowing.
   d. recognizing familiar objects.

5. The nurse is discussing self-care measures with the client who takes L-Dopa for Parkinson's disease. The nurse advises the client to
   a. avoid high-protein foods.
   b. take a multivitamin daily.
   c. eat foods high in vitamin B6.
   d. adjust the dose according to symptoms.

6. The central nervous system is comprised of the
   a. sympathetic and parasympathetic systems.
   b. autonomic nervous system.
   c. cranial and spinal nerves.
   d. brain and spinal cord.

7. The right side of the brain specializes in
   a. analysis.
   b. perception of the physical environment.
   c. verbal communication.
   d. reading.

8. The sympathetic system causes
   a. bladder evacuation.
   b. increasing gastrointestinal activity.
   c. increased heart rate.
   d. slowing heart rate.

9. A Glasgow Coma Scale of 3 indicates a
   a. fully oriented client.
   b. client who is confused.
   c. client who can respond.
   d. client in deep coma.

10. Cushing's triad or reflex refers to
    a. bradycardia, widening pulse pressure, and respiratory irregularities.
    b. bradycardia, narrowing pulse pressure, and increased respiratory rate.
    c. tachycardia, widening pulse pressure, and respiratory irregularities.
    d. tachycardia, narrowing pulse pressure, and increased respiratory rate.

Sensory System

Key Terms

Match the following terms with their correct definitions.

___ 1. Affect

___ 2. Afferent nerve pathways

___ 3. Arousal

___ 4. Astigmatism

___ 5. Awareness

___ 6. Cerumen

___ 7. Chalazion

___ 8. Cognition

___ 9. Conductive hearing loss

___10. Conjunctivitis

___11. Consciousness

___12. Disorientation

___13. Efferent nerve pathways

___14. Hallucination

___15. Hyperopia

___16. Illusion

___17. Judgment

___18. Keratitis

a. Expression of mood or feeling.

b. Condition characterized by the inability of sound waves to reach the inner ear.

c. Ability to evaluate alternatives to arrive at an appropriate course of action.

d. Condition in which the inner ear or cochlear portion of cranial nerve VIII is abnormal or diseased.

e. Change in the perception of sensory stimuli; can affect any of the senses.

f. Dizziness

g. Repetitive and involuntary movement of the eyeballs.

h. Inability of the eyes to focus in the same direction.

i. State of awareness of self, others, and the surrounding environment.

j. Inaccurate perception or misinterpretation of sensory stimuli.

k. Sensorineural hearing loss associated with aging.

l. Descending spinal cord pathways that transmit sensory impulses from the brain.

m. Inflammation of the conjunctiva.

n. Asymmetric focus of light rays on the retina.

o. State of excessive and sustained multisensory stimulation manifested by behavior change and perceptual distortion.

p. Intellectual ability to think.

q. Capacity to perceive sensory impressions through thoughts and actions.

r. Nearsightedness.

___19. Myopia

___20. Nystagmus

___21. Orientation

___22. Perception

___23. Presbycusis

___24. Presbyopia

___25. Sensation

___26. Sensorineural hearing loss

___27. Sensory deficit

___28. Sensory deprivation

___29. Sensory overload

___30. Sensory perception

___31. Strabismus

___32. Stye

___33. Tinnitus

___34. Vertigo

s. Ability to receive and process stimuli received through the sensory organs.

t. State of mental confusion in which awareness of time, place, self, and/or situation is impaired.

u. Ascending spinal cord pathways that transmit sensory impulses to the brain.

v. A sensory perception that occurs in the absence of external stimuli and is not based on reality.

w. Earwax.

x. Farsightedness.

y. Perception of self in relation to the surrounding environment.

z. State of reduced sensory input from the internal or external environment, manifested by alterations in sensory perception.

aa. Ability to receive sensory impressions and, through cortical association, relate the stimuli to past experiences and to form an impression of the nature of the stimulus.

bb. State of wakefulness and alertness.

cc. Cyst of the meibomian glands.

dd. Ability to experience, recognize, organize, and interpret sensory stimuli.

ee. Inflammation of the cornea.

ff. Inability of the lens of the eye to change curvature to focus near objects.

gg. Pustular inflammation of an eyelash follicle or sebaceous gland on the eyelid margin.

hh. Ringing sound in the ear.

Abbreviation Review

Write the meaning or definition of the following abbreviations and acronyms.

1. ANS _____

2. BAER _____

3. CNS _____

4. CT _____

5. ERG _____

6. IOL _____

7. IOP _____

8. LOC _____

9. MRI _____

10. PNS _____

11. TDD _____

12. UPSIT _____

Exercises and Activities

1. In what ways is an intact, functioning sensory system important for an individual?

   _____

   _____

   _____

   a. How would you differentiate perception and cognition?

      _____

      _____

   b. Describe aspects of the hospital environment that can distort a client's perception of time.

      _____

      _____

      (1) How can hospitalization contribute to sensory overload?

          _____

          _____

      (2) How can hospitalization contribute to sensory deficit?

          _____

          _____

   c. A nursing assistant tells you, "F.D. doesn't seem to be very alert this morning. I tried to help her eat her breakfast, but she just kept staring, not smiling at me or saying anything. It was like I wasn't even there." List the components of cognition, and circle the ones that are altered in F.D. today.

      (1) _____   (4) _____

      (2) _____   (5) _____

      (3) _____   (6) _____

   d. Write two questions that the nurse could ask a client to determine immediate, recent, and remote memory.

      Immediate   (1) _____

                         (2) _____

      Recent   (1) _____

                         (2) _____

      Remote   (1) _____

                         (2) _____

2. Label the diagram of the eye using the terms listed below.

Anterior chamber

Ciliary body

Conjunctiva

Cornea

Fovea centralis

Iris

Lens

Optic disk

Optic nerve

Posterior chamber

Pupil

Retina

Sclera

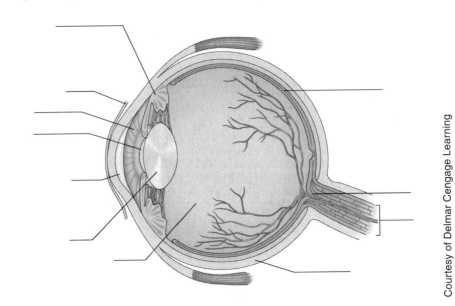

Courtesy of Delmar Cengage Learning

a. Name each structure that light passes through to reach the optic nerve.

_____

_____

b. Identify the structures of the ear on the following diagram. Draw a circle around the middle ear.

Auricle

Cochlea

Cranial nerve VIII

Eustachian tube

External auditory
   canal

Incus

Malleus

Round window

Semicircular canals

Stapes

Tympanic membrane

Ear Disorders
Acoustic neuroma
Ménière's disease
Otosclerosis
Otitis media
Otitis externa

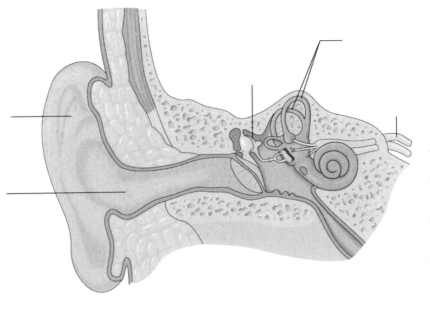

Courtesy of Delmar Cengage Learning

c. Draw a line from each disorder in the box to the part of the ear that it affects.

d. What changes occur in the following components of the sensory system with aging?

Hearing: _____

_____

Vision: _____

_____

Touch: _____

_____

e. Identify each of these common terms by the correct medical term.

Earwax _____

Eardrum _____

Nearsighted _____

Swimmer's ear _____

Dizziness _____

Pinkeye _____

3. What interventions might help a hospitalized client with a visual impairment?

_____

_____

_____

a. Identify safety measures for a client with vertigo.

_____

_____

b. Your friend tells you she must be "legally blind" because she cannot even see the first letter on the eye chart without her glasses. Is she correct?

_____

_____

c. List symptoms a client would experience with the following disorders and the treatment.

	Symptoms	Treatment
Ménière's disease		
Retinal detachment		
Glaucoma		
Cataracts		

d. A 3-year-old child has been pulling on his ear and crying. His mother thinks he may have another ear infection. The term for a middle ear infection is _____.
What other symptoms might the child have with this infection? Briefly describe surgical management that may be used for this disorder.

_____
_____
_____
_____
_____
_____

4. A new client has recently arrived at a long-term care facility for a brief stay following discharge from the hospital. The nursing assistant tells you, "J.D. doesn't do anything I ask. I'm not sure he can hear me."

a. Describe behaviors that might indicate a hearing loss in a client.

_____
_____
_____

b. After reviewing the chart and assessing J.D., you determine that he has a moderate hearing loss and uses a hearing aid, which was left at the hospital. What interventions can assist you and your client to communicate until the hearing aid is retrieved?

_____
_____
_____
_____

c. During morning care, the nursing assistant notices that J.D.'s eyelids are crusted over and his eyes look reddened. You are concerned that he may have conjunctivitis. What other symptoms might be present?

_____
_____
_____
_____

(1) Identify special precautions the nurse takes to prevent the spread of conjunctivitis.

_____
_____

(2) When providing care to the eye, describe the personal protective equipment the nurse uses.

_____
_____

d. J.D. seems to have a poor appetite. When you ask, he tells you that nothing tastes very good. What changes occur in taste and smell with aging? How can these changes cause nutrition problems?

_____

_____

_____

_____

5. C.W. is going to have cataract surgery on her left eye. She asks the nurse to explain the procedure to her. What should the nurse include in the explanation to C.W.?

_____

_____

_____

   a. The surgeon will also use an IOL for C.W. What does this mean?

   _____

   _____

   b. What types of eye drops are given pre-operatively to C.W. and why?

   _____

   _____

   c. The care plan includes a nursing diagnosis of Risk for Injury. What activities should the nurse include when teaching C.W. about going home after the procedure?

   _____

   _____

6. E.G. is a diabetic. He complains of inability to see in his right eye to the opthamologist. Upon examination, the opthamologist determines E.G. has had a retinal detachment. What causes retinal detachment?

_____

_____

_____

   a. The opthamologist plans to do scleral buckling. Explain this in terms that E.G. can understand.

   _____

   _____

   b. E.G. is anxious about having surgery on his eye. List nursing interventions that will reduce his anxiety.

   _____

   _____

Self-Assessment Questions

Circle the letter that corresponds to the best answer.

1. A nurse caring for a client recovering from surgery notes that he is still very drowsy from medication. This client is exhibiting an alteration in
   a. affect.
   b. arousal.
   c. sensation.
   d. cognition.

2. The nurse is performing a physical assessment on a client with a diagnosis of acoustic neuroma affecting cranial nerves VII and VIII. Which of these findings will the nurse anticipate?
   a. Tinnitus and ear pain
   b. Conductive hearing loss
   c. Facial weakness and vertigo
   d. Loss of hearing and nystagmus

3. The nurse observes the client turning his head to use peripheral vision when talking with her. The nurse recalls that this may occur with
   a. cataracts.
   b. presbyopia.
   c. retinal detachment.
   d. macular degeneration.

4. The nurse is providing home care for an older adult client. Family members tell the nurse that the client is showing changes in speech patterns and habits. The nurse tells them that these changes may indicate
   a. hearing loss.
   b. disorientation.
   c. sensory overload.
   d. normal effects of aging.

5. The nurse is admitting a client to a long-term care facility following a stroke. Because the client also has a diagnosis of glaucoma, the physician orders
   a. antibiotics.
   b. mydriatic drops.
   c. topical anesthetic.
   d. pilocarpine drops.

6. Your client, who is newly diagnosed with open-angle glaucoma, asks you why this could cause blindness. You reply that
   a. increased pressure within the eye causes a detachment of the retina.
   b. an increase in fluid in the front of the eye damages the lens, causing loss of vision.
   c. the fluid in the eye puts pressure on the neurons of the retina, which destroys them.
   d. an inflammatory response in the posterior chamber of the eye damages the optic nerve.

7. An inaccurate perception of sensory stimuli is called
    a. arousal.
    b. orientation.
    c. an illusion.
    d. a hallucination.

8. A state of reduced sensory input from the external environment is called
    a. sensory deficit.
    b. sensory deprivation.
    c. sensory overload.
    d. disorientation.

9. One factor contributing to sensory overload is
    a. pain.
    b. blindness.
    c. use of sedatives.
    d. glaucoma.

10. In sensorineural hearing loss
    a. the problem may be cerumen buildup.
    b. the tympanic membrane may be perforated.
    c. the ossicles may be fixed.
    d. cranial nerve VIII may be abnormal.

Endocrine System

Key Terms

Match the following terms with their correct definitions.

c 1. Agranulocytosis

m 2. Autosomal

t 3. Chvostek's sign

n 4. Cretinism

a 5. Dawn phenomenon

o 6. Endocrine

b 7. Exophthalmos

e 8. Glucagon

u 9. Glycosuria

x 10. Goiter

l 11. Gynecomastia

p 12. Hirsutism

d 13. Hormone

v 14. Hyperglycemia

f 15. Hypoglycemia

z 16. Hypovolemia

h 17. Iatrogenic

a. Early morning glucose elevation produced by the release of growth hormone.

b. Marked protrusion of the eyeballs resulting from increased orbital fluid behind the eyeballs.

c. Acute condition causing a severe reduction in the number of granulocytes (basophils, eosinophils, and neutrophils).

d. Substance that initiates or regulates activity of another organ, system, or gland in another part of the body.

e. Hormone secreted by the alpha cells of the pancreas, which stimulates release of glucose by the liver.

f. Low blood glucose.

g. Descriptor for a symptom that begins and ends abruptly.

h. Caused by treatment or diagnostic procedures.

i. Hormone produced and secreted by the beta cells in the islets of Langerhans of the pancreas.

j. Increased urination.

k. Sharp flexion of the wrist and ankle joints, involving muscle twitching or cramps.

l. Abnormal enlargement of one or both breasts in males.

m. Pertaining to a condition transmitted by a nonsex chromosome.

n. Congenital condition due to a lack of thyroid hormones causing defective physical development and mental retardation.

o. Group of cells secreting substances directly into the blood or lymph circulation and affecting another part of the body.

p. Excessive body hair in a masculine distribution.

q. Severe hypothyroidism in adults.

_i_18. Insulin

r. In response to hypoglycemia, the release of glucose-elevating hormones (epinephrine, cortisol, glucagon), which produces a hyperglycemic state.

_v_19. Ketone

s. Carpal spasm caused by inflating a blood pressure cuff above the client's systolic pressure and leaving it in place for 3 minutes.

_aa_20. Ketonuria

t. Abnormal spasm of the facial muscles in response to a light tapping of the facial nerve.

_cc_21. Lipodystrophy

u. Presence of excessive glucose in the urine.

_q_22. Myxedema

v. Elevated blood glucose.

_q_23. Paroxysmal

w. Acidic by-product of fat metabolism.

_bb_24. Polydipsia

x. Enlargement of the thyroid gland.

_y_25. Polyphagia

y. Increased hunger.

_j_26. Polyuria

z. Abnormally low circulatory blood volume.

_r_27. Somogyi phenomenon

aa. Presence of ketones in the urine.

_k_28. Tetany

bb. Excessive thirst.

_s_29. Trousseau's sign

cc. Atrophy or hypertrophy of subcutaneous fat.

Abbreviation Review

Write the meaning or definition of the following abbreviations and acronyms.

1. ACTH _____
2. ADA _____
3. ADH _____
4. CATT _____
5. CVA _____
6. DKA _____
7. FBS _____
8. FSH _____
9. GDM _____
10. GH _____
11. GTT _____
12. HHNS _____
13. IDDM _____
14. IFG _____
15. IGT _____
16. LH _____
17. MSH _____
18. NIDDM _____
19. PTH _____
20. PTU _____
21. PVD _____

22. RAIU _____

23. SIADH _____

24. TSH _____

25. VMA _____

Exercises and Activities

1. Write the name of each unidentified endocrine gland in the diagram and at least one of its functions.

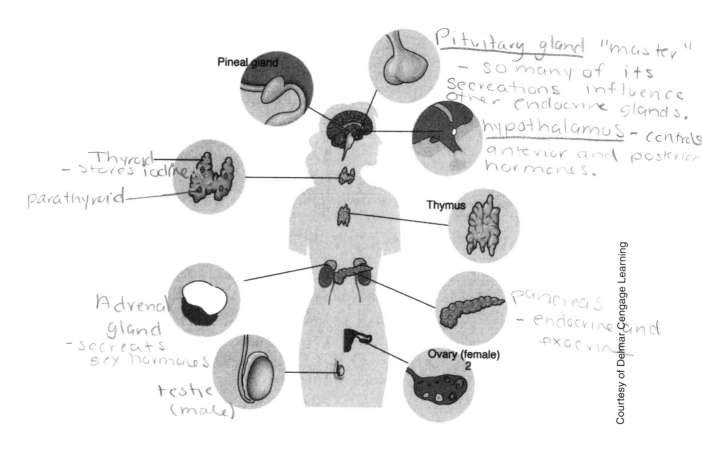

Pineal gland

Pituitary gland "master"
– so many of its secreations influence other endocrine glands.
hypothalamus – controls anterior and posterior hormones.

Thyroid
– stores iodine
parathyroid

Thymus

Adrenal gland
– secreats sex hormones

pancreas
– endocrine and exocrin

testie (male)

Ovary (female) 2

Courtesy of Delmar Cengage Learning

a. How does negative feedback affect hormone production?

_____

_____

b. Name the hormone(s) responsible for each of these functions.

_____ Increases metabolic rate.

_____ Prolongs the sympathetic nervous response to stress.

_____ Increases blood glucose (two).

_____ Stimulates growth.

_____ Regulates electrolyte and fluid homeostasis.

_____ Stimulates milk secretion with pregnancy.

_____ Alters blood calcium concentration (two).

_____ Stimulates uterine contractions.

c. What factors make assessment of the endocrine system difficult?

_____

_____

2. List signs/symptoms for the following disorders. Briefly describe treatment for the adult client.

	Signs/Symptoms	*Treatment*
Acromegaly		
Diabetes insipidus		
Hyperthyroidism		
Hypothyroidism		
Addison's disease		

3. List several risk factors for type 2 diabetes.

(1) _____

(2) _____

(3) _____

(4) _____

(5) _____

(6) _____

a. Which of these clients would be diagnosed with diabetes mellitus?

Client A: Has a random blood sugar of 150, asymptomatic.

Client B: Has a fasting blood sugar of 130.

Client C: Two hours after GTT, has a blood sugar of 180.

b. Compare the etiology and management of type 1 and type 2 diabetes.

	Type 1	*Type 2*
Etiology		
Management		

c. Your client was recently diagnosed with type 1 diabetes. He was an avid bicyclist before his diagnosis and is eager to return to competitive racing next season. What guidelines should he follow?

_____

_____

d. Your client with type 1 diabetes describes feeling ill with a mild case of flu. How does he manage his diabetes while he is ill?

_____

_____

e. Compare signs and symptoms for the following acute complications of diabetes.

Hypoglycemia: _____

_____

DKA: _____

_____

HHNS: _____

_____

f. List several long-term complications of diabetes.

1. _____   5. _____
2. _____   6. _____
3. _____   7. _____
4. _____   8. _____

g. What special concerns are associated with older adults who are diabetic?

_____

_____

h. Polydipsia, polyphagia, and polyuria are classic signs of diabetes. Explain why they occur.

_____

_____

4. N.L., a 25-year-old special education teacher with one toddler at home, has developed a problem with acne and hirsutism, and an irregular menstrual cycle. Although N.L. readily admits that feeling tired by the end of the school day is typical for her, lately the weariness seems to start earlier and earlier. Last week she even felt a little weak. Her family has mentioned to her that she seems to be unusually moody. Physically, her face is looking more full, but she has not gained any weight to account for it. An examination indicates N.L. may have Cushing's syndrome.

a. What is the normal function of the adrenal gland?

_____

_____

b. Describe the causes of adrenal hyperfunction.

_____

_____

c. What other physical and psychological signs and symptoms could N.L. be experiencing?

_____

_____

_____

_____

d. Following a discovery of a growth on her left adrenal gland, N.L. was scheduled for an adrenalectomy. What nursing observations will be needed following her surgery?

_____

_____

e. How does having increased levels of corticosteroids affect wound healing?

_____

_____

f. If steroid therapy is prescribed, what client teaching would you include?

_____

_____

_____

_____

5. Using Table 43–1 in the text, describe the onset and duration for the types of insulin.

Type of Insulin	Onset	Duration
Very short-acting		
Short-acting		
Intermediate-acting		
Long-acting		
Pre-mixed		

6. Insulin injection sites need to be rotated to prevent _____.

7. Insulin is available as U-100 and U-500. What does this mean?

   _____

   _____

   _____

8. L.B., a nurse on the unit, complains of heart palpitations and her pulse is 140 beats per minute. She sees her physician who is concerned that L.B. may have hyperthyroidism. What other symptoms are common with hyperthyroidism?

   _____

   _____

   _____

   a. What laboratory and diagnostic tests are used to determine hyperthyroidism?

      _____

      _____

   b. L.B. is worried about a thyroid storm as it is an emergency. What can you tell her about that?

      _____

      _____

   c. Although L.B. is a nurse, she admits it has been a long time since she studied the thyroid gland. She would like to know what treatments are used for hyperthyroidism. Can you explain that for her?

      _____

      _____

   d. The physician decides to treat L.B. initially with antithyroid medication. What teaching about dietary restrictions should be included for L.B.?

      _____

      _____

   e. Eventually the physician plans for L.B. to have radioactive iodine administered. Explain this procedure and the safety precautions that must be used with this treatment.

      _____

      _____

Self-Assessment Questions

Circle the letter that corresponds to the best answer.

1. While reviewing the nursing care for a client who had a removal of the parathyroid glands, the student nurse recalls that a major function of this gland is to
   a. regulate the concentration of blood calcium.
   b. assist the thyroid in regulation of metabolism.
   c. produce a sympathetic nervous response to stress.
   d. stimulate production of stress hormones by the adrenals.

2. The nurse is reviewing care with the nursing student for a client with SIADH. The nurse explains that an important part of the therapeutic management of this syndrome is
   a. frequent oral care.
   b. water restriction and diuretics.
   c. sodium restriction and IV fluids.
   d. monitoring for signs of infection.

3. A client who was diagnosed previously with type 2 diabetes is now using insulin. Two hours before dinner, the client exhibits diaphoresis, pallor, and anxiety, with a blood glucose of 90. This client would benefit most by
   a. eating two packets of sugar quickly.
   b. asking the physician to adjust the insulin dosage.
   c. having a small glass of juice and an ounce of cheese.
   d. trying to remain calm, because anxiety produces the other symptoms.

4. The nurse is performing an assessment on a client with a diagnosis of Addison's disease. Which of the following signs or symptoms would the nurse anticipate?
   a. Bronze coloring and fatigue
   b. Muscle tremors and insomnia
   c. Positive Trousseau's and Chvostek's signs
   d. Moon face and purple striae on the abdomen

5. A nurse is caring for a client following a thyroidectomy. To monitor for the most serious complication of this surgery, the nurse will
   a. monitor the serum calcium levels.
   b. perform voice checks every 2 to 4 hours.
   c. check for respiratory distress and bleeding.
   d. notify the physician of a sore throat or hoarseness.

6. The hormone that decreases blood calcium is
   a. parathyroid hormone.
   b. cortisol.
   c. somatostatin.
   d. calcitonin.

7. The hormone that stimulates gluconeogenesis is
   a. parathyroid hormone.
   b. cortisol.
   c. somatostatin.
   d. calcitonin.

8. A diagnostic test that may be completed to check adrenal function is
   a. FBS
   b. ADH
   c. VMA
   d. RAIU

9. A diagnostic test that may be completed to check thyroid function is
   a. FBS
   b. ADH
   c. VMA
   d. RAIU

10. All are functions of insulin except
    a. stimulation of release of glucose by the liver.
    b. promotion of glucose conversion to glycogen.
    c. conversion of fatty acids to fat.
    d. stimulation of protein synthesis within tissue.

Key Terms

Match the following terms with their correct definitions.

___ 1. Abortion

___ 2. Amenorrhea

___ 3. Contraception

___ 4. Cystocele

___ 5. Dysmenorrhea

___ 6. Dyspareunia

___ 7. Endometriosis

___ 8. Hematuria

___ 9. Hesitancy

___10. Impotence

___11. Infertility

___12. Menopause

___13. Menorrhagia

___14. Metrorrhagia

___15. Nocturia

___16. Oligomenorrhea

___17. Orchiectomy

___18. Polymenorrhea

___19. Postvoid residual

___20. Priapism

___21. Prolapsed uterus

___22. Rectocele

a. Painful intercourse.

b. Inability or diminished ability to produce offspring.

c. Termination of pregnancy before the age of fetal viability, usually 24 weeks.

d. Menstrual periods that are abnormally frequent, generally less than every 21 days.

e. Production of sperm.

f. Awakening at night to void.

g. Spasmodic contraction of the anal or bladder sphincter, causing pain and a persistent urge to empty the bowel or bladder.

h. Surgical resection of the vas deferens.

i. Downward displacement of the bladder into the anterior vaginal wall.

j. Absence of menstruation.

k. Difficulty initiating the urinary stream.

l. Cessation of menstruation.

m. Prolonged erection that does not occur in response to sexual stimulation.

n. Downward displacement of the urethra into the vagina.

o. Growth of endometrial tissue on structures outside of the uterus, within the pelvic cavity.

p. Vaginal bleeding between menstrual periods.

q. Measure taken to prevent pregnancy.

r. Downward displacement of the uterus into the vagina.

s. A material used to hold tissue in place or support tissue.

t. Painful menstruation.

u. Blood in the urine.

v. Excessively heavy menstrual flow.

___23. Spermatogenesis

w. Inability of an adult male to have an erection firm enough, or to maintain it long enough, to complete sexual intercourse.

___24. Stent

x. Decreased menstrual flow.

___25. Tenesmus

y. Urine that remains in the bladder after urination.

___26. Urethrocele

z. Removal of a testis.

___27. Vasectomy

aa. Anterior displacement of the rectum into the posterior vaginal wall.

Abbreviation Review

Write the meaning or definition of the following abbreviations, acronyms, and symbols.

1. ACS _____

2. AFP _____

3. AP _____

4. B&O _____

5. BPH _____

6. BSE _____

7. CIS _____

8. CPAP _____

9. D&C _____

10. DES _____

11. DICC _____

12. ERT _____

13. FBD _____

14. FSH _____

15. GIFT _____

16. hCG _____

17. IVF-ER _____

18. IUD _____

19. IVP _____

20. KUB _____

21. LH _____

22. NP _____

23. PAP _____

24. PID _____

25. PMS _____

26. PSA _____

27. STD _____

28. TSE _____

29. TSS _____
30. TULIP _____
31. TURP _____
32. UTI _____
33. VCD _____
34. ZIFT _____

Exercises and Activities

1. Label the following diagrams of the male and female reproductive systems.

   a. Female reproductive system

   Cervix

   Clitoris

   Fallopian tube

   Fimbriae

   Ovary

   Symphysis pubis

   Urethra

   Urinary bladder

   Uterus

   Vagina

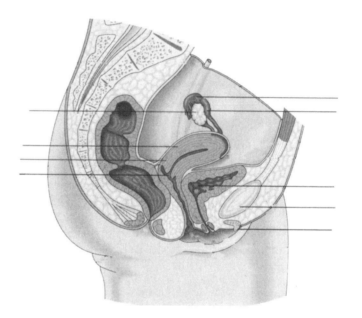
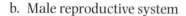

   b. Male reproductive system

   Cowper's glands

   Ejaculatory duct

   Epididymis

   Glans penis

   Prepuce (foreskin)

   Prostate gland

   Scrotum

   Seminal vesicle

   Testis

   Urethra

   Vas deferens

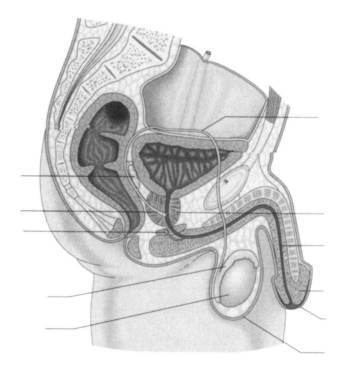

Courtesy of Delmar Cengage Learning

Courtesy of Delmar Cengage Learning

2. Describe the life cycle of an ovum from the time it ripens until implantation occurs (with pregnancy) and the influence of hormones.

   a. What changes take place if implantation does not occur?

   b. How are sperm produced and released?

3. Compare the following breast lesions: cyst, fibroadenoma, and carcinoma.

	Shape	Mobility	Tenderness	Erythema	Retraction
Cyst					
Fibroadenoma					
Carcinoma					

   a. M.C., a 31-year-old woman in your clinic, tells you that a close friend of hers was just diagnosed with breast cancer. Although M.C. occasionally has breast and pelvic exams done at the clinic, she has never really wanted to learn breast self-examination until now. How will you instruct her to perform BSE? What will you tell her about the frequency and timing for BSE?

   b. List nine risk factors for breast cancer.

(1) _____ (6) _____

(2) _____ (7) _____

(3) _____ (8) _____

(4) _____ (9) _____

(5) _____

4. What are the risk factors and symptoms for testicular cancer?

a. How would you describe the testicular self-exam (TSE) to your male client?

_____

_____

5. Compare the signs/symptoms and the primary treatment for the following disorders.

	Signs/Symptoms	Treatment
Pelvic inflammatory disease		
Orchitis		
Ovarian cancer		
Prostate cancer		
Prolapsed uterus		

a. List several risk factors for cervical cancer.

(1) _____

(2) _____

(3) _____

(4) _____

b. How does toxic shock syndrome develop?

_____

_____

6. A female client has determined that she would like to use the rhythm method of contraception. What information will she need? What might be the risks/side effects and advantages of this method?

_____

_____

_____

a. Which methods of contraception require the client to be seen by a health care provider?

_____

_____

b. List methods of contraception that may offer some protection against STDs.

_____

_____

7. K.V., a 48-year-old office administrator, has an appointment today at your clinic. Over the past few months, she has noticed that her menstrual cycle is changing. She has also noticed feeling some nervousness and mood swings. At first she attributed her symptoms to a recent promotion and increased responsibility. Now K.V. is also having occasional "hot flashes" that wake her up at night. She is here for a Pap smear and wants to talk about hormone replacement therapy.

a. What physical changes occur with menopause?

_____

_____

b. What subjective and objective data will be obtained during the assessment?

_____

_____

_____

c. List advantages and disadvantages of hormone replacement therapy.

_____

_____

_____

_____

d. What steps can K.V. take to maintain or improve her health?

_____

_____

_____

e. K.V. states, "Well, at least I won't be needing any more pelvic exams now." What will you tell your client? How does her risk for breast cancer change?

_____

_____

_____

8. I.O., age 38, has avoided routine health care as she generally feels healthy. She noticed her menses becoming heavier. At the beginning of her next menstrual cycle, she noticed extremely heavy flow with blood clots. I.O. sees a physician for a pelvic examination. What equipment should the nurse prepare for this examination?

_____

_____

_____

a. The physician recommends a D&C procedure for I.O What does this mean and how would you explain it to I.O.?

_____

_____

b. The physician also does an endometrial biopsy on the tissue removed. The results come back for endometrial cancer. What treatment options are there for this condition?

_____

_____

c. I.O. opts to have a total abdominal hysterectomy and bilateral salpingo-opherectomy. I.O. states that she will no longer feel like a woman because of the loss of child-bearing ability. How should the nurse respond?

_____

_____

d. I.O. asks the nurse about her ability to have sexual relations with her husband after the surgery. What information should the nurse provide to I.O.?

_____

_____

e. Since I.O. had a surgically induced menopause, what information should the nurse include about osteoporosis?

_____

_____

f. When I.O. is discharged home, what information should be included in her discharge instructions regarding activity?

_____

_____

Self-Assessment Questions

Circle the letter that corresponds to the best answer.

1. An early screening tool is available for all but which of the following cancers of the reproductive system?
   a. Breast cancer
   b. Ovarian cancer
   c. Cervical cancer
   d. Prostate cancer

2. A female client has been recently diagnosed with infertility related to a hormone imbalance. To treat infertility for this client, the physician orders
   a. Clomid.
   b. Norplant.
   c. Progesterone.
   d. Depo-Provera.

3. A client has just had a modified mastectomy for breast cancer. To help the client adjust to the loss of her breast, the nurse will
   a. expect the client to assume self-care after the surgery.
   b. assess breath sounds and vital signs and provide O_2 as needed.
   c. encourage the client to look at the surgical site when she is ready.
   d. assist the client to do active ROM exercises to strengthen the affected side.

4. The nurse is assessing a client with a diagnosis of fibroid tumors. The nurse anticipates that this client may report pelvic pressure, abdominal enlargement, bleeding between menstrual periods, and an excessively heavy menstrual flow called
   a. hematuria.
   b. menorrhagia.
   c. hematemesis.
   d. dysmenorrhea.

5. A 45-year-old male client is having a routine physical examination. For this client, the most useful screening method to detect prostate cancer is
   a. a rectal examination performed annually.
   b. a serum PSA test.
   c. observation of symptoms such as hematuria.
   d. monthly self-exam for painless lumps in the testes.

6. A male client with which of the following conditions would require immediate surgery?
   a. Varicocele
   b. Cryptorchidism
   c. Prostatic hypertrophy
   d. Torsion of the spermatic cord

7. The hormone that stimulates ovulation is
   a. follicle-stimulating hormone.
   b. luteinizing hormone.
   c. estrogen.
   d. progesterone.

8. Spermatogenesis is regulated by
   a. the testis.
   b. FSH.
   c. LH.
   d. testosterone.

9. A client with fibrocystic breast disease has a green, sticky discharge from one of her breasts. It would be recommended that she
   a. eliminate protein from her diet.
   b. eliminate fats from her diet.
   c. eliminate caffeine products from her diet.
   d. just ignore it.

10. Metrorrhagia is
    a. vaginal bleeding between menstrual periods.
    b. excessively heavy menstrual periods.
    c. a green-yellow vaginal discharge.
    d. excessively long menstrual flow.

Sexually Transmitted Infections

Key Terms

Match the following terms with their correct definitions.

_____ 1. Abstinence

_____ 2. Asymptomatic

_____ 3. Chancre

_____ 4. Exposure

_____ 5. Incidence

_____ 6. Incubation period

a. Frequency of disease occurrence.

b. Clean, painless, syphilitic, primary ulcer appearing 2 to 6 weeks after infection at the site of body contact.

c. Contact with an infected person or agent.

d. Interval between exposure to an infectious disease and the first appearance of symptoms.

e. Refraining from sexual intercourse or mucous membrane–to–mucous membrane contact.

f. Without symptoms.

Abbreviation Review

Write the meaning or definition of the following abbreviations and acronyms.

1. AIDS _____

2. CMV _____

3. ELISA _____

4. HBV _____

5. HIV _____

6. HPV _____

7. HSV _____

8. NIAID _____

9. PID _____

10. RPR _____

11. STI _____

12. VDRL _____

Exercises and Activities

1. Describe the role of the nurse in the identification and treatment of sexually transmitted infections (STI).

   _____

   _____

   _____

   a. What information would be gathered in the client interview?

   _____

   _____

   b. List signs and symptoms frequently noted in the client with an STI.

   _____

   _____

   c. How can the nurse help the client feel more comfortable during the interview and physical assessment?

   _____

   _____

2. What factors have contributed to an increase in the frequency of STIs?

   _____

   _____

   _____

   a. Why is education important in prevention of STIs?

   _____

   _____

   b. You are asked to help prepare an educational program for high school–age students on prevention of STIs. What topics will you include?

   _____

   _____

   _____

   c. What would you advise the students to do if they feel they have been exposed to an STI?

   _____

   _____

3. Describe the signs and symptoms and treatment for each of the following STIs.

	Signs/Symptoms	Treatment
Genital herpes		
Gonorrhea		
Genital warts		
Trichomoniasis		

a. Why are STIs more dangerous for female clients?

_____

_____

4. R.S., a 23-year-old single male client, is being seen at the clinic for a small painless ulcer on the end of his penis. He first noticed it last week and thought it would go away, but when it did not he decided to get it checked. R.S. admits having sexual relations with three different partners within the past several months. He says he probably should be using condoms, but his current girlfriend is on birth control pills. R.S. denies burning on urination, penile discharge, fever, rash, or other symptoms. Assessment findings include regional lymphadenopathy. Results on VDRL and FTA-ABS (fluorescent treponemal antibody absorption) tests indicate syphilis.

a. List signs and symptoms for each stage of syphilis.

Primary: _____

_____

Secondary: _____

_____

Latent: _____

_____

Tertiary: _____

_____

b. What stage of syphilis is R.S. probably in? _____

Which stage is most contagious? _____

What medication will be used to treat R.S.? _____

c. Why is syphilis called "the great imitator"?

_____

_____

d. What information does R.S. need about follow-up care, sexual activity, and risk for STIs?

_____

_____

5. B.W. sees her physician because of a grayish-white vaginal discharge. B.W. admits to attending a party and having unprotected sex with a friend of a friend a few weeks ago. The physician performs a pelvic examination and orders the following laboratory tests: VDRL, cultures, and urine specimens. Explain why these tests would be necessary.

_____

_____

_____

a. The cultures came back positive for chlamydia and gonorrhea. What antibiotics are commonly prescribed as a treatment for these conditions?

_____

_____

b. What should the nurse include in the patient teaching about these antibiotics?

_____

_____

c. B.W. asks the nurse if spermicides would helps prevent getting future STIs. How should the nurse respond?

_____

_____

6. Using the following terms, fill in the blanks regarding hepatitis B.

bacteria   failure   heath care   hepatic

inflammation   jaundice   series   virus

Hepatitis B is caused by _____ , not by _____ .
Symptoms of HBV include liver _____ , _____ ,
fatigue, and nausea. Untreated hepatitis B may progress to _____
cancer and hepatic _____ . Treatment of HBV may be prevented by
a _____ of three intramuscular injections. The CDC recommends
vaccinations for newborns, _____ workers, and high-risk groups.

Self-Assessment Questions

Circle the letter that corresponds to the best answer.

1. A female client with genital warts is receiving treatment to have them removed. When instructing the client about this STI, the nurse emphasizes that the client
   a. will need frequent Pap smears.
   b. must complete the entire antibiotic therapy.
   c. should avoid sexual activity until she is cured.
   d. will probably not have a recurrence, because the warts were removed.

2. A nursing student explains to new parents that an antibiotic ointment is put in the eyes of all newborns to prevent ophthalmia neonatorum, caused by
   a. syphilis.
   b. gonorrhea.
   c. trichomoniasis.
   d. cytomegalovirus.

3. Between 80% and 100% of adults have developed antibodies to
   a. CMV.
   b. chlamydia.
   c. hepatitis B.
   d. genital herpes.

4. A male client is diagnosed with secondary syphilis. While assessing this client, the nurse is likely to note
   a. seizures and stroke symptoms.
   b. a single chancre, usually near the tip of the penis.
   c. burning on urination and a discharge from the penis.
   d. a skin rash of small brownish sores, including on the palms and soles.

5. The nurse is instructing a client about preventing STIs. Which of these statements by the client indicates a need for additional teaching?
   a. "I won't get STIs if I use a latex condom."
   b. "Even if I have an STI, I may not have any symptoms."
   c. "If I have an STI, my partner and I both need treatment."
   d. "Hepatitis B is the only STI I can be vaccinated against."

6. Factors that have caused an increased number of clients with STIs include all but which of the following?
   a. Increased alcohol and drug use
   b. Use of nonbarrier methods of birth control
   c. Greater awareness of how STIs are transmitted
   d. Increased numbers of teens engaging in sexual activity

7. The nurse is providing care for a client with genital herpes. The nurse remembers that this STI is
   a. contagious even if there are no symptoms present.
   b. curable if diagnosed early and treated with acyclovir.
   c. contagious only when blisters are present in the perineal area.
   d. caused by HSV type 1, which also causes "fever blisters" on the lips.

8. Vesicles on the penis may be indicative of
   a. genital herpes.
   b. gonorrhea.
   c. trichomoniasis.
   d. syphilis.

9. Petechial lesions may be indicative of
   a. genital herpes.
   b. gonorrhea.
   c. trichomoniasis.
   d. syphilis.

10. The infection known as the "silent STI" is
    a. genital warts.
    b. herpes.
    c. chlamydia.
    d. syphilis.

Integumentary System

Key Terms

Match the following terms with their correct definitions.

_e_ 1. Alopecia

_n_ 2. Angiogenesis

_t_ 3. Angioma

_u_ 4. Blanching

_o_ 5. Cyanosis

_d_ 6. Debride

_m_ 7. Ecchymosis

_v_ 8. Erythema

_cc_ 9. Eschar

_jj_ 10. Exudate

_s_ 11. Friction

_gg_ 12. Granulation tissue

_dd_ 13. Hemorrhagic exudate

_b_ 14. Hemostasis

_f_ 15. Hyperthermia

_w_ 16. Hypothermia

_l_ 17. Inflammation

_i_ 18. Ischemia

a. Pigmented areas in the skin; commonly known as birthmarks or moles.

b. Cessation of bleeding.

c. Abnormal paleness of the skin, seen especially in the face, conjunctiva, nail beds, and oral mucous membranes.

d. To remove dead or damaged tissue or foreign material from a wound.

e. Partial or complete baldness or loss of hair.

f. Condition in which the core body temperature rises above 106°F.

g. Pinpoint hemorrhagic spots on the skin.

h. Discharge that is clear with some blood tinge; seen with surgical incisions.

i. Local and temporary decrease in blood supply.

j. Disruption in the integrity of body tissue.

k. Distended sebaceous gland filled with sebum.

l. Body's defensive adaptation to tissue injury; involves both vascular and cellular responses.

m. Large, irregular hemorrhagic area on the skin; also called a bruise.

n. Formation of new blood vessels.

o. Bluish discoloration of the skin and mucous membranes observed in lips, nail beds, and earlobes.

p. Abnormal growth of scar tissue that is elevated, rounded, and firm with irregular, clawlike margins.

q. Permanent dilation of groups of superficial capillaries and venules; commonly known as spider veins.

r. Yellowing of the skin, mucous membranes, and sclera of the eyes.

r 19. Jaundice

p 20. Keloid

x 21. Keratin

bb 22. Lipoma

ee 23. Melanin

a 24. Nevi (Nevus)

c 25. Pallor

g 26. Petechiae

y 27. Purulent exudate

ii 28. Sanguineous

k 29. Sebaceous cyst

aa 30. Sebum

h 31. Serosanguineous exudate

ff 32. Serous exudate

hh 33. Shearing

q 34. Telangiectasia

z 35. Vitiligo

j 36. Wound

s. Force of two surfaces moving against one another.

t. Benign vascular tumor involving skin and subcutaneous tissue.

u. White color of the skin when pressure is applied.

v. Reddish hue to the skin that may be caused by inflammation of tissues or by sunburn.

w. A condition in which the core body temperature drops below 95°F.

x. Tough, fibrous protein produced by cells in the epidermis called keratinocytes.

y. Discharge that occurs with severe inflammation accompanied by infection; also called pus.

z. Depigmentation of the skin caused by destruction of melanocytes; appears as milk-white patches on the skin.

aa. Oily substance secreted by the sebaceous glands of the skin.

bb. Benign tumor consisting of mature fat cells.

cc. Dry, dark, leathery scab composed of denatured protein.

dd. Discharge that has a large component of red blood cells.

ee. Pigment that gives skin its color.

ff. Discharge composed primarily of serum; is watery in appearance and has low protein level.

gg. Delicate connective tissue consisting of fibroblasts, collagen, and capillaries.

hh. Force exerted against the skin by movement or repositioning.

ii. An exudate that is clear with some blood tinge.

jj. Material, fluids, and cells discharged from cells or blood vessels.

Abbreviation Review

Write the meaning or definition of the following abbreviations and acronyms.

1. ABCD _____

2. AGF _____

3. FAF _____

4. MRSA _____

5. MDI _____

6. NPUAP _____

7. ROM _____

8. SPF _____

9. TPN _____

10. USDHHS _____

11. VAC _____

Exercises and Activities

1. Why is healthy, intact skin important for an individual?

   _____

   _____

   _____

   a. On the following diagram, identify the three layers of the skin and label at least two structures in each layer.

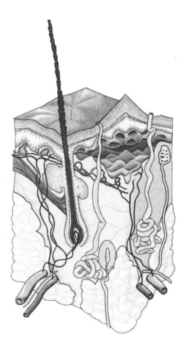

Courtesy of Delmar Cengage Learning

   b. You are caring for a 25-year-old client and a 72-year-old. How would you expect the skin, hair, and nails of your older client to differ from those of your younger client?

   Skin: _____

   _____

   Hair: _____

   _____

   Nails: _____

   _____

2. A client tells you that she has noticed several small blisters on her left side that are painful. List several questions that you will ask her to gather information about this problem.

(1) _____

(2) _____

(3) _____

(4) _____

(5) _____

(6) _____

(7) _____

(8) _____

a. In the first column, identify the seven parameters assessed during the physical examination of the skin. In the second column, write two abnormal findings for each parameter.

Assessment Parameters	Abnormal Findings
(1)	
(2)	
(3)	
(4)	
(5)	
(6)	
(7)	

b. Think of a client you have cared for recently who had a wound, skin lesion, or pressure sore. Use the following diagram to mark the location of the skin problem. Describe its size, shape, appearance, and any drainage. Was it painful? If so, include the type and severity of any pain.

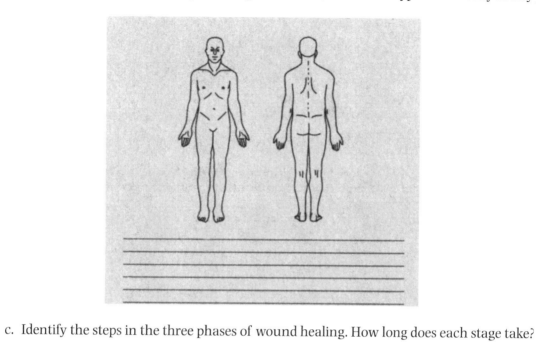

Courtesy of Delmar Cengage Learning

c. Identify the steps in the three phases of wound healing. How long does each stage take?

First phase (primary intention): _____

_____

Second phase (secondary intention): _____

_____

Third phase (tertiary intention): _____

_____

d. How does infection slow down the healing process?

_____

_____

_____

3. Two nursing assistants are moving an elderly client up in bed. By sliding the client along the sheets, they cause shearing, which leads to skin breakdown. Why are elderly clients more susceptible to skin breakdown?

_____

_____

_____

a. What is it about moving the client in bed improperly that can cause skin breakdown?

_____

_____

b. What are the risk factors for a pressure ulcer?

_____

_____

c. The next morning, the nurse notices a new reddish patch of skin on the client's sacrum measuring 4 by 6 cm. When the nurse presses on it, the redness does not blanch. What has happened?

_____

_____

_____

d. List nursing interventions that can help prevent pressure ulcers.

_____

_____

_____

_____

e. Where are venous ulcers usually found on a client? Draw and label a venous ulcer on the preceding diagram.

_____

_____

_____

4. List symptoms that a client might experience with the following disorders and at least two nursing–medical interventions for each.

	Symptoms	*Nursing–Medical Interventions*
Carbuncle		
Herpes zoster (shingles)		
Scabies		
Psoriasis		

a. What is the significance of a fourth-degree burn?

_____

_____

_____

b. Identify the goals of treatment after a client with extensive burns is stabilized.

_____

_____

_____

c. What factors make good nutrition difficult for a burn victim?

_____

_____

_____

_____

5. Identify each of these commonly used words by the correct medical term.

Mole _____

Bed sore _____

Birthmark _____

Athlete's foot _____

Cold sore _____

Shingles _____

Pus _____

6. L.N., a 27-year-old client, was in her usual state of good health until 3 days ago when her husband noticed a lesion on her right shoulder. She remembers having a mole there but says it is now bigger and looks darker. Her skin is very fair, and although she does not tan well, she has always loved being in the sun. In fact, she earned money for 2 years in college as a lifeguard. The nurse describes the lesion as having a smooth surface, elevated, with an irregular border, 6 mm in diameter, and bluish gray in color.

a. What type of skin lesion might this be?

_____

b. What are the ABCDs of skin cancer?

A: _____

B: _____

C: _____

D: _____

c. Identify risk factors for skin cancer.

_____

_____

d. L.N. may have malignant melanoma. What medical–surgical interventions would be used for this disease?

_____

_____

_____

e. After L.N. has the melanoma removed, she asks you if she can get skin cancer again. What will you tell her?

_____

_____

_____

f. On the older adult client, where are skin cancers often found?

_____

_____

_____

_____

_____

7. J.J. was camping when the campfire got out of control. He attempted to put it out but the fire flared up in a gust of wind. J.J. received burns on his face, arms, hands, and chest. His eyebrows are singed off. He complains of severe pain when he arrives in the emergency room with a hoarse voice. The nurse immediately applies oxygen to J.J. What is the rationale for this?

_____

_____

_____

a. The nurse used 100% humidified air. Why would the nurse select this volume of oxygen and why would the nurse include humidity?

_____

_____

b. As the nurse examines J.J.'s burns, she uses a chart similar to Figure 46–9 in the text. Using that chart, what percentage of burns did J.J. receive?

_____

_____

c. The burns on his face have blisters, the one on his right hand is red like a sunburn, and the one on his left forearm is black. Describe the degree of burns to each of these sites:

Face _____

Right hand _____

Left forearm _____

d. What types of shock does the nurse anticipate with J.J.'s burns?

_____

_____

e. J.J. may require skin grafting o the burn on his left forearm. Describe the four types of skin grafts.

(1) _____

(2) _____

(3) _____

(4) _____

f. How does the nurse prevent contractures during the recovery phase for J.J.?

_____

_____

Self-Assessment Questions

Circle the letter that corresponds to the best answer.

1. The nurse is performing a visual inspection of the skin on a client with psoriasis. With this skin disorder, the nurse would note
   a. red patches covered with thick silvery scales.
   b. large round lesions with a pale center that itch.
   c. painful red lesions with blisters around the trunk.
   d. clusters of vesicles in a linear pattern on the extremities.

2. While assessing the skin of an elderly client, the nurse notes an increased number of melanocytes on the face of the client. The nurse recognizes that this is
   a. a precursor for melanoma.
   b. a normal finding in an older adult.
   c. a local reaction to topical creams and ointments.
   d. a result of a disease process causing a loss of subcutaneous tissue.

3. The nurse is doing teaching with clients about skin cancer. The nurse explains that the major risk factor for skin cancer is
   a. exposure to the sun.
   b. genetic predisposition.
   c. previous radiation therapy.
   d. not using an adequate sun screen lotion.

4. The nursing student is caring for a client with AIDS who has developed mycosis fungoides, a type of malignant disease with skin manifestations. The instructor tells the student that the skin lesions with this disease are
   a. treated with surgical removal and radiation.
   b. caused by a fungus that destroys the epidermis.
   c. similar in appearance to psoriasis in the early stages.
   d. an inflammatory condition of the epidermal and dermal skin layers.

5. A student is preparing to care for a client with third-degree burns on the thorax and arms. The student nurse recalls that third-degree burns
   a. are more painful than second-degree burns.
   b. will develop eschar within 2 to 3 days.
   c. are often associated with muscle and bone damage.
   d. damage the epidermis and dermis and are partial thickness.

6. The nurse is performing a physical assessment on a newly admitted client. The nurse pinches up a fold of skin on the client and observes how quickly and easily it returns to its normal position. This assesses for
   a. moisture.
   b. skin integrity.
   c. skin sensation.
   d. hydration status.

7. A young child has been diagnosed with head lice after the school nurse finds nits on the hair. The nurse will instruct the parents to wash or dry-clean clothing and linens and to apply
   a. Kwell.
   b. Zovirax.
   c. Micatin.
   d. a topical antibiotic.

8. The client has third-degree full-thickness burns resulting from an industrial explosion. After the initial period of stabilization, the nurse is aware that the most serious complication will be
   a. pain.
   b. scarring.
   c. infection.
   d. respiratory depression.

9. Which of the following is true in vitiligo?
    a. Areas of redness are present.
    b. Melanocytes are destroyed.
    c. Pustules can be present.
    d. There is increased melanin.
10. When checking for skin vascularity, an abnormal finding could be
    a. cyanosis.
    b. jaundice.
    c. erythema.
    d. telangiectasia.

Immune System

Key Terms

Match the following terms with their correct definitions.

___ 1. Acquired immunodeficiency syndrome

___ 2. Allergen

___ 3. Allogeneic

___ 4. Anaphylaxis

___ 5. Angioedema

___ 6. Antibodies

___ 7. Antigen

___ 8. Autoimmune disorder

___ 9. Autologous

___10. Cellular immunity

___11. Diplopia

___12. Enzyme-linked immunosorbent assay

___13. Exacerbation

___14. Histamine

___15. Human immunodeficiency virus

___16. Human leukocyte antigen

___17. Humoral immunity

___18. Hypersensitivity

a. A donor of the same species.

b. Type of acquired immunity involving T-cell lymphocytes.

c. Excessive reaction to a stimulus.

d. Disease wherein the body identifies its own cells as foreign and activates mechanisms to destroy them.

e. Type of antigen commonly found in the environment.

f. Body's ability to protect itself from foreign agents or organisms.

g. Progressively fatal disease that destroys the immune system and the body's ability to fight infection; caused by the human immunodeficiency virus.

h. Drooping upper eyelid.

i. Test that measures copies of HIV RNA.

j. Basic screening test currently used to detect antibodies to HIV.

k. A type I systemic reaction to allergens.

l. From the same organism (person).

m. Substance released during allergic reactions.

n. Body's reaction to substances identified as nonself.

o. Decrease or absence of symptoms of a disease.

p. Allergic reaction causing raised pruritic, red, non-tender wheals on the skin; also called hives.

q. Treatment to suppress or enhance immunological functioning.

r. Allergic reaction consisting of edema of subcutaneous layers and mucous membranes.

___19. Immune response

___20. Immunity

___21. Immunotherapy

___22. Opportunistic infection

___23. Ptosis

___24. Remission

___25. Seroconversion

___26. Urticaria

___27. Viral load test

___28. Western blot test

s. Double vision.

t. Proteins that react with antigens to neutralize or destroy them.

u. Type of immunity dominated by antibodies.

v. Confirmatory test used to detect HIV infection.

w. Any substance identified by the body as nonself.

x. Increase in the symptoms of a disease.

y. Retrovirus that causes AIDS.

z. Antigen present in human blood.

aa. Infection in persons with a defective immune system that rarely causes harm in healthy individuals.

bb. Evidence of antibody formation in response to disease or vaccine.

Abbreviation Review

Write the meaning or definition of the following abbreviations, acronyms, and symbols.

1. ADC _____

2. AFB _____

3. CIN _____

4. CMV _____

5. DMARD _____

6. ELISA _____

7. EMG _____

8. ESR _____

9. HARRT _____

10. HBV _____

11. HCV _____

12. HDV _____

13. HIV _____

14. HPV _____

15. IgG _____

16. IgM _____

17. KS _____

18. LE _____

19. MAC _____

20. MDR-TB _____

21. MG _____

22. NHL _____

23. NIAID _____

24. NNRTI _____

25. NRTI _____

26. OHL _____

27. PCP _____

28. PCR _____

29. PPD _____

30. RA _____

31. RF _____

32. RNA _____

33. ROM _____

34. SLE _____

35. SPF _____

36. WBC _____

Exercises and Activities

1. How does our immune system protect us against foreign agents or organisms?

   _____

   _____

   _____

   a. Compare active and passive acquired immunity and give two examples of each.

   _____

   _____

   _____

   _____

   b. What factors could depress an individual's immune response?

   _____

   _____

   _____

   c. List several symptoms that a client may experience with an immune system disorder.

   (1) _____

   (2) _____

   (3) _____

   (4) _____

   (5) _____

   (6) _____

d. Identify several physical assessment findings that the nurse would note during physical examination of the client with an immune disorder.

(1) _____

(2) _____

(3) _____

(4) _____

(5) _____

(6) _____

(7) _____

(8) _____

e. What is the difference between an "allergen" and an "antibody"?

_____

_____

2. Briefly describe the cause of each type of allergic reaction.

Type I: _____

_____

_____

Type II: _____

_____

_____

Type III: _____

_____

_____

Type IV: _____

_____

_____

a. Circle the three examples of type I allergic reactions in the following list.

Transfusion reaction	Poison ivy contact dermatitis
Food allergy	Hay fever
Transplant rejection	Anaphylaxis

b. Describe the signs and symptoms of an anaphylactic reaction.

_____

_____

_____

c. What nursing interventions are appropriate for a client with anaphylaxis?

_____

_____

_____

3. Compare the typical manifestations and treatment for each of the following immunological disorders.

	Manifestations	*Treatment/Intervention*
Systemic lupus erythematosus		
Myasthenia gravis		
Toxoplasmosis		
Kaposi's sarcoma		

a. What lifestyle modifications might you recommend for a client with SLE?

_____

_____

_____

4. Describe disease progression, from a client's exposure to HIV until AIDS is diagnosed.

_____

_____

_____

a. List several opportunistic infections that are often noted in clients with HIV/AIDS.

(1) _____   (6) _____

(2) _____   (7) _____

(3) _____   (8) _____

(4) _____   (9) _____

(5) _____   (10) _____

b. Describe signs and symptoms of HIV-wasting syndrome. How are symptoms controlled?

_____

_____

_____

c. Compare the differences between a cold and an allergy by filling in the following table.

Signs and Symptoms	Cold	Allergy
Cough		
Aches and pains		
Itchy eyes		
Sneezing		
Sore throat		
Runny nose		
Stuffy nose		
Fever		

d. A friend confides that she may have been exposed to HIV but is afraid to go for testing. How would you address her fears?

_____

_____

e. A nurse received a needlestick injury from a needle used on an unknown person in the emergency department. What actions should the nurse take?

_____

_____

5. A.L., a 34-year-old artist, has been having increasing pain in her hands and knees for some time now. Mornings are really the worst for her, and some days the pain has made it difficult to work. She thought maybe she had a little osteoarthritis like her mother, but A.L.'s symptoms seem different. At first, her fingers hurt, but now it has spread to her wrists and knees. She has also noticed some nodules on her elbows. During an assessment, you note that her hands feel warm and are showing characteristic signs of rheumatoid arthritis.

a. What triggers the onset of rheumatoid arthritis in an individual?

_____

_____

b. What other symptoms might A.L. experience?

_____

_____

c. How is rheumatoid arthritis different from osteoarthritis?

_____

_____

d. List signs of rheumatoid arthritis that would be noted during an assessment.

_____

_____

e. A.L. tells you she cannot quit working, but sometimes her hands are so stiff and painful. She is ready to try anything that might help. What medications might be used to control her disease and symptoms?

_____

_____

f. List three goals for this client.

(1) _____

(2) _____

(3) _____

g What will you advise A.L. about her diet and activity?

_____

_____

_____

_____

_____

_____

_____

_____

Self-Assessment Questions

Circle the letter that corresponds to the best answer.

1. The nurse is doing teaching with a client who has had a severe allergic reaction to a substance. The nurse will emphasize to the client that because of this reaction, it is **most** important for him to
   a. wear a Medic Alert tag.
   b. get tested for environmental allergies.
   c. know the signs and symptoms of anaphylaxis.
   d. avoid all situations in which the offending substance might be present.

2. A nurse is performing a physical assessment on a 27-year-old female client admitted with a diagnosis of systemic lupus erythematosus. Which of the following manifestations would the nurse anticipate?
   a. Muscle weakness and fatigue
   b. Fatigue, weight loss, and anemia
   c. Facial rash and painful, swollen joints
   d. Movable, subcutaneous skin nodules

3. A client who received penicillin has developed flushing, facial swelling, and dyspnea. The first medication to be administered is:
   a. epinephrine.
   b. corticosteroids.
   c. an antihistamine.
   d. a different antibiotic.

4. A nurse is caring for a 35-year-old client diagnosed with rheumatoid arthritis. The nurse explains to the client that she may experience periods of remission in the disease alternating with periods of
   a. sensitization.
   b. exacerbation.
   c. susceptibility.
   d. inflammation.

5. The primary modes of transmission for HIV infection include all but which of the following?
   a. Urine
   b. Blood
   c. Amniotic fluid
   d. Vaginal secretions

6. A client has received a transplanted kidney. To minimize transplant rejection, this client is most likely to be
   a. given antibiotics prophylactically.
   b. placed in reverse isolation for 2 weeks.
   c. placed on immunosuppressive medications.
   d. monitored for weight loss, fever, and swelling and redness at the transplant site.

7. CD4 T-cells are also known as
   a. killer cells.
   b. suppressor cells.
   c. helper cells.
   d. plasma cells.

8. If a client has raised pruritic, red, nontender wheals on the skin, the wheals are
   a. cysts.
   b. an erythemic rash.
   c. Kaposi's sarcoma.
   d. urticaria.

9. Which is not a classic deformity of rheumatoid arthritis?
   a. Charcot
   b. Boutonniere
   c. Ulnar drift
   d. Swan-neck

10. Which is a pulmonary opportunistic fungal infection (present in bird droppings) of advanced HIV disease?
    a. *Pneumocystis carinii* pneumonia
    b. Histoplasmosis
    c. Tuberculosis
    d. Mycobacterium avium complex

Mentall Illness

Key Terms

Match the following terms with their correct definitions.

___ 1. Abuse

___ 2. Actively Suicidal

___ 3. Affect

___ 4. Anger-control assistance

___ 5. Anxiety

___ 6. Anxiolytic

___ 7. Auditory hallucination

___ 8. Brief dynamic therapy

___ 9. Cognitive-behavioral therapy

___ 10. Command Hallucination

___ 11. Crisis

___ 12. Cycling

___ 13. Delusion

___ 14. Depression

a. Laboratory test done to determine whether the client's lithium level is within a therapeutic range.

b. Antianxiety medication.

c. Constantly scanning the environment for potentially dangerous situations.

d. Treatment of mental and emotional disorders through psychological rather than physical methods.

e. Stressor that forces an individual to respond and/or adapt in some way.

f. Condition wherein an individual has a distorted view of self, is unable to maintain satisfying personal relationships, and is unable to adapt to the environment.

g. Bond or connection between two people that is based on mutual trust.

h. Procedure whereby clients are treated with pulses of electrical energy sufficient to cause brief convulsions or seizures.

i. Rapid, intense speech.

j. Perception by an individual that someone is talking when no one in fact is there.

k. Treatment approach aimed at helping a client identify stimuli that cause the client's anxiety, develop plans to respond to those stimuli in a nonanxious manner, and problem-solve when unanticipated anxiety-provoking situations arise.

l. Incident involving some type of violation to the client.

m. Therapy focused on uncovering unconscious memories and processes.

n. Reliving of an original trauma as though the individual were currently experiencing it.

____15. Domestic violence

____16. Electroconvulsive therapy

____17. Empathy

____18. Euphoric

____19. Flashback

____20. Genuineness

____21. Hallucination

____22. Hypervigilant

____23. Hypomania

____24. Mania

____25. Mental disorder

____26. Mental illness

____27. Mood

____28. Neglect

____29. Paradoxical reaction

____30. Physically aggressive

____31. Pressured speech

____32. Psychoanalysis

____33. Psychosis

____34. Psychotherapy

____35. Rapport

o. Mild form of mania without significant impairment.

p. State wherein an individual experiences feelings of extreme sadness, hopelessness, and helplessness.

q. Perception by an individual that someone is present when no one is.

r. Short-term psychotherapy that focuses on resolving core conflicts deriving from personality and living situations.

s. Perception that something is present when it is not.

t. Extremely elevated mood with accompanying agitated behavior.

u. Acquired resistance to the effects of a drug.

v. Descriptor of an individual who threatens to or actually harms someone.

w. State wherein a person feels a strong sense of dread, frequently accompanied by physical symptoms of increased heart and respiratory rates and elevated blood pressure in the absence of a specific source or reason for the emotions or responses.

x. Ability to perceive and relate to another's personal experience.

y. Aggression and violence involving family members.

z. Descriptor of an individual intent upon hurting or killing self and who is in imminent danger of doing so.

aa. Acceptance of an individual as is and in a nonjudgmental manner.

bb. Perception an individual has of a voice or voices telling the individual to do something, usually to him/herself and/or someone else.

cc. Overreaction to minor sounds or noises.

dd. Confinement of a client to a single room.

ee. Clinically significant behavior or psychological syndrome or pattern that occurs in an individual and is associated with present distress or disability or with a significantly increased risk of suffering, death, pain, disability, or an important loss of freedom (APA, 1994).

ff. Alteration in mood between depression and mania.

gg. Outward manifestation of the way an individual is feeling.

hh. Subjective report of the way an individual is feeling.

ii. Opposite effect of that which would normally be expected.

___36. Respect

___37. Seclusion

___38. Serum lithium level

___39. Startle response

___40. Suicidal ideation

___41. Tolerance

___42. Trust

___43. Verbally aggressive

___44. Visual hallucination

___45. Word salad

jj. Nursing intervention aimed at facilitating the expression of anger in an adaptive and nonviolent manner.

kk. False belief that misrepresents reality.

ll. State wherein an individual has lost the ability to recognize reality.

mm. Characterized by elation out of context to the situation.

nn. Thought of hurting or killing oneself.

oo. Ability to rely on an individual's character and ability.

pp. Sincerity.

qq. Descriptor of an individual who says things in a loud and/or intimidating manner.

rr. Combination of words that is nonsensical and meaningless to others.

ss. Situation in which a basic need of the client is not being provided.

Abbreviation Review

Write the meaning or definition of the following abbreviations, acronyms, and symbols.

1. ABA _____

2. ADHD _____

3. APA _____

4. APS _____

5. CPS _____

6. DBSA _____

7. DSM-IV _____

8. ECT _____

9. EPS _____

10. FVPF _____

11. GAD _____

12. ICU _____

13. MAOI _____

14. NCADV _____

15. NMS _____

16. OCD _____

17. OTC _____

18. PCP _____

19. PTSD _____

20. SSRI _____

21. TD _____

Exercises and Activities

1. Describe the characteristics of a person that you feel demonstrates mental health.

   _____

   _____

   _____

2. What is the role of the nurse in the mental health field?

   _____

   _____

   _____

   _____

3. List the essential components of a therapeutic relationship.

   (1) _____   (4) _____

   (2) _____   (5) _____

   (3) _____

4. How can the nurse develop a trusting relationship with the client?

   _____

   _____

   _____

5. Compare the symptoms for a client with mild anxiety, moderate anxiety, and severe anxiety.

   _____

   _____

   _____

6. What nursing interventions are important for the client experiencing panic anxiety?

   _____

   _____

   _____

7. Review Table 48-1 in your text, and list several of the most common side effects of antianxiety medications.

   (1) _____   (4) _____

   (2) _____   (5) _____

   (3) _____   (6) _____

8. How does cognitive-behavioral therapy work in the treatment of anxiety disorders?

   _____

   _____

   _____

9. The nursing management of anxiety includes using the acronym CALM. What does each letter represent?

C _____

A _____

L _____

M _____

10. Identify methods the nurse can use to help a client achieve stress reduction or relaxation.

_____

_____

_____

11. How would you assess a client for potential for aggression?

_____

_____

_____

12. What techniques can be used with the client who is angry?

_____

_____

_____

13. List behavioral clues that might indicate a client is suicidal.

(1) _____   (5) _____

(2) _____   (6) _____

(3) _____   (7) _____

(4) _____   (8) _____

14. Identify the goals of psychosocial and clinical treatment for the client with schizophrenia.

_____

_____

_____

15. What factors make it difficult to treat clients with schizophrenia?

_____

_____

_____

16. Your client has been prescribed Thorazine, a phenothiazine drug. What information will you include in client teaching about this medication?

_____

_____

_____

a. One set of side effects to Thorazine is tardive dyskinesia. Explain what tardive dyskinesia is and what signs the nurse observes the client for.

_____

_____

17. What assessment findings might alert the health care team to abuse or neglect in a client?

    _____

    _____

    _____

18. What information should be reported if child abuse is suspected?

    _____

    _____

    _____

19. Nine months ago, S.D. and her husband lost their 4-month-old baby boy from sudden infant
    death syndrome (SIDS). Since then, S.D. has felt overwhelmed with guilt and grief over the loss.
    She returned to her secretarial job a month after the death but left again when she could not seem
    to keep her mind on her work. S.D. no longer enjoys visits with friends or gardening, a favorite
    hobby. She has lost several pounds and has trouble making even simple decisions. S.D. sometimes
    feels that if she were a stronger person, she could pull herself out of her sadness and move on.
    Her husband and friends shared her grief at first but now think she needs to get on with her life.
    After all, she still has C., their beautiful 6-year-old daughter.

    a. What signs and symptoms of depression do you see in S.D.?

    _____

    _____

    _____

    _____

    b. List other symptoms that may be noted in a client with depression.

    _____

    _____

    c. Describe medical and pharmacological treatments for depression.

    _____

    _____

    _____

    d. S.D. was started in outpatient therapy and will be taking Paxil, a selective serotonin reuptake
       inhibitor antidepressant, to help with her symptoms. List possible side effects she may expe-
       rience.

    (1) _____   (7) _____

    (2) _____   (8) _____

    (3) _____   (9) _____

    (4) _____   (10) _____

    (5) _____   (11) _____

    (6) _____   (12) _____

    e. Why would a dietary consult be helpful for S.D.?

    _____

    _____

f. What information will you include in client teaching about Paxil?

_____

_____

_____

20. R.N., age 26, is hospitalized with bipolar disorder. He is extremely manic. R.N. is agitated, and pacing the floors. He admits to being awake for 72 hours straight. His family brought him to the hospital because he was playing the stereo loudly all night, took all the money in the savings account, and went to the maximum limit on his credit card buying more stereo equipment, an electric guitar, and music. His speech is rambling. he asked the nurse several times if he looked hot or sexy. Which of R.N.'s statement's supports the diagnosis of manic phase?

_____

_____

_____

a. The physician prescribed Lithium as a treatment for R.N. What is the therapeutic serum level of Lithium?

_____

_____

b. How does salt intake affect Lithium levels?

_____

_____

c. What laboratory values need to be monitored in clients taking Lithium?

_____

_____

d. Identify a nursing diagnosis that would be appropriate for a client in this state.

_____

_____

Self-Assessment Questions

Circle the letter that corresponds to the best answer.

1. The nurse is performing an assessment on a client who is taking lithium carbonate for bipolar disorder. The nurse notes that the client has anorexia, headache, tinnitus, and confusion. Which of these findings may indicate lithium toxicity?
   a. Tinnitus
   b. Anorexia
   c. Headache
   d. Confusion

2. One of the first symptoms that may be noted in the client with depression is a
   a. change in sleeping patterns.
   b. decrease in job performance.
   c. sudden change in personal appearance or hygiene.
   d. preoccupation with death or dying.

3. A child diagnosed with ADHD is maintained during the school year on Ritalin, a central nervous system stimulant. Because of the side effects associated with this medication, the parent is advised to monitor the child for
   a. lethargy.
   b. weight loss.
   c. nosebleeds.
   d. increased urination.

4. A nurse has been assigned to care for a client who is identified as being actively suicidal. The highest priority for the nurse will be to
   a. maintain the safety of the client.
   b. supervise the client's medication.
   c. initiate a therapeutic relationship.
   d. document behaviors that indicate self-harm potential.

5. The nurse is discharging a client who is taking Nardil, a monoamine oxidase inhibitor, for depression. The client is advised to avoid decongestants to prevent which serious drug–drug reaction?
   a. Liver toxicity
   b. Agranulocytosis
   c. Atrial fibrillation
   d. Hypertensive crisis

6. Which is *not* a component in a therapeutic nurse–client relationship?
   a. Sincerity
   b. Respect
   c. Rapport
   d. Attribute finding

7. Consistency is an element of
   a. trust.
   b. rapport.
   c. respect.
   d. empathy.

8. A fearful and irrational client's anxiety level may be classified as
   a. mild.
   b. moderate.
   c. severe.
   d. panic.

9. Therapy focused on uncovering unconscious memories is called
   a. psychotherapy.
   b. psychoanalysis.
   c. cognitive-behavioral.
   d. memory recovery.

10. Which is not a potential side effect of mirtazapine (Remeron)?
    a. Drowsiness
    b. Dry mouth
    c. Weight loss
    d. Dizziness with position change

Substance Abuse

Key Terms

Match the following terms with their correct definitions.

___ 1. Abuse

___ 2. Addiction

___ 3. Behavioral tolerance

___ 4. Codependent

___ 5. Confabulation

___ 6. Cross-tolerance

___ 7. Dependence

___ 8. Detoxification

___ 9. Hallucination

___10. Intoxication

___11. Johnsonian intervention

___12. Misuse

___13. Opisthotonos

___14. Relapse

a. Reliance on a substance to such a degree that abstinence causes functional impairment, physical withdrawal symptoms, and/or psychological craving for the substance.

b. Decreased sensitivity to other substances in the same category.

c. Use of a legal substance for which it was not intended or exceeding the recommended dosage of a drug.

d. Misuse or excessive or improper use of a substance, the absence of which does not cause withdrawal symptoms.

e. Phenomenon whereby a smaller amount of substance will elicit the desired psychic effects.

f. Symptoms produced when a substance on which an individual has dependence is no longer used by that individual.

g. A drug, legal or illegal, that may cause physical or mental impairment.

h. Compensatory adjustments of behavior made under the influence of a particular substance.

i. A reversible effect on the central nervous system soon after the use of a substance.

j. Description for people who live based on what others think of them.

k. Return to a previous behavior or condition.

l. Elimination of a substance from a person's body.

m. The making up of information to fill in memory gaps.

n. Reliance on a substance to such a degree that abstinence causes functional impairment, physical withdrawal symptoms, and/or psychological craving for the substance.

___15. Reverse Tolerance

o. A complete arching of the body with only the head and feet on the bed.

___16. Substance

p. A confrontational approach to a client with a substance problem that lessens the chance of denial and encourages treatment before the client "hits bottom."

___17. Synthesiasis

q. Hearing colors and seeing sounds.

___18. Teratogenic

r. Decreased sensitivity to subsequent doses of the same substance; an increased dose of the substance is needed to produce the same desired effect.

___19. Tolerance

s. Causing abnormal development of the embryo.

___20. Withdrawal

t. Perceiving things that are not present in reality.

Abbreviation Review

Write the meaning or definition of the following abbreviations and acronyms.

1. AA _____
2. ADHD _____
3. AWS _____
4. CNS _____
5. DEA _____
6. DET _____
7. DETOX _____
8. DMT _____
9. DSM-IV _____
10. FAE _____
11. FAS _____
12. LSD _____
13. MADD _____
14. MAOI _____
15. MDMA _____
16. NA _____
17. NIAAA _____
18. NIDA _____
19. PCP _____
20. ROM _____
21. SADD _____
22. SIDS _____

Exercises and Activities

1. Describe the factors that might predispose an individual to substance abuse.

   Individual factors: _____

   _____

   Family patterns: _____

   _____

   Lifestyle: _____

   _____

   Environmental factors: _____

   _____

   Developmental factors: _____

   _____

   a. What interpersonal skills can protect an individual from substance abuse?

   _____

   _____

   b. How would you differentiate abuse from addiction?

   _____

   _____

2. List diagnostic testing that can be performed to detect drug and alcohol use.

   _____

   _____

   _____

3. What objective data might be noted on assessment of the client with substance abuse?

   _____

   _____

   _____

   _____

4. How would you characterize an individual who is codependent?

   _____

   _____

   _____

   a. What is the goal of treatment?

   _____

   _____

5. Identify four problems associated with substance misuse in the elderly.

    (1) _____

    (2) _____

    (3) _____

    (4) _____

6. List indicators of substance abuse in the adolescent.

    _____

    _____

    _____

7. What action would you take if you realized a coworker was impaired?

    _____

    _____

    _____

    a. Describe how you might identify a coworker who is diverting drugs in the workplace.

    _____

    _____

8. Identify the goals of the peer assistance program.

    (1) _____

    (2) _____

    (3) _____

    (4) _____

9. D.P. considers herself a typical college sophomore who just enjoys a good party. She did not do much drinking until she went away to school. College seemed like the perfect place to meet new people, study hard during the week, and party hard on the weekends. It was not as if she had to drive anywhere; there was always a party nearby. Last year, D.P. drank only on Friday or Saturday. Now she starts in the middle of the week and is binge-drinking most weekends. Her grades are slipping, but not bad enough to get her kicked out of school yet. The campus police caught her drunk in public (DIP) a few times, and the college has required her to go into counseling. But if she had not broken her foot last weekend falling down the stairs after one of her binges, her parents still would not know.

    a. What signs and symptoms indicate that D.P. has a problem with alcohol?

    _____

    _____

    _____

    b. List the physical and psychological effects of alcohol on the individual.

    _____

    _____

    _____

c. At the urging of her parents and college officials, D.P. will be starting in an outpatient counseling program. If D.P. experiences minor alcohol withdrawal symptoms, what might these include?

(1) _____ (4)_____ (7) _____

(2) _____ (5)_____ (8) _____

(3) _____ (6)_____ (9) _____

d. List four drugs that are often used to treat the symptoms of alcohol withdrawal in a client.

(1) _____ (3) _____

(2) _____ (4) _____

e. Identify problems that are associated with long-term alcohol use.

_____

_____

_____

f. What information on life skills and coping mechanisms would you include in client education with D.P.?

_____

_____

_____

_____

_____

_____

g. D.P. said that she used to take aspirin with her alcohol to avoid a hangover. Why is this combination dangerous?

_____

_____

h. When D.P.'s parents discovered her excessive alcohol use, they worked with a counselor to effect a Johsonian intervention. What is this?

_____

_____

i. D.P. agrees to take disulfiram as a part of her treatment. What information about this medication should she receive?

_____

_____

10. S.B.'s mother suspects that he is using illicit street drugs. S.B. agreed to diagnostic testing to prove his innocence. What tests are done to diagnose substance abuse?

_____

_____

_____

a. The nurse explains during the testing that having a positive test result does not necessarily prove drug use. How is this so?

_____

_____

b. Give an example of a false positive result.

_____

_____

c. How are newborns tested for the effects of drugs that their mothers used before they were born?

_____

_____

11. M.A. is a member of the wrestling team and wants to be part of the next Olympic wrestling team. He would like to increase both his strength and performance. He is considering the use of anabolic steroids and he asks you about them. What would you tell him about the effects of these drugs?

_____

_____

_____

a. How dos the Olympic Committee rule on the use of steroids?

_____

_____

b. What effect would taking steroids have on M.A. physically and emotionally?

_____

_____

c. If M.A. were to take steroids, what is the process for withdrawing from their use?

_____

_____

d. List some examples of when steroid use is indicated in the medical care of an individual.

_____

_____

Self-Assessment Questions

Circle the letter that corresponds to the best answer.

1. The nurse is performing a physical assessment on a client admitted with a diagnosis of alcohol withdrawal syndrome. Which of the following findings would indicate stage 2 (major) withdrawal?
    a. Confabulation
    b. Hallucinations
    c. Global confusion
    d. Delirium tremens

2. An example of a schedule I drug is
   a. opium.
   b. morphine.
   c. marijuana.
   d. amphetamine.

3. The nurse at the substance abuse treatment center is caring for a client who had been using phencyclidine. The nurse recalls that treatment for the client will include
   a. monitoring for seizures.
   b. confrontation to control behaviors.
   c. use of disulfiram (Antabuse) as a deterrent.
   d. observing for signs of physical dependence.

4. A sign that a client with substance abuse is achieving social and family recovery occurs when the client
   a. is able to return to work.
   b. develops a relationship with a higher power.
   c. learns to resist social pressure to use the substance.
   d. receives and accepts professional treatment for detoxification.

5. Which of the following physical manifestations would the nurse associate with fetal alcohol syndrome in the newborn?
   a. Hydrocephalus
   b. Growth retardation
   c. Cleft lip and palate
   d. Erythema toxicum neonatorum

6. Reliance on a substance to such a degree that abstinence causes functional impairment is called
   a. intoxication.
   b. abuse.
   c. dependence.
   d. tolerance.

7. Alcohol use can be detected for less than
   a. 1 day.
   b. 2 days.
   c. 3 days.
   d. 4 days.

8. Excessive and prolonged alcohol intake can cause
   a. heat exhaustion.
   b. excessive thiamine.
   c. constipation.
   d. liver problems.

9. Clients using disulfiram should refrain from using
   a. mouthwash.
   b. deodorant.
   c. toothpaste.
   d. shaving cream.

10. A medication to decrease the craving of amphetamines is called
    a. dextroamphetamine sulfate.
    b. bromocriptine mesylate.
    c. ascorbic acid.
    d. acetaminophen.

The Older Adult

Key Terms

Match the following terms with their correct definitions.

b 1. Activities of daily living

h 2. Ageism

e 3. Delirium

g 4. Dementia

a 5. Gerontological nursing

f 6. Gerontologist

d 7. Gerontology

c 8. Polypharmacy

a. Specialty within nursing that addresses and advocates for the special care needs of older adults.

b. Basic care activities that include mobility, bathing, hygiene, grooming, dressing, eating, and toileting.

c. Problem of clients taking numerous prescription and over-the-counter medications for the same or various disease processes, with unknown consequences from the resulting combinations of chemical compounds and cumulative side effects.

d. Study of the effects of normal aging and age-related diseases on human beings.

e. Cognitive changes or acute confusion of rapid onset (less than 6 months).

f. Specialist in gerontology in advanced practice nursing, geriatric psychiatry, medicine, and social services.

g. Organic brain pathology characterized by losses in intellectual functioning and a slow onset (longer than 6 months).

h. Stereotyping of older adults.

Abbreviation Review

Write the meaning or definition of the following abbreviations and acronyms.

1. AARP _____
2. AD _____
3. ANA _____
4. BBA _____
5. BPH _____
6. CHF _____
7. CMS _____

8. COPD _____

9. ERT _____

10. HCFA _____

11. NCOA _____

12. OBRA _____

13. ORIF _____

14. PPS _____

15. PSA _____

16. PVD _____

17. RTI _____

18. RUGS _____

19. SNF _____

20. SSA _____

21. THA _____

22. UTI _____

Exercises and Activities

1. What changes have occurred in U.S. demographics related to the aging population?

   _____

   _____

   _____

2. How are attitudes toward aging changing in the United States?

   _____

   _____

   _____

3. Describe the financial challenges that Americans are facing for elder-care services.

   _____

   _____

   _____

4. Your client, who is approaching retirement, tells you that he is not worried about future health care expenses because he will have Medicare and Medicaid coverage once he reaches 65. What would you tell him?

   _____

   _____

   _____

5. Describe a biological theory of aging.

   _____

   _____

   _____

a. Describe a psychological theory of aging.

_____

_____

6. Why is it important to identify individual strengths in the older client?

_____

_____

_____

7. What is polypharmacy and why is it a danger to the health of the older client?

_____

_____

_____

8. List normal physiological changes that occur with aging in each of the following systems.
   Urinary: _____

_____

   Cardiovascular: _____

_____

   Gastrointestinal: _____

_____

   Nervous system: _____

_____

   Integumentary system: _____

_____

9. What physical and lifestyle changes cause the older client to be more susceptible to lung infection?

_____

_____

_____

   a. Identify three interventions that can help older adults have healthier respiratory systems and ultimately healthier lifestyles.

_____

_____

10. What sensory alterations can cause safety issues for the older client?

_____

_____

_____

11. Describe at least four nursing interventions for the client with each of the following disorders.

Peripheral vascular disease

(1) _____

(2) _____

(3) _____

(4) _____

Chronic CHF

(1) _____

(2) _____

(3) _____

(4) _____

Alzheimer's disease

(1) _____

(2) _____

(3) _____

(4) _____

12. Your client is taking digoxin for chronic congestive heart failure. What are your nursing responsibilities for the safe administration of this medication?

_____

_____

_____

13. V.S. is a 76-year-old former engineer who has been admitted to the long-term care facility. Divorced years ago, he was living in a retirement community until symptoms of advancing Parkinson's disease required him to have more care. V.S. had done well on his own, always maintaining a sense of humor. He had regular health checkups and screening, walked outside daily until last year, quit smoking many years ago, and had been active in his retirement community. V.S. did find it difficult, however, to get food and never enjoyed cooking, so he lost a few pounds recently. His son lives several hours away and is unable to provide the care V.S. now requires.

a. Identify the strengths that have helped V.S. maintain his optimal level of functioning.

_____

_____

b. What impairments will you anticipate with this client related to his Parkinson's disease?

_____

_____

c. V.S. will need assistance with ADL. What activities are included in ADL?

(1) _____   (4) _____   (6) _____

(2) _____   (5) _____   (7) _____

(3) _____

d. How can you help V.S. with his ADL while still encouraging his independence and self-esteem?

_____

_____

_____

_____

e. Several days after his admission, you notice that V.S. seems a little confused. What can cause problems with mentation?

_____

_____

_____

f. The nursing assistant says V.S. has been experiencing urinary incontinence. What problems could this indicate? Identify interventions that might help.

_____

_____

_____

g. How can adequate nutrition be maintained as swallowing becomes more difficult?

_____

_____

_____

h. V.S. spends most of his time in his room, rarely leaving or socializing with other residents in the facility. Why is social interaction important and what can you do to support him?

_____

_____

_____

Self-Assessment Questions

Circle the letter that corresponds to the best answer.

1. The nurse is reviewing assessment data for an older client recently admitted to a long-term care facility. Which of the following is an <u>unexpected</u> finding and may indicate pathology?
   a. Kyphosis
   b. Cognitive changes
   c. Dyspnea on exertion or stress
   d. Decrease in deep tendon reflexes

2. The physician prescribes nonsteroidal antiinflammatory drugs (NSAIDs) for an older client with degenerative arthritis. Because of the side effects of NSAIDs, the nurse will teach the client and family to monitor for
   a. pruritus.
   b. fluid retention.
   c. muscle weakness.
   d. gastrointestinal distress. (G.I.)

3. The <u>most common</u> endocrine disorder in the older client is
   a. hypothyroidism. ← Hormones
   b. diabetes mellitus. ✓
   c. Cushing's disease.
   d. diabetes insipidus.

also part of the endocrine system

4. An older client has been admitted to an acute care setting following a fracture of the hip. To prevent friction and shearing damage to the skin of this client, the nursing assistants are instructed to
   a. use plastic or rubber sheet protectors. ✗
   b. monitor for nutrition and weight loss. → encourage protien + fluids
   c. use a turning sheet for positioning in the bed. ✓
   d. keep the head of the bed elevated 45 degrees.

5. Which of the following is a correct statement about the financing of elder care?
   a. Medicare does not pay for hearing aids, prescription drugs, or glasses. —true
   b. Routine medical checkups and health screening tests are covered by Medicare.
   POOR! c. Medicaid was developed to pay for long-term care for most Americans after age 65.
   d. Costs for elder care have been generally stable since the Balanced Budget Act of 1997.

6. The miscoding of enzymes that causes changes in DNA is the basis of a theory of aging related to
   a. somatic mutation.
   b. cross-linkage.
   c. immunity.
   d. stress.

7. The psychosocial view of aging that states that roles and responsibilities change throughout one's lifetime, and life satisfaction depends on maintaining involvement is the basis of _____ theory.
   Pg 1601 in book
   a. programmed
   b. continuity
   c. disengagement
   d. activity

8. An older adult who has not had a bowel movement in 2 days should be
   a. given an enema.
   b. treated with stool softeners.   if this fails
   c. watched an extra day.
   d. introduced to dietary changes and/or an exercise regimen.

9. As the older adult ages, systolic and diastolic blood pressure tends to
   a. rise.
   b. decrease.
   c. rise and decrease respectively.
   d. have no changes.

10. What common electrolyte should be monitored when the client is taking diuretics and digoxin?
    a. Chloride
    b. Potassium ✳
    c. Creatinine
    d. Glucose

Ambulatory, Restorative, and Palliative Care in Community Settings

**Chapter
51**

Key Terms

Match the following terms with their correct definitions.

___ 1. Adult day care

___ 2. Age-appropriate care

___ 3. Ambulatory care

___ 4. Assisted living

___ 5. Disability

___ 6. Extended care facility

___ 7. Handicap

___ 8. Hospice

___ 9. Impairment

___ 10. Long-term care

___ 11. Managed care

___ 12. Minimum data set

___ 13. Outcomes and Assessment Information Set

___ 14. Palliative care

___ 15. Rehabilitation

a. Lack of ability to complete activities in a normal manner.

b. Facility providing care for a long period of time.

c. Centers that provide services for adults who are unable to stay alone but who do not need 24-hour care.

d. Care provided through the dying and grieving processes.

e. Abnormal psychological or physical anomaly or anatomic loss that prevents normal functioning.

f. Nursing care that considers the client's physical, emotional, mental, and spiritual developmental level.

g. A community-based nursing home licensed for skilled or intermediate care.

h. An assessment tool for assessing a client's physical and psychosocial functioning used by Medicare.

i. Care that addresses chronic diseases that are not responsive to a cure.

j. A facility providing diagnostic and medical treatment and preventative care on an outpatient basis.

k. Therapy to assist individuals in reaching their optimal level of functioning.

l. Care where case management, individual, or team control provides cost savings.

m. Physical or mental inability to function normally and be self-sustaining.

n. An interdisciplinary program that focuses on the performance potential.

o. Facility that combines housing and services for persons requiring assistance with ADLs.

___16. Reportable conditions

___17. Respite care

___18. Restorative care

___19. Telehealth

___20. Urgent care center

p. A tool that determines the care given and reimbursement required.

q. An electronic information service.

r. A break provided to caregivers.

s. Facility designed for efficient treatment of acute illnesses.

t. Diseases or injuries that the government requires be reported to the appropriate authority or agency.

Abbreviation Review

Write the meaning or definition of the following abbreviations and acronyms.

1. ADL _____

2. CMS _____

3. ECF _____

4. FAM _____

5. FIM _____

6. HIPAA _____

7. MDS _____

8. OASIS _____

9. OBRA _____

10. SHIP _____

11. UDS _____

Exercises and Activities

1. What are some advantages to providing care outside of a hospital setting?

_____

_____

_____

2. What type of facilities provides ambulatory care services?

_____

_____

_____

3. What are some of the legal issues that nurses face when working in ambulatory care?

_____

_____

_____

4. Review the three goals of rehabilitative care.

_____

_____

_____

5. Long-term care facilities use the MDS to develop the plan of care. Identify areas of client assessment in an MDS.

   _____

   _____

   _____

6. Who participates in an interdisciplinary team and what are their roles?

   _____

   _____

   _____

7. Explain how FIM and FAM scores are used to document disabilities.

   _____

   _____

   _____

8. How is the professional type of home care different from that of technical care?

   _____

   _____

   _____

9. What do nurses teach their clients about in home care settings?

   _____

   _____

   _____

10. How is palliative care different from hospice care?

   _____

   _____

   _____

Self-Assessment Questions

Circle the letter that corresponds to the best answer.

1. Which of the following actions prevents the nurse from a legal action in a clinic setting?
   a. Having the client sign an informed consent before a biopsy is obtained
   b. Keeping a work list of all appointments by the door of each room
   c. Telling another coworker about a suspected child abuse client
   d. Helping to conduct a physical on a 14-year-old without the parent present

2. Which of the following team members of the long-term care facility assists clients with relearning how to dress themselves?
   a. Pharmacist
   b. Physical therapist
   c. Occupational therapist
   d. Social worker

3. Which of the following best describes respite care?
    a. The client who receives IV antibiotics for pneumonia in the hospital
    b. The client receiving physical therapy following a hip replacement in a nursing home
    c. The client who attends adult day care for socializations
    d. The client whose caregiver attends a wedding out of state for two days

4. Identify which source of funding is used to help clients pay for extended care following joint replacement surgery.
    a. Medicare part A
    b. Medicare part B
    c. Medical Assistance
    d. Medicaid

5. A.B., age 87, had another large heart attack. Her sons do not feel as though she can live in her large four-bedroom farm three miles from town any longer. A.B. is unable to do laundry, drive a car, or shop for groceries any longer without becoming severely short of breath. She is able to maintain her ADLs but very slowly. What sort of facility should the family consider for A.B. as she agrees to move out of her home?
    a. Long-term care facility
    b. Skilled nursing facility
    c. Respite care
    d. Assisted living

Responding to Emergencies

Key Terms

Match the following terms with their correct definitions.

____ 1. Chain of custody

____ 2. Disaster

____ 3. Emergency

____ 4. Emergency Medical Technician

____ 5. Emergency nursing

____ 6. Glasgow Coma Scale

____ 7. Paramedic

____ 8. Shock

____ 9. Trauma

____ 10. Triage

a. Medical or surgical condition requiring immediate or timely intervention to prevent permanent disability or death.

b. Neurological screening test that measures a client's best verbal, motor, and eye response to stimuli.

c. Documentation of the transfer of evidence (of a crime) from one worker to the next in a secure fashion.

d. Condition of profound hemodynamic and metabolic disturbance characterized by inadequate tissue perfusion and inadequate circulation to the vital organs.

e. Classification of clients to determine priority of need and proper place of treatment.

f. Health care professional trained to provide basic lifesaving measures prior to arrival at the hospital.

g. Specialized health care professional trained to provide advanced life support to the client requiring emergency interventions.

h. Care of clients who require emergency interventions.

i. Wound or injury.

j. A situation or event of greater magnitude than an emergency that has unforeseen, serious, or immediate threats to public health.

Abbreviation Review

Write the meaning or definition of the following abbreviations and acronyms.

1. ABC _____

2. ARS _____

3. CDC _____

4. CPR _____

  5. ED _____

  6. EMS_____

  7. EMT_____

  8. LOC _____

  9. MVC _____

10. RDD _____

11. RICE _____

12. SOP _____

13. VHF _____

Exercises and Activities

  1. Describe the role of the nurse in emergency care.

  _____

  _____

  _____

  _____

  2. List the "golden rules" of emergency care or first aid.

  (1) _____   (5) _____

  (2) _____   (6) _____

  (3) _____   (7) _____

  (4) _____

  3. Why do hospitals and emergency care organizations use triage systems for evaluating clients?

  _____

  _____

  _____

  4. How does the Good Samaritan Law protect the client and the caregiver?

  _____

  _____

  _____

  5. Identify two common causes for each type of shock.

  Hypovolemic: Anaphylactic:

  (1) _____   (1) _____

  (2) _____   (2) _____

  Cardiogenic: Neurogenic:

  (1) _____   (1) _____

  (2) _____   (2) _____

  Septic: Obstructive:

  (1) _____   (1) _____

  (2) _____   (2) _____

6. How can the nurse assess the neurological status of a client?

_____

_____

_____

7. Compare the medical treatment and at least three nursing interventions for each of the following categories of emergencies.

	Medical Treatment	Nursing Interventions
Abdominal		1. 2. 3.
Cardiopulmonary		1. 2. 3.
Musculoskeletal		1. 2. 3.
Neurological		1. 2. 3.

8. Describe the immediate care for the client with an ocular injury.

_____

_____

_____

9. Following examination and x-rays, a client is diagnosed with a sprain to the right ankle. How would you explain the RICE treatment for this client to use at home?

_____

_____

_____

10. Identify the special needs of sexual assault victims. What tests and medications may be included in their care?

_____

_____

_____

11. A child has taken several of her grandparent's acetaminophen tablets. What is the pharmacological treatment for this and how will it be administered?

_____

_____

_____

12. F.L., a 73-year-old grandparent, had joined her son, daughter-in-law, and two of their children for a day at their county fair and music festival. Although she was drinking what she thought was adequate fluid, as the afternoon continued F.L. developed a headache, mild weakness, and nausea. She was sure the feelings would pass with a short rest. However, she soon developed symptoms of heat stroke and was transported to the community hospital 5 miles away.

   a. Compare signs and symptoms for heat cramps, heat exhaustion, and heat stroke.

   _____

   _____

   b. What subjective and objective data would be collected on admission to the emergency facility?

   _____

   _____

   c. Describe immediate medical and pharmacological treatment that would be used with F.L.

   _____

   _____

   d. Identify nursing interventions that would be appropriate for this client.
      (1) _____
      (2) _____
      (3) _____
      (4) _____
      (5) _____

   e. A medication that F.L. had been using for a short time had contributed to her susceptibility to heat injury. What precautions could you suggest for her to prevent heat injury in the future?

   _____

   _____

   _____

   _____

   _____

   _____

13. A school bus crash brings 25 victims of the high school band into the emergency department. The charge nurse rapidly sets up three stations to care for the victims. They are emergent, urgent, and nonurgent. What do these terms mean?

   Emergent: _____

   Urgent: _____

   Nonurgent _____

   a. Place a number 1 beside those who would be placed in the emergent group, a number 2 by those who are urgent, and a number 3 by those who are nonurgent. Then, using red, yellow, and green designations for the severity of the injuries, indicate which color tag would be applied to the victims.

Group   *Severity*

_____   _____   B.A., the tuba player with complaints of shortness of breath

_____   _____   J.J., the drummer complaining of abdominal pain with vomiting

_____   _____   E.E., the trombonist with a compound fracture of her left arm

_____   _____   J.H., a trumpet player with a broken finger

_____   _____   K.N., a pregnant flute player with vaginal bleeding

_____   _____   K.R., a saxophonist with a broken nose and facial lacerations

_____   _____   K.W., a clarinetist with lacerations to her hands

_____   _____   M.D., another trumpet player who is unconscious

b. J.Z., another trumpet player, is in cardiac arrest and the nurse begins CPR. What personal protective equipment should the nurse be using?

_____

_____

c. B.P., another flute player, complains of neck pain and numbness in her legs. What is the first action the nurse takes with her and why?

_____

_____

(1) What position should the nurse place B.P. in and why?

_____

_____

d. M.D. remains unconscious, She has clear liquid leaking from her ears and nose. What might this indicate?

_____

_____

e. The nurse applies a sterile dressing to E.E.'s wounds while she waits for an orthopedist to attend to her. What factors need to be included when assessing the neurovascular status of E.E.'s hand?

_____

_____

f. K.R.'s scalp laceration continues to bleed profusely. How should the nurse address this injury?

_____

_____

g. Following the suturing of K.W.'s lacerations, the physician orders a Td injection. What is the rationale for this?

_____

_____

Self-Assessment Questions

Circle the letter that corresponds to the best answer.

1. A client arrives at a busy emergency room with a compound fracture of the right leg. Using the principles of hospital triage, the nurse assesses this condition as
   a. urgent.
   b. emergent.
   c. nonurgent.
   d. life threatening.

2. A client arrives in the emergency room with active bleeding from an abdominal wound and multiple leg wounds. Assessment indicates the client is in shock. The first priority for the health care team will be to
   a. notify the next of kin.
   b. determine the precipitating events.
   c. control active bleeding as quickly as possible.
   d. determine whether airway and breathing are adequate.

3. A client is brought into the emergency room after falling from a roof. Because a spinal cord injury is suspected, this client is at risk for
   a. traumatic shock.
   b. neurogenic shock.
   c. cardiogenic shock.
   d. anaphylactic shock.

4. Late signs of increased intracranial pressure include dilated pupils, widened pulse pressure, spontaneous emesis, and
   a. tremors.
   b. dyspnea.
   c. headache.
   d. hiccups.

5. Emergency personnel arrive at the scene of a two-car accident on the shoulder of a busy interstate highway. One car has a victim who appears trapped inside and unconscious. The first priority for the emergency personnel will be to
   a. ensure their own safety.
   b. call for additional help if needed.
   c. remove the victim from immediate danger.
   d. determine whether the injuries are life threatening.

6. The client arrives at the emergency room with a neighbor following a bee sting. Assessment findings include edema in the throat, difficulty breathing, hypotension, and tachycardia. Medical treatment for this client will most likely include
   a. digoxin.
   b. epinephrine.
   c. fluid replacement.
   d. a broad-spectrum antibiotic.

7. Using the disaster triage approach, which would be an example of an injury categorized with a delayed priority?
   a. Chest wound
   b. Crush injury
   c. Burns
   d. Open fracture of the femur

8. Which is *not* nonurgent in triage?
   a. Contusion
   b. Persistent vomiting and diarrhea
   c. Sprain
   d. Minor fracture

9. Which is *not* a type of distributive shock?
   a. Septic
   b. Anaphylactic
   c. Obstructive
   d. Neurogenic

10. Which is a sign of the compensatory stage of shock?
    a. Hypoactive bowel sounds
    b. Cell death
    c. Multiple organ failure
    d. Lack of peripheral pulses

Integration

Chapter 53

Exercises and Activities

Exercise: Myocardial Infarction

An overweight 52-year-old man presented to the emergency department about 4 hours after moving bricks from his garden. He is pale, slightly dyspneic, and diaphoretic. He states, "It just started off feeling heavy in my chest but now it hurts so bad." He points to his lower sternal area as the location of the pain. The client indicates he has been a smoker but quit 3 years ago. He is currently on one medication, an oral hypoglycemic.

1. List the etiological risk factors for myocardial infarction.

   _____

   _____

   _____

   _____

2. What are the risk factors for this client?

   _____

   _____

   _____

   _____

3. Develop a pathoflow diagram identifying the symptoms the client may have been experiencing on admission and relate the pathophysiology of myocardial infarction to the symptoms.

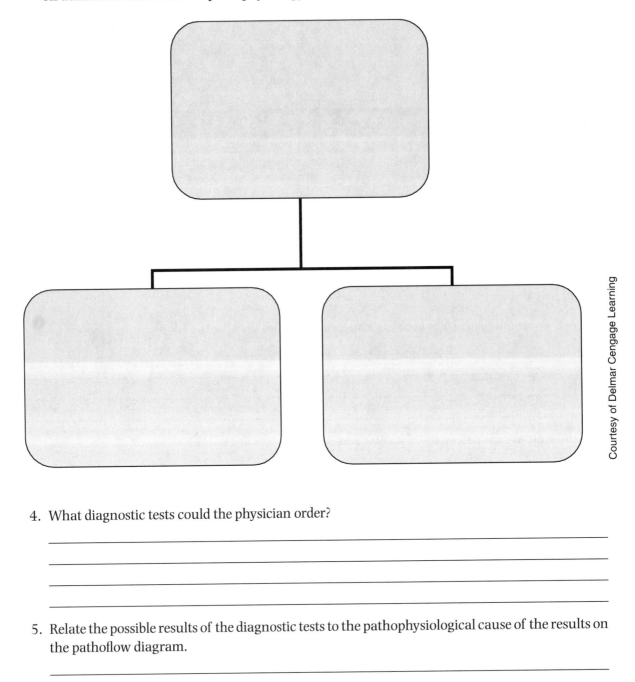

Courtesy of Delmar Cengage Learning

4. What diagnostic tests could the physician order?

_____

_____

_____

_____

5. Relate the possible results of the diagnostic tests to the pathophysiological cause of the results on the pathoflow diagram.

_____

_____

_____

_____

6. What education would be included in the discharge teaching for the client's care? Include materials and resources to be used.

   _____
   _____
   _____
   _____
   _____

7. Identify three nursing diagnoses appropriate to this client.
   (1) _____
   (2) _____
   (3) _____

   a. Identify one goal per diagnosis for the client.
      (1) _____
      (2) _____
      (3) _____

   b. Identify at least three strategies with rationales for each goal.
      (1) (a)_____
          (b)_____
          (c)_____
      (2) (a)_____
          (b)_____
          (c)_____
      (3) (a)_____
          (b)_____
          (c)_____

Exercise: Chronic Obstructive Pulmonary Disease

A 62-year-old woman presented to the emergency room with a complaint of increasing shortness of breath. She is a restless, thin, frail woman and indicates she has lost 15 pounds within the last 3 months. She states, "My shortness of breath has gotten worse. I could walk around the neighborhood but now I can't even walk around the block. I can't get my breath." The client indicates she has been a pack-a-day smoker for 40 years and quit 2 months ago due to the shortness of breath. She takes no medications but complains of a chronic cough that produces clear sputum. She denies chest pain and any significant medical history.

1. List the etiological risk factors for chronic obstructive pulmonary disease.

   _____
   _____
   _____
   _____

2. What are the risk factors for this client?

_____

_____

_____

3. Develop a pathoflow diagram identifying the symptoms the client may have been experiencing on admission and relate the pathophysiology of myocardial infarction to the symptoms.

Courtesy of Delmar Cengage Learning

4. What diagnostic tests could the physician order?

_____

_____

_____

_____

5. Relate the possible results of the diagnostic tests to the pathophysiological cause of the results on the pathoflow diagram.

_____

_____

_____

_____

6. The client is obviously dyspenic with the exertion of talking and requests that oxygen be applied. The nurse explains that this would be contraindicated in her condition. Why is that so?

_____

_____

_____

7. What education would be included in the discharge teaching for the client's care? Include materials and resources to be used.

_____

_____

_____

_____

_____

_____

_____

_____

_____

_____

8. Identify three nursing diagnoses appropriate to this client.
   (1) _____
   (2) _____
   (3) _____

   a. Identify one goal per diagnosis for the client.
      (1) _____
      (2) _____
      (3) _____

   b. Identify at least three strategies with rationales for each goal.
      (1) (a)_____
          (b)_____
          (c)_____
      (2) (a)_____
          (b)_____
          (c)_____
      (3) (a)_____
          (b)_____
          (c)_____

Exercise: Shock

A 21-year-old male was involved in a motor vehicle collision. In the field his vital signs were heart rate of 120, blood pressure 102/68, and respirations of 28; an IV of lactated ringers is started. In the emergency room his vital signs are heart rate 130, blood pressure 90/70, and respirations 38. The client is pale and restless and complains of severe abdominal pain and difficulty breathing.

1. List the etiological risk factors for *all* types of shock.

_____
_____
_____
_____
_____
_____
_____
_____

2. What are the risk factors for this client?

_____
_____
_____
_____

3. Develop a pathoflow diagram identifying the symptoms the client may have been experiencing on admission and relate the pathophysiology of myocardial infarction to the symptoms.

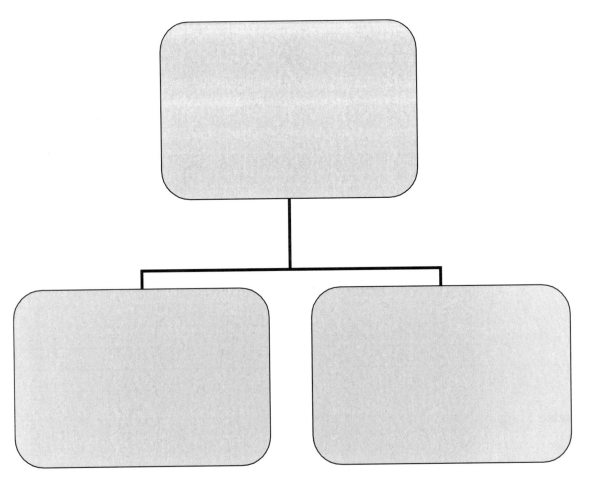

Courtesy of Delmar Cengage Learning

4. What diagnostic tests could the physician order?

_____
_____
_____
_____

5. Relate the possible results of the diagnostic tests to the pathophysiological cause of the results on the pathoflow diagram.

_____
_____
_____
_____

6. What education would be included in the discharge teaching for the client's care? Include materials and resources to be used.

_____
_____
_____
_____
_____

7. Identify three nursing diagnoses appropriate to this client.
   (1) _____
   (2) _____
   (3) _____

   a. Identify one goal per diagnosis for the client.
      (1) _____
      (2) _____
      (3) _____

   b. Identify at least three strategies with rationales for each goal.
      (1) (a)_____
          (b)_____
          (c)_____
      (2) (a)_____
          (b)_____
          (c)_____
      (3) (a)_____
          (b)_____
          (c)_____

Prenatal Care

Key Terms

Match the following terms with their correct definitions.

____ 1. Abortion

____ 2. Age of viability

____ 3. Amenorrhea

____ 4. Amnion

____ 5. Anticipatory guidance

____ 6. Ballottement

____ 7. Blastocyst

____ 8. Braxton-Hicks contractions

____ 9. Chadwick's sign

___10. Chloasma

___11. Chorion

___12. Coitus

___13. Colostrum

___14. Copulation

___15. Cotyledon

___16. Couvade

___17. Decidua

a. Delivery after 24 weeks' gestation but before 38 weeks (full term).

b. False pregnancy.

c. Sexual act that delivers sperm to the cervix by ejaculation of the erect penis.

d. Gestational age at which a fetus could live outside the uterus, generally considered to be 24 weeks.

e. Descriptor for a pregnancy between 38 and 42 weeks' gestation.

f. Rebounding of the floating fetus when pushed upward though the vagina or abdomen.

g. Fetal vessel connecting the pulmonary trunk to the aorta.

h. Structure that connects the fetus to the placenta.

i. Absence of menses.

j. Loss of pregnancy before the age of viability, usually considered to be 24 weeks.

k. White, creamy substance covering the fetus's body.

l. Information, teaching, and guidance given to a client in anticipation of an expected event.

m. Darkening of the skin of the forehead and around the eyes; also called "mask of pregnancy."

n. Fecal material stored in the fetal intestines.

o. Practice of eating substances not considered edible and that have no nutritive value such as laundry starch, dirt, clay, and freezer frost.

p. Delivery after 42 weeks' gestation.

q. Fertilized ovum.

___18. Ductus arteriosus

___19. Ductus venosus

___20. Fertilization

___21. Foramen ovale

___22. Fundus

___23. Funic souffle

___24. Goodell's sign

___25. GP/TPAL

___26. Gravida

___27. Hegar's sign

___28. Implantation

___29. Lanugo

___30. Leopold's maneuvers

___31. Linea nigra

___32. Meconium

___33. Morula

___34. Multigravida

___35. Multipara

___36. Nesting

___37. Nulligrava

___38. Nullipara

r. Condition of being pregnant for the first time.

s. Lowering of blood pressure in a pregnant woman when lying supine due to compression of the vena cava by the enlarged, heavy uterus.

t. Inner fetal membrane originating in the blastocyst.

u. Sexual act that delivers sperm to the cervix by ejaculation of the erect penis.

v. Flap opening in the atrial septum that allows only right to left movement of blood.

w. Condition of having delivered once after 24 weeks' gestation.

x. Thick substance surrounding and protecting the vessels of the umbilical cord.

y. Care of a woman during pregnancy, before labor.

z. Outer fetal membrane formed from the trophoblast.

aa. Irregular, painless uterine contractions felt by the pregnant woman toward the end of pregnancy.

bb. Mental and physical preparation for childbirth; synonymous with Lamaze.

cc. Purplish blue color of the cervix and vagina noted at about week 8 of pregnancy.

dd. Development of physical symptoms by the expectant father such as fatigue, depression, headache, backache, and nausea.

ee. Pregnancy, regardless of duration, including present pregnancy.

ff. Descriptor for when the mother feels the fetus move, about 16 to 20 weeks' gestation.

gg. The mammalian conceptus in the postmorula stage.

hh. Hemodilution caused by the increased maternal blood volume.

ii. Membranous vascular organ connecting the fetus to the mother, which produces hormones to sustain a pregnancy, supplies the fetus with oxygen and food, and transports waste products out of the fetal system.

jj. Reddish streaks frequently found on the abdomen, thighs, buttocks, and breasts; also called stretch marks.

kk. Series of specific palpations of the pregnant uterus to determine fetal position and presentation.

ll. Top of the uterus.

____39. Para

____40. Physiologic anemia
of pregnancy

____41. Pica

____42. Placenta

____43. Polyhydramnios

____44. Postterm

____45. Prenatal care

____46. Preterm

____47. Primigravida

____48. Primipara

____49. Pseudocyesis

____50. Psychoprophylaxis

____51. Quickening

____52. Striae gravidarum

____53. Supine hypotensive syndrome

____54. Teratogen

____55. Term

____56. Umbilical cord

____57. Uterine souffle

____58. Vernix caseosa

____59. Wharton's jelly

____60. Zygote

mm. Dark line on the abdomen from umbilicus to symphysis during pregnancy.

nn. Agent such as radiation, drugs, viruses, and other microorganisms capable of causing abnormal fetal development.

oo. Sound of blood pulsating through the uterus and placenta.

pp. Condition of being pregnant two or more times.

qq. Branch of the umbilical vein that enters the inferior vena cava.

rr. Condition of having delivered twice or more after 24 weeks' gestation.

ss. Embedding of a fertilized egg into the uterine lining.

tt. Antibody-rich yellow fluid secreted by the breasts during the last trimester of pregnancy and first 2 to 3 days after birth; gradually changes to milk.

uu. Fine hair covering the fetus's body.

vv. Softening of the cervix noted about week 8 of pregnancy.

ww. Condition of never having been pregnant.

xx. Softening of the uterine isthmus about week 6 of pregnancy.

yy. Gravida, para/term, preterm, abortions, living.

zz. Condition of having delivered (given birth) after 24 weeks' gestation, regardless of whether infant is born alive or dead or number of infants born.

aaa. Subdivision on the maternal side of the placenta.

bbb. Union of an ovum and a sperm.

ccc. Sound of blood pulsating through the umbilical cord; rate the same as the fetal heartbeat.

ddd. Surge of energy late in pregnancy when the pregnant woman organizes and cleans the house.

eee. Condition of never having delivered an infant after 24 weeks' gestation.

fff. The endometrium after implantation of the trophoblast.

ggg. A solid mass of cells formed by cleavage of a zygote.

hhh. Excessive amniotic fluid.

Abbreviation Review

Write the meaning or definition of the following abbreviations, acronyms, and symbols.

1. ASPO _____

2. AWHONN _____

3. BOW _____

4. BPD _____

5. C-H _____

6. C-R _____

7. DES _____

8. EDB _____

9. EDD _____

10. GP/TPAL _____

11. GFR _____

12. hCG _____

13. Hgb F _____

14. hPL _____

15. ICEA _____

16. LMP _____

17. NAACOG _____

18. OTC _____

19. PBI _____

Exercises and Activities

1. What is the importance of prenatal care for the woman and her baby?

   _____
   _____
   _____
   _____

2. List several factors that can affect the development of the fetus.

   (1) _____   (5) _____

   (2) _____   (6) _____

   (3) _____   (7) _____

   (4) _____   (8) _____

3. Your client is a 23-year-old with insulin-dependent diabetes who is hoping to become pregnant within the next year. Why is it important for her to begin preconception care now?

   _____
   _____
   _____

4. Describe the physiological changes and symptoms that occur with pregnancy in the following systems.

   Cardiovascular: _____

   _____

Respiratory: _____

_____

Musculoskeletal: _____

_____

Gastrointestinal: _____

_____

Urinary: _____

_____

5. Draw a line under each of the "probable" signs of pregnancy, and draw a circle around those that are "positive" signs.

Amenorrhea	Abdominal enlargement	Chadwick's sign
Funic souffle	Breast tenderness	Braxton-Hicks contractions
Fatigue	Goodell's sign	Fetus visualization
Quickening	Uterine enlargement	Uterine souffle
Ballottement	Chloasma	Hegar's sign
Positive pregnancy test	Morning sickness	Linea nigra
Fetal heartbeat	Fetal movement by examiner	

6. List four developmental tasks of pregnancy.

(1) _____

(2) _____

(3) _____

(4) _____

7. How does the father or support person prepare for the birth of the baby?

_____

_____

8. What causes each of these common discomforts? Identify two or more interventions that can help to relieve each one.

	Cause	*Interventions*
Nausea/vomiting		
Constipation		
Ankle edema		
Dyspnea		
Leg cramps		
Dizziness/fainting		

9. F.M. is a 29-year-old mother of two children, ages 3 and 7, and is now 34 weeks pregnant. F.M. tells you that she wants to do everything she can to prepare her children for the birth of their new baby brother or sister. What suggestions can you give her?

_____

_____

_____

10. The nurse asks you to review the warning signs for hypertension/preeclampsia with F.M. before she leaves today. What information will you include?

_____

_____

11. Convert each of the following to the abbreviated form (G_P_/T_P_A_L_) for these clients.

(1) _____   Second pregnancy, one child at home who was born at 38 weeks

(2) _____   First pregnancy (now at 22 weeks)

(3) _____   Pregnant for the third time; the first pregnancy ended in a miscarriage at 11 weeks; the second ended with a full-term birth; one living child at home

(4) _____   Nulligravida

(5) _____   Second pregnancy with twins; first pregnancy resulted in twins born at 34 weeks, who are doing well

12. Using Naegele's rule, calculate the EDB for each of the following:

LMP July 9   EDB_____

LMP December 22   EDB_____

LMP February 1   EDB_____

LMP May 15   EDB_____

13. S.B. is a 23-year-old child-care worker who is pregnant for the second time. She tells you that her first child, a 3-year-old boy, was born prematurely at 34 weeks but is doing well now. S.B. says that she was so young when she had her first baby that she didn't feel ready. She had no prenatal care until late in the pregnancy. S.B. would have preferred to become pregnant next year rather than now. However, this time she really wants to take care of herself and have a full-term, healthy baby.

a. You write on the prenatal assessment form that S.B. is G__P__/T__P__A__L__.
The date of her LMP was June 12, so you note that her EDB is _____.

b. S.B. appears to be completing the first developmental task of pregnancy because:

_____

_____

c. S.B. is about nine weeks pregnant now. When you ask about any discomforts that she may be experiencing, she tells you that she is having some heartburn and mood swings. You advise her to:

_____

_____

d. Besides a thorough health history, what else will the first visit include?

_____

_____

e. S.B. has a few questions for you. Can you help?

"How soon can you hear the baby's heartbeat?" _____

"How big is the baby right now?" _____

"When will I feel the baby move?" _____

"How often do I have to come to the clinic?" _____

"I want to know if it's a boy or a girl. Can I get an ultrasound to find out?" _____

f. S.B. returns for one of her follow-up prenatal visits when she is 28 weeks pregnant.

What would you expect for a fundal height measurement at this time? _____

What is the approximate weight gain you would expect by this time? _____

What other tests will probably be done at this visit?

_____

_____

g. You mention the childbirth classes your hospital offers. S.B. says, "I've been through this once already, so I don't see how going to classes would really help me. Nothing helps labor, anyway." What would you tell her about the benefits of attending a prepared childbirth class?

_____

_____

_____

_____

_____

_____

14. Write in the possible cause for each warning sign in pregnancy.

Warning Sign	Possible Cause
Vaginal bleeding (any), bloody show	
Sudden gush of fluid from the vagina	
Persistent vomiting	
Sever continuous headache	
Swelling of face, hands, legs, feet when rising in the morning	
Visual disturbances: blurring, double vision, flashes of light, spots before eyes	
Dizziness	
Fever over 100°F	
Pain in abdomen or cramping	
Epigastric pain	
Irritating vaginal discharge	
Dysuria	
Oliguria	
Noticeable reduction or absence of fetal movement	

Self-Assessment Questions

Circle the letter that corresponds to the best answer.

1. The nurse measuring the fundal height of a client who is 20 weeks pregnant finds it at the level of her umbilicus. The nurse determines that this
   a. is a normal finding.
   b. is greater than expected.
   c. indicates oligohydramnios.
   d. requires an immediate ultrasound.

2. You review lab work on your client, who is 32 weeks pregnant. You note that she has a hematocrit of 34%. This is most likely caused by
   a. iron deficiency anemia.
   b. poor dietary intake of protein.
   c. placental transport of blood to the fetus.
   d. hemodilution from an increase in plasma.

3. When the client complains about the Braxton-Hicks contractions she is experiencing, the nurse explains that their purpose is to
   a. soften and dilate the cervix.
   b. help her to practice breathing techniques.
   c. help with uterine and placental circulation.
   d. improve the abdominal muscle tone for delivery.

4. A client has gone into labor at 23 weeks of gestation. The nurse understands that this is below the age of viability for the infant because
   a. there is an absent suck/swallow reflex.
   b. alveoli are insufficient for air exchange.
   c. the infant has fetal hemoglobin present.
   d. the fetus has passed meconium in utero.

5. A client in the prenatal clinic is scheduled to have the following tests during her pregnancy. Which of these would be used to screen for possible birth defects?
   a. Venereal Disease Research Laboratory
   b. Rubella titer
   c. Coomb's test
   d. Alpha-fetoprotein

6. A nurse is reviewing data for her client, a 37-year-old primigravida who is now at 35 weeks' gestation. Her blood pressure today is 150/85, and she is complaining of mild edema in her legs. You determine that according to her usual blood pressure of 120/68, this is
   a. high and needs to be reported.
   b. a typical increase in the last month of pregnancy.
   c. abnormal only if the client also has edema in her hands and face.
   d. a result of a later maternal age in an otherwise normal pregnancy.

7. Fathers who smoke and mothers who do not
   a. have lower-birth-weight infants.
   b. have infants who are unaffected.
   c. have large-for-gestational age infants.
   d. have normal-weight infants.

8. The trophoblast secretes _____ during the early pregnancy.
   a. estrogen
   b. progesterone
   c. hPL
   d. hCG

9. The fetal stage of development from the beginning of week 3 through week 8 is called
   a. germinal stage.
   b. embryonic stage.
   c. fetal stage.
   d. cephalo stage.

10. At what week of fetal development is lanugo only on the shoulders and upper back?
   a. Week 28
   b. Week 32
   c. Week 36
   d. Week 40

Complications
of Pregnancy

Key Terms

Match the following terms with their correct definitions.

____ 1. Abortion

____ 2. Abruptio placenta

____ 3. Amniocentesis

____ 4. Biophysical profile

____ 5. Early deceleration

____ 6. Eclampsia

____ 7. Ectopic pregnancy

____ 8. Euglycemia

____ 9. HELLP syndrome

____10. Hydatidiform mole

____11. Hydramnios

____12. Hyperemesis gravidarum

____13. Incompetent cervix

____14. Kernicterus

a. Pregnancy in which the fertilized ovum is implanted outside the uterine cavity.

b. Reduction in fetal heart rate that begins after the uterus has begun contraction and increases to the baseline level after the uterine contraction has ceased.

c. Assessment of five variables: fetal breathing movement, fetal movements of body or limbs, fetal tone (flexion/extension of extremities), amniotic fluid volume, and reactive NST.

d. Termination of a pregnancy before viability of the fetus, usually 24 weeks.

e. Withdrawal of amniotic fluid to obtain a sample for specimen examination.

f. Abnormality of the placenta wherein the chorionic villi become fluid-filled, grapelike clusters; the trophoblastic tissue proliferates; and there is no viable fetus.

g. Deficiency in the amount of amniotic fluid.

h. Reduction in fetal heart rate that begins early with the contraction and virtually mirrors the uterine contraction.

i. Excessive fetal growth characterized by a fetus weighing more than 4,000 g (8.8 lb).

j. Reduction in fetal heart rate that has no relationship to contractions of the uterus.

k. Normal blood glucose level.

l. Premature separation, from the wall of the uterus, of normally implanted placenta.

m. Convulsion occurring in pregnancy-induced hypertension.

n. Pregnancy-induced hypertension with liver damage characterized by hemolysis, elevated liver enzymes, and low platelet count.

___15. Late deceleration

___16. Macrosomia

___17. Miscarriage

___18. Modified biophysical profile

___19. Oligohydramnios

___20. Placenta previa

___21. Preeclampsia

___22. Tocolysis

___23. Variable deceleration

o. Spontaneous abortion.

p. Excessive vomiting during pregnancy.

q. Condition in which the placenta forms over or very near the internal cervicalos.

r. Excess amount of amniotic fluid.

s. Descriptor for when the cervix begins to dilate, usually during the second trimester.

t. Phase of pregnancy-induced hypertension prior to convulsions.

u. Severe neurological damage resulting from a high level of bilirubin (jaundice).

v. Process of stopping labor with medications.

w. Assessment of the NST and amniotic fluid volume to determine fetal wellness.

Abbreviation Review

Write the meaning or definition of the following abbreviations, acronyms, and symbols.

1. CMV _____

2. CST _____

3. CVS _____

4. D&C _____

5. DIC _____

6. EDB _____

7. EFM _____

8. FAST _____

9. FBPP _____

10. FHR _____

11. FHT _____

12. GDM _____

13. hCG _____

14. HELLP _____

15. hPL _____

16. HSV-2 _____

17. IUGR _____

18. L/S _____

19. $MgSO_4$ _____

20. MSAFP _____

21. NST _____

22. PG _____

23. PlH _____

24. PKU _____

25. RhoGam _____

26. SGA _____

27. TORCH _____

28. VST _____

Exercises and Activities

1. What role does fetal assessment play during pregnancy?

   _____

   _____

2. If a pregnancy is determined to be high-risk, what monitoring may be used to assess fetal well-being?

   _____

   _____

3. List several abnormal conditions that can be detected with ultrasound.

   (1) _____ (4) _____

   (2) _____ (5) _____

   (3) _____ (6) _____

4. Describe a "normal" finding for a nonstress test.

   _____

   _____

5. Describe a "normal" finding for a contraction stress test.

   _____

   _____

   _____

6. Identify the variables that are assessed with a biophysical profile.

   (1) _____

   (2) _____

   (3) _____

   (4) _____

   (5) _____

7. What information is obtained with each of the following tests? What is the expected change in laboratory values as the pregnancy progresses?

   MSAFP: _____

   Estriol: _____

   hPL: _____

   L/S ratio: _____

8. M.W. is identified as being high-risk with her current pregnancy because her last pregnancy resulted in a fetal demise 2 years ago. She has been advised to check fetal activity daily at home. How will you instruct M.W. to use the Cardiff method to monitor fetal well-being? Include warning signs.

_____

_____

_____

9. J.C., who is 32 weeks pregnant, was involved in an automobile accident. You will be assessing her for fetal well-being. What are the advantages of external fetal monitoring for this client?

_____

_____

_____

10. S.L. is a 39-year-old, G2 P1, being seen for her first prenatal visit. She is concerned about possible genetic problems with this pregnancy because of her age and a family history of birth defects. What tests could be done to reassure S.L.? When could each test be done?

_____

_____

_____

11. Briefly describe the signs and symptoms and the medical–surgical management for the following obstetrical disorders.

	Signs/Symptoms	Medical–Surgical Management
Incompetent cervix		
Ectopic pregnancy		
Hydatidiform mole		

   a. What follow-up care is important to the client with hydatidiform mole?

_____

_____

   b. How would you explain the difference between placenta previa and abruptio placenta?

_____

_____

   c. List several obstetrical disorders that can lead to DIC.

(1) _____   (5) _____

(2) _____   (6) _____

(3) _____   (7) _____

(4) _____

d. How can abruptio placenta lead to DIC?

_____

_____

e. What effect can each of the following disorders have on the fetus?

Maternal PKU: _____

Rubella: _____

CMV: _____

Herpes genitalis: _____

12. What clients are at risk of developing PIH?

_____

_____

_____

a. List the classic symptoms for PIH.

(1) _____

(2) _____

(3) _____

b. What are the three major goals of treatment for the client with PIH?

(1) _____

(2) _____

(3) _____

13. C.A., a 21-year-old primigravida, is diagnosed with PIH. Because her symptoms are mild at present, she can remain at home. What will you tell C.A. about home management for PIH?

_____

_____

_____

a. What factors might lead to hospitalization for C.A.?

_____

_____

14. M.A., a 23-year-old client, G1 P0, is O negative. Her husband is O positive. Will M.A. need RhoGAM during this pregnancy? If so, why?

_____

_____

_____

a. If this client is to receive RhoGAM, when would it be given?

_____

_____

_____

15. D.P. is a 24-year-old client with diabetes mellitus, type 1, diagnosed when she was a teenager. Her obstetric history includes two previous pregnancy losses, including a miscarriage last year. D.P. has poorly controlled diabetes as evidenced by high glucose levels and evidence of retinopathy. When asked, she admits she has not returned to her physician for diabetes management in "a long time." She is now approximately 10 weeks pregnant at her first prenatal visit. D.P. will be monitored closely for glucose levels and fetal well-being.

   a. What effect will the pregnancy have on D.P.'s diabetes?

   _____
   _____
   _____

   b. In what ways might her diabetes affect the pregnancy?

   _____
   _____
   _____

   c. What are the risks for the fetus related to D.P.'s diabetes?

   _____
   _____
   _____

   d. D.P. tells you that she is very motivated to have a healthy baby with this pregnancy. What will she need to do to take care of herself while she is pregnant?

   _____
   _____
   _____

   e. How will the fetus be monitored during the pregnancy?

   _____
   _____
   _____

   f. How would preconception counseling have benefited D.P.?

   _____
   _____
   _____

16. Fill in the table, which identifies high risk factors in pregnancy.

General	Obstetrical	Medical	Other

17. E.O., age 40, is a primipara and is at 16 weeks gestation. The obstetrician decided to recommend amniocentesis for E.O. Describe amniocentesis in terms that E.O. may understand.

   a. Describe how normal amniotic fluid looks.

   _____

   _____

   _____

   b. What laboratory tests are done on amniotic fluid? What are the tests for?

   _____

   _____

   _____

18. N.W. has been nauseated and vomiting into her second trimester of pregnancy. Why would the physician be concerned if N.W. were to become dehydrated?

   _____

   _____

   _____

   a. What types of medical treatment are indicated for hyperemesis gravidarum?

   _____

   _____

   _____

   b. What signs and symptoms could N.W. exhibit if she were dehydrated?

   _____

   _____

   _____

Self-Assessment Questions

Circle the letter that corresponds to the best answer.

1. You have been assigned to care for a client who is suspected of having HELLP syndrome as a result of PIH. You recall that this indicates your client may have all but which of the following complications?
   a. Hyperglycemia
   b. Lysing of red blood cells
   c. Decreased platelets
   d. Increased liver enzymes

2. The nurse is caring for a client with PIH who is receiving $MgSO_4$, a central nervous system depressant. To counteract respiratory depression that may occur with this medication, the nurse will be prepared to administer
   a. Narcan.
   b. Apresoline.
   c. epinephrine.
   d. calcium gluconate.

3. The nurse is caring for a client who is a 31-year-old multigravida diagnosed with gestational diabetes mellitus. Because of the effects of this disorder on the pregnancy, the nurse would anticipate a finding of
   a. macrosomia.
   b. hyporeflexia.
   c. oligohydramnios.
   d. peripheral edema.

4. The student is observing a fetal biophysical profile on her client, who is 35 weeks pregnant. The student recalls that this test should demonstrate fetal breathing and movement, fetal tone, amniotic fluid pockets, and
   a. a negative CST.
   b. a reactive NST.
   c. a negative Coombs' test.
   d. mild uterine contractions.

5. The nurse is caring for a client in active labor. The fetus is in a cephalic presentation at +2 station. With each contraction, the fetal heart rate is dropping after the acme of the contraction before returning to its baseline rate. The nurse determines that these are late decelerations caused by
   a. head compression.
   b. breech presentation.
   c. uteroplacental insufficiency.
   d. umbilical cord compression.

6. A nurse is performing an assessment on a client who is 33 weeks pregnant with a diagnosis of placenta previa. Which of the following findings will the nurse anticipate?
   a. Painless bleeding
   b. Abdominal rigidity
   c. Uterine tenderness
   d. Bright red bleeding

7. A general high-risk factor in pregnancy is that the client
   a. has diabetes.
   b. has had preeclampsia.
   c. has had a Cesarean birth.
   d. is unmarried.

8. The time of quickening is
   a. 8 to 12 weeks.
   b. 12 to 16 weeks.
   c. 16 to 20 weeks.
   d. 20 to 24 weeks.

9. When habitual abortions are caused by an incompetent cervix, it can be treated by
   a. a D&C.
   b. cerclage.
   c. a salpingectomy.
   d. induction of labor.

10. In an attempt to accelerate fetal lung maturity, a drug such as _____ may be given to the mother.
    a. betamethasone
    b. heparin
    c. methotrexate
    d. magnesium sulfate

The Birth Process

Key Terms

Match the following terms with their correct definitions.

_____ 1. Acme

_____ 2. Amniotomy

_____ 3. Augmentation of labor

_____ 4. Bloody show

_____ 5. Braxton-Hicks contractions

_____ 6. Cephalopelvic disproportion

_____ 7. Cervical dilation

_____ 8. Cesarean birth

_____ 9. Crowning

_____ 10. Decrement

_____ 11. Duration

_____ 12. Dysfunctional labor

_____ 13. Dystocia

_____ 14. Effacement

a. Relationship of fetal body parts to one another, either flexion or extension.

b. Length of one contraction, from the beginning of the increment to the conclusion of the decrement.

c. Thin, fibrous membrane-covered space between skull bones.

d. Injection of a local anesthetic into the pudendal nerve to provide perineal, external genitalia, and lower vaginal anesthesia.

e. Condition in which the fetal head will not fit through the mother's pelvis.

f. Contractions that do not cause the cervix to dilate.

g. Unique ability of the muscle fibers of the uterus to remain shortened to a small degree after each contraction.

h. Labor with problems of the contractions or of maternal bearing down.

i. Expulsion of cervical secretions, blood-tinged mucus, and the mucous plug that blocked the cervix during pregnancy.

j. Relationship of the fetal presenting part to the ischial spines.

k. Relationship of the identified landmark on the presenting part to the four quadrants of the mother's pelvis.

l. Metal instruments used on the fetal head to provide traction or to provide a method of rotating the fetal head to an occiput-anterior position.

m. Condition of the umbilical cord being wrapped around the baby's neck.

n. Onset of regular contractions of the utuerus that cause cervical changes between 20 and 37 weeks' gestation.

____15. Engagement

____16. Episiotomy

____17. External version

____18. False labor

____19. Ferguson's reflex

____20. Fetal attitude

____21. Fetal lie

____22. Fetal position

____23. Fetal presentation

____24. Fontanelle

____25. Forceps

____26. Frequency

____27. Fundus

____28. Increment

____29. Induction of labor

____30. Intensity

____31. Interval

____32. Lightening

____33. Macrosomia

____34. Molding

____35. Nuchal cord

____36. Precipitate birth

____37. Precipitate labor

____38. Presenting part

o. Long, difficult, or abnormal labor caused by any of the four major variables (4 Ps) that affect labor.

p. Rotation of the fetal head back to be in normal alignment with the shoulders after delivery of the fetal head.

q. Incision in the perineum to facilitate passage of the baby.

r. Top of the uterus.

s. Medication that inhibits uterine contractions.

t. Peak of a contraction.

u. Stimulation of uterine contractions before contractions begin spontaneously for the purpose of birthing an infant.

v. Spontaneous, involuntary urge to bear down during labor.

w. Thinning of the cervix.

x. Artificial rupture of the membranes.

y. Irregular, intermittent contractions felt by the pregnant woman toward the end of pregnancy.

z. Manipulation of the fetus through the mother's abdomen to a presentation facilitating birth.

aa. Condition of the widest diameter of the fetal presenting part (head) entering the inlet to the true pelvis.

bb. Determined by the fetal lie and the part of the fetus that enters the pelvis first.

cc. Strength of the contraction at the acme.

dd. Enlargement of the cervical opening from 0 to 10 cm (complete dilation).

ee. Relationship of the cephalocaudal axis of the fetus to the cephalocaudal axis of the mother, either longitudinal or transverse.

ff. Increasing intensity of a contraction.

gg. Excessive fetal growth characterized by a fetus weighing more than 4,000 g (8.8 lb).

hh. Labor lasting less than 3 hours from the onset of contractions to the birth of the infant.

ii. Condition in which the umbilical cord lies below the presenting part of the fetus.

jj. Part of the fetus in contact with the cervix.

kk. Time from the beginning of one contraction to the beginning of the next contraction.

ll. Stimulation of uterine contractions after spontaneously beginning but having unsatisfactory progress of labor.

___39. Preterm birth

___40. Preterm labor

___41. Prolapsed cord

___42. Pudendal block

___43. Restitution

___44. Rupture of membranes

___45. Station

___46. Suture

___47. Tocolytic agent

___48. Uterine retraction

mm. Birth of an infant through an incision in the abdomen and uterus.

nn. Membranous area where sutures meet on the fetal skull.

oo. When the largest diameter of the fetal head is past the vulva.

pp. Resting period between two contractions.

qq. Decreasing intensity of a contraction.

rr. Descent of the fetus into the pelvis, causing the uterus to tip forward, relieving pressure on the diaphragm.

ss. Birth occurring suddenly and unexpectedly without a CNM/physician present to assist.

tt. Birth that takes place before the end of the 37th week of gestation.

uu. Shaping of the fetal head to adapt to the mother's pelvis during labor.

vv. Rupture of the amniotic sac.

Abbreviation Review

Write the meaning or definition of the following abbreviations and acronyms.

1. 4 Ps _____

2. AROM _____

3. CNM _____

4. CPD _____

5. FHR _____

6. LDRP _____

7. LMA _____

8. LMP _____

9. LMT _____

10. LOA _____

11. LOP _____

12. LOT _____

13. LSA _____

14. LSP _____

15. LST _____

16. PROM _____

17. RMA _____

18. RMP _____

19. RMT _____

20. ROA _____

21. ROM _____

22. ROP _____

23. ROT _____

24. RSA _____

25. RSP _____

26. RST _____

27. SROM _____

28. VBAC _____

Exercises and Activities

1. Briefly describe how each of these four variables affects labor.

   Passage: _____

   _____

   Passenger: _____

   _____

   Powers: _____

   _____

   Psyche: _____

   _____

   a. How do nursing interventions support the psyche of a client in labor?

   _____

   _____

   _____

   b. List six signs of impending labor.

   (1) _____   (4) _____

   (2) _____   (5) _____

   (3) _____   (6) _____

   c. How do contractions differ in true versus false labor?

   _____

   _____

   d. What are the expected changes for each of the following during labor?

   Temperature: _____

   Pulse: _____

   Respirations: _____

   Blood pressure: _____

   White blood cell count: _____

   Gastrointestinal (GI) system: _____

Copyright © 2011 Delmar Cengage Learning

2. For the following diagram, identify the fetal presentation, lie, attitude, and position.

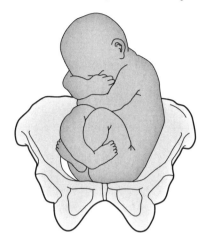

Draw an X over the place on the diagram where you would listen for the FHR.

Fetal presentation _____

Fetal lie _____

Fetal attitude _____

Fetal position _____

3. Complete the following statements.
    a. The first stage of labor ends when the _____.
    b. The delivery of the placenta occurs at the end of the _____ stage of labor.
    c. A client is pushing during the _____ stage of labor.
    d. Transition is part of the _____ stage of labor.
    e. The shortest stage of labor is the _____ stage.
    f. The second stage of labor ends with the _____.

4. On the following graph, draw in the labor pattern using the descriptions given.

Frequency: 2 1/2 minutes

Duration: 50 seconds

Intensity: moderate

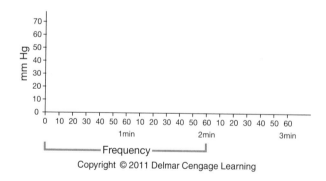

Copyright © 2011 Delmar Cengage Learning

5. List two nursing interventions to support your client for each stage/phase of labor.

First stage:

Latent	1.	
	2.	
Active	1.	
	2.	
Transition	1.	
	2.	
Second stage	1.	
	2.	

6. Identify nursing interventions to support the mother and baby during the fourth stage of labor.

_____

_____

7. Using the following time lines, compare the length of each stage/phase of labor for the primigravida and the multigravida.

Primigravida   5 hr   10 hr   15 hr   20 hr

Multigravida   5 hr   10 hr   15 hr   20 hr

8. List risk factors for preterm labor.

(1) _____

(2) _____

(3) _____

(4) _____

(5) _____

9. S.S. and J.S. have just arrived at the birthing unit for the delivery of their first child. S.S. is anxious and uncomfortable during her contractions. J.S. is excited about the birth and eager to help S.S. They attended all the childbirth classes but haven't been practicing the breathing and relaxation techniques. Describe nursing activities and interventions that can help S.S. and J.S. to feel welcome and comfortable during admission.

_____

_____

_____

a. List questions you could ask S.S. to obtain information about her labor.

(1) _____

(2) _____

(3) _____

(4) _____

b. What information will be collected in the admission assessment?

_____

_____

_____

c. What effect can S.S.'s anxiety have on her labor?

_____

_____

d. S.S. needs support with her breathing techniques. How will you instruct S.S. and J.S. in the first technique?

_____

_____

e. S.S. had hoped for an unmedicated birth but is feeling overwhelmed with her contractions. A regional block is offered to her. List advantages and disadvantages of an epidural block for S.S.

Advantages	*Disadvantages*
_____	_____
_____	_____
_____	_____
_____	_____

10. Describe nursing actions for the immediate care of the newborn.

_____

_____

_____

_____

11. What are the five variables assessed with the Apgar score?

(1) _____   (4) _____

(2) _____   (5) _____

(3) _____

12. If the birth involves the use of forceps or is vacuum assisted, how might the infant be affected?

_____

_____

_____

13. How can you promote maternal/infant bonding after delivery?

_____

_____

_____

14. C.R., a 29-year-old, G3 P2, arrives on the birthing unit early in the morning with her husband. She tells you that she was awakened this morning with a contraction. She tells you that she had short labors with her last delivery. C.R. is full term and her pregnancy has been uneventful so far. Her membranes have ruptured. An assessment is completed and her physician has been notified.

a. Because C.R. is in the active phase of labor, how often will you check her vital signs, FHR, and contractions?

_____

_____

_____

b. If C.R. experiences a precipitate labor, what are the possible complications for her and the fetus?

_____

_____

c. C.R.'s labor is progressing well, but the FHR on the monitoring strip indicates that the fetal heart rate has dropped. C.R. is advised she may have a Cesarean delivery. List several indications for a Cesarean birth.

(1) _____

(2) _____

(3) _____

(4) _____

(5) _____

(6) _____

d. What preoperative procedures and support will be initiated for C.R.?

_____

_____

e. Following surgery with a horizontal uterine incision, the infant is suctioned, warmed, and assessed. Calculate the infant's Apgar score at 1 minute and 5 minutes.

	1 minute	5 minutes
Heart rate	96	126
Respiratory rate	Weak cry	Good cry
Muscle tone	Some flexion	Good flexion
Reflex irritability	Grimace	Crying
Color	Hands and feet blue	Body pink, extremities blue

Score

f. The next day, C.R. tells you she's just happy the baby is okay, but they had always hoped to have four children. Does this mean she has to have another Cesarean birth if she gets pregnant again?

_____

_____

_____

_____

_____

15. What is the difference between cephalic presentation and a breech presentation?

_____

_____

a. What are the three types of breech presentations?

_____

_____

16. What infection control practices do nurses use during labor and delivery?

_____

_____

17. B.K. is in active labor with her second child. She feels the need to push. As she begins to push, the nurse notes that the umbilical cord is protruding before head emerges. What actions should the nurse take immediately?

_____

_____

_____

Self-Assessment Questions

Circle the letter that corresponds to the best answer.

1. The fetus of a laboring client is noted to be macrosomic. The nurse realizes that this may predispose this client to a longer, more difficult labor known as
   a. dystocia.
   b. hypertonia.
   c. uterine inertia.
   d. dysfunctional labor.

2. The nurse is caring for a laboring client who will be having an amniotomy. The first nursing action following this procedure will be to
   a. test the fluid with nitrazine paper.
   b. assess the fetal heart rate for 1 minute.
   c. assess the mother's vital signs and level of comfort.
   d. perform a vaginal exam to determine the dilation and effacement.

3. A client in labor is using breathing techniques to deal with the discomfort. The client is using slow, deep chest breathing, which is no longer effective to deal with the pain of her contractions. The nurse will advise this client to
   a. take Demoral IM.
   b. try pant-blow breathing.
   c. use relaxation techniques.
   d. advance to shallow breathing.

4. A nurse caring for a client in labor identifies a prolapsed cord occurring with the spontaneous rupture of membranes. Which of the following positions will the nurse utilize with this client?
   a. Supine
   b. Lithotomy
   c. Modified Sims'
   d. Reverse Trendelenburg

5. The risks to the fetus in a breech delivery include all but which of the following?
   a. Fluid aspiration
   b. Precipitate birth
   c. Cord compression
   d. Head becoming stuck

6. The nurse is monitoring oxytocin augmentation with a client whose membranes have ruptured but who has exhibited poor labor progress. For this client, the goal for oxytocin administration is to promote
   a. cervical ripening.
   b. hypotonic uterine contractions.
   c. contractions every 2 to 3 minutes, 45 to 60 seconds in length, of moderate intensity.
   d. contractions lasting 90 seconds with a uterine resting tone of at least 20 mm Hg.

7. When is labor induced after membrane rupture with a near-term pregnancy?
   a. 6–12 hours
   b. 12–24 hours
   c. 24–36 hours
   d. 36–48 hours

8. The position that improves labor progression is
   a. prone.
   b. supine.
   c. side-lying.
   d. dorsal recumbent.

9. The client is alert and talkative and the cervix is dilated 3 cm. The client is in the _____ phase.
   a. latent
   b. active
   c. transition
   d. focusing

10. Which mechanism of labor generally occurs during the first stage?
    a. Internal rotation
    b. Expulsion
    c. Extension
    d. Flexion

Postpartum Care

Key Terms

Match the following terms with their correct definitions.

___ 1. Afterpains

___ 2. Attachment

___ 3. Bonding

___ 4. Claiming process

___ 5. Colostrum

___ 6. Disseminated intravascular coagulation

___ 7. Dyspareunia

___ 8. Engorgement

___ 9. Engrossment

___ 10. Entrainment

___ 11. Involution

___ 12. Let-down reflex

___ 13. Lochia

___ 14. Mastitis

a. Term for the first 6 weeks after the birth of an infant.

b. Neurohormonal reflex that causes milk to be expressed from the alveoli into the lactiferous ducts.

c. Incomplete return of the uterus to its prepregnant size and consistency.

d. Painful intercourse.

e. Long-term process that begins during pregnancy and intensifies during the postpartum period that establishes an enduring bond between parent and child and develops through reciprocal (parent to child and child to parent) behaviors.

f. Return of the reproductive organs, especially the uterus, to their prepregnancy size and condition.

g. Uterine/vaginal discharge after childbirth; initially bright red, then changing to a pink or pinkish brown, then to a yellowish white.

h. Newborn from birth to 28 days of life.

i. Discomfort caused by the contracting uterus after the infant's birth.

j. Infection following childbirth occurring between the birth and 6 weeks postpartum.

k. Formation of a clot due to an inflammation in the wall of the vessel.

l. Distention and swelling of the breasts in the first few days following delivery.

m. Abnormal stimulation of the clotting mechanism causing small clots throughout the vascular system and widespread bleeding internally, externally, or both.

n. Rapid process of attachment, parent to infant, that takes place during the sensitive period, the first 30 to 60 minutes after the birth.

___15. Metritis

___16. Neonate

___17. Oophoritis

___18. Postpartum blues

___19. Postpartum depression

___20. Postpartum hemorrhage

___21. Postpartum psychosis

___22. Puerperal (postpartum) infection

___23. Puerperium

___24. Salpingitis

___25. Subinvolution

___26. Thrombophlebitis

o. Inflammation of the fallopian tube.

p. Blood loss of more than 500 mL after the third stage of labor or 1,000 mL following a Cesarean birth.

q. Inflammation of the breast, generally during breast-feeding.

r. Condition more severe than postpartum depression and characterized by delusions and thoughts of self-harm or infant harm.

s. Process whereby a family identifies the infant's likeness to and differences from family members, and the infant's unique qualities.

t. Inflammation of the ovary.

u. Yellowish breast fluid rich in antibodies and high in protein.

v. Mild transient condition of emotional liability and crying for no apparent reason, which affects up to 80% of women who have just given birth and lasts about 2 weeks.

w. Parents' intense interest in and preoccupation with the newborn.

x. Inflammation of the uterus, including the endometrium and parametrium.

y. Infant's ability to move in rhythm to the parent's voice.

z. Condition similar to postpartum blues but which is more serious, intense, and persistent.

Abbreviation Review

Write the meaning or definition of the following abbreviations, acronyms, and symbols.

1. CNM _____
2. DIC _____
3. DVT _____
4. hCG _____
5. hPL _____
6. MSH _____
7. PPD _____
8. RhoGAM _____

Exercises and Activities

1. How do the parents and family members establish attachment with the infant?

_____
_____
_____

a. What behaviors by the infant are important in bonding and attachment?

_____

_____

_____

b. Describe nursing actions and interventions that can facilitate bonding.

_____

_____

c. J.B. expresses concern about how her 2-year-old daughter will react to the new baby. She does not feel they really prepared her for the birth. The daughter will be arriving with Dad in a little while. What guidance could you give J.B.?

_____

_____

_____

_____

_____

2. Briefly describe physiological changes that occur during the postpartum period in each of the following.

Uterus: _____

_____

Breasts: _____

_____

GI system: _____

_____

Urinary system: _____

_____

Musculoskeletal system: _____

_____

Blood values: _____

_____

a. What changes would the nurse anticipate in vital signs within the first 24 hours?

_____

_____

_____

b. How do prolactin and oxytocin affect the postpartum client?

_____

_____

_____

c. R.L. tells you that she will not need to use birth control for quite a while because she plans to breastfeed her newborn son for a year. What information would you share with her?

_____

_____

3. What are the main tasks for the mother in each phase of maternal restoration and adaptation according to Rubin?

Taking-in phase: _____

_____

Taking-hold phase: _____

_____

Letting-go phase: _____

_____

a. List several nursing actions or interventions that can facilitate the taking-hold phase.

(1) _____

(2) _____

(3) _____

(4) _____

(5) _____

(6) _____

b. Identify what each letter represents in the acronym BUBBLE for postpartum assessment.

B _____

U _____

B _____

B _____

L _____

E _____

c. What other subjective and objective information is collected during the assessment?

_____

_____

d. List factors that cause discomfort in the postpartum client.

_____

_____

e. J.A. tells you during your assessment that she is having a lot of pain "in my bottom." What comfort measures can you offer or suggest?

_____

_____

_____

_____

4. How do postpartum blues differ from postpartum depression?

_____

_____

_____

  a. Describe why postpartum psychosis is a medical emergency.

  _____

  _____

5. Identify factors that predispose the postpartum client to infection.

_____

_____

  a. You are helping to discharge your client, T.Z., and her new baby today. The nurse asks you to review the signs and symptoms of postpartum infection with T.Z. before she goes home. What information will you include?

  _____

  _____

6. C.V. had a normal pregnancy and vaginally delivered a healthy girl. C.V. asks the nurse when she will get her figure back. Describe the process of involution in terms C.V. can understand.

_____

_____

_____

  a. C.V. asks when her vaginal discharge will end. Describe the changes that occur in the lochia.

  _____

  _____

  _____

  b. C.V. also wants to know how soon her menses will resume. How should the nurse respond?

  _____

  _____

  _____

7. D.P. is a 17-year-old single mother, G1 P1, who has delivered an apparently healthy baby girl 3 hours ago with a Cesarean birth. D.P.'s mother is with her in the room and is holding the baby. She smiles and tells you this is their second grandchild. There is no information about the father of the baby. You notice that your client is very tired and is dozing on and off.

  a. What additional assessment is necessary for D.P. because she had a Cesarean birth?

  _____

  _____

  _____

b. What special concerns may be related to D.P.'s age?

_____

_____

_____

c. After D.P. has rested, you ask her if she would like to feed the baby. D.P. tells you that she would like to try to breastfeed, but she does not have any milk yet. What will you tell her?

_____

_____

_____

_____

d. The next day, D.P. has been encouraged to walk some and begin caring for herself and her baby. A few hours later, you notice D.P. is still lying in bed. She tells you she is too tired and too uncomfortable to get up. Why is it important for her to become more active? How can you help D.P. to balance her need for rest and activity?

_____

_____

_____

e. What observations might tell you whether D.P. is adapting to her new role as mother?

_____

_____

_____

_____

_____

_____

8. Describe the infection control practices that the nurse uses in postpartum care.

_____

_____

_____

9. Explain why Rh immune globulin is used following the birth.

_____

_____

10. Postpartum hemorrhage is a serious complication of childbirth. Identify causes of postpartum hemorrhage.

_____

_____

a. What medications may be given in the event of postpartum hemorrhage and why?

_____

_____

_____

Self-Assessment Questions

Circle the letter that corresponds to the best answer.

1. While assessing the postpartum client, the nurse makes the following findings. Which of these findings would *not* be expected during the first 24 hours after delivery?
   a. Diaphoresis
   b. Bradycardia
   c. Positive Homans' sign
   d. Temperature of 99.8°F

2. The nursing student is caring for a 39-year-old client who has given birth to her first baby. The student tells her instructor that the mother seems a little anxious and unsure of herself with her infant. She asks for help with infant care. The instructor reminds the student that this is
   a. typical behavior for an older mother.
   b. part of the taking-hold phase for the mother.
   c. a sign that the client is still in the taking-in phase.
   d. an indication of the mother's having a problem relating to her infant.

3. The nurse is assessing a postpartum client 2 days after delivery. The nurse notes that the fundus is firm, 2 cm below the umbilicus, she has lochia rubra with occasional small clots, and some edema of the perineum. The nurse will
   a. chart normal findings.
   b. medicate for uterine atony.
   c. note signs of puerperal infection.
   d. alert the CNM/physician to possible subinvolution.

4. The postpartum client is predisposed to urinary tract infection by all except which of the following factors?
   a. Urinary stasis after birth
   b. Trauma to the bladder and urethra
   c. Catheterization during labor or surgery
   d. Voiding every 2 hours after delivery

5. A new mother is breastfeeding her infant. At 3 days postpartum, she tells you her breasts are enlarged, warm, and tender. She also has a tingling or burning sensation in her nipples and a low-grade fever. The nurse advises the mother to
   a. use a breast pump to increase her comfort.
   b. discontinue breastfeeding and notify her CNM/physician.
   c. continue nursing the infant, because these are expected changes.
   d. supplement the infant with formula until her breasts return to normal size.

6. A behavior indicating that a toddler is adapting to a new infant in the home is:
   a. thumb sucking.
   b. bed wetting.
   c. hostility.
   d. independence.

7. The client's lochia is pinkish brown. This is called
    a. lochia rubra.
    b. lochia serosa.
    c. lochia alba.
    d. lochia drainage.

8. A laceration through the skin, mucous membrane, muscle, and rectal sphincter is considered
    _____ degree.
    a. first
    b. second
    c. third
    d. fourth

9. Oxytocin causes
    a. tingling and burning.
    b. milk expression.
    c. increased glucose levels.
    d. ovulation.

10. A mother who cares lovingly for her infant but is unable to feel love is experiencing _____
    postpartum depression.
    a. mild
    b. moderate
    c. severe
    d. transient

Newborn Care

Key Terms

Match the following terms with their correct definitions.

____ 1. Appropriate for gestational age

____ 2. Caput succedaneum

____ 3. Cephalhematoma

____ 4. Circumcision

____ 5. Cold stress

____ 6. Conduction

____ 7. Convection

____ 8. Cryptorchidism

____ 9. Down syndrome

____10. Epispadias

____11. Epstein's pearls

____12. Evaporation

____13. Foremilk

____14. Hallux varus

____15. Hindmilk

a. Maintenance of body temperature.

b. Whitish fluid secreted by a newborn's nipples.

c. Loss of heat when water is changed to a vapor.

d. Failure of one or both testes to descend.

e. Saclike protrusion along the vertebral column filled with cerebrospinal fluid, meninges, nerve roots, and spinal cord.

f. Production of heat.

g. Environment in which the newborn can maintain internal body temperature with minimal oxygen consumption and metabolism.

h. Infant's weight is above the 90th percentile for gestational age.

i. Metabolism of brown fat; process unique to the newborn.

j. Infant's weight falls below the 10th percentile for gestational age.

k. Small, whitish yellow epithelial cysts found on the hard palate.

l. Edema of the newborn's scalp that is present at birth, may cross suture lines, and is caused by head compression against the cervix.

m. Follows foremilk; is higher in fat content, leading to weight gain; and is more satisfying.

n. First few hours after birth wherein the newborn makes changes to and stabilizes respiratory and circulatory functions.

o. Collection of blood between the periosteum and the skull of a newborn; appears several hours to a day after birth, does not cross suture lines, and is caused by the rupturing of the periosteal bridging veins due to friction and pressure during labor and delivery.

___16. Hydrocele

___17. Hyperbilirubinemia

___18. Hypospadias

___19. Kernicterus

___20. Large for gestational age

___21. Meningocele

___22. Myelomeningocele

___23. Neonatal transition

___24. Neutral thermal environment

___25. Nonshivering thermogenesis

___26. Ophthalmia neonatorum

___27. Phimosis

___28. Pseudomenstruation

___29. Radiation

___30. Small for gestational age

___31. Spina bifida occulta

___32. Syndactyly

___33. Talipes equinovarus

___34. Thermogenesis

___35. Thermoregulation

___36. Witch's milk

p. Infant's weight falls between the 90th and 10th percentile for gestational age.

q. Placement of the great toe farther from the other toes.

r. Inflammation of the newborn's eyes that results from passing through the birth canal when a gonorrheal or chlamydial infection is present.

s. Congenital deformity in which the foot and ankle are twisted inward and cannot be moved to a midline position; also known as club foot.

t. Saclike protrusion along the vertebral column filled with cerebrospinal fluid and meninges.

u. Loss of heat by direct contact with a cooler object

v. Fluid around the testes in the scrotum.

w. Surgical removal of the prepuce (foreskin) that covers the glans penis.

x. Placement of the urinary meatus on the underside of the penis.

y. Condition wherein the opening in the foreskin is so small that it cannot be pulled back over the glans.

z. Loss of heat by transfer to cooler near objects, but not through direct contact.

aa. Excessive heat loss.

bb. Failure of the vertebral arch to close.

cc. Blood-tinged mucous discharge from the vagina of a newborn, caused by the withdrawal of maternal hormones.

dd. Watery first milk from the breast, high in lactose, like skim milk, and effective in quenching thirst.

ee. Loss of heat by the movement of air.

ff. Excess of bilirubin in the blood.

gg. Severe neurological damage resulting from a high level of bilirubin (jaundice).

hh. Congenital chromosomal abnormality; also called trisomy 21.

ii. Fusion of two or more fingers or toes.

jj. The placement of the urinary meatus on the top of the penis.

Key Terms Regarding Physical Characteristics of Newborns

____ 1. Acrocyanosis

____ 2. Erythema toxicum neonatorum

____ 3. Lanugo

____ 4. Meconium

____ 5. Milia

____ 6. Molding

____ 7. Mongolian spots

____ 8. Nevus flammeus

____ 9. Nevus vascularis

____10. Telangiectactic nevi

____11. Vernix caseosa

a. Shaping of the fetal head to adapt to the mother's pelvis during labor.

b. Large patches of bluish skin on the buttocks of dark-skinned infants.

c. Birthmark of enlarged superficial blood vessels, elevated and red in color.

d. Large purplish birthmark usually found on the face or neck that does not blanch with pressure.

e. Birthmarks of dilated capillaries that blanch with pressure; also called storkbites.

f. Pink rash with firm, yellow-white papules or pustules found on the chest, abdomen, back, and/or buttocks of a newborn.

g. White, pinhead-size distended sebaceous glands on cheeks, nose, and chin.

h. Blue coloring of hands and feet.

i. Fine, downy hair covering the fetus's body.

j. White, creamy substance covering a fetus's body.

k. First bowel movement of a newborn.

Abbreviation Review

Write the meaning or definition of the following abbreviations, acronyms, and symbols.

1. AAFP _____

2. AAP _____

3. ACIP _____

4. AGA _____

5. CPAP _____

6. FAS _____

7. HBIG _____

8. Hep B _____

9. IDM _____

10. ISAM _____

11. LGA _____

12. PKU _____

13. RDS _____

14. REM _____

15. SIDS _____

16. SGA _____

17. TTN _____

Exercises and Activities

1. List the four factors that help to initiate breathing in the newborn.

   (1) _____   (3) _____

   (2) _____   (4) _____

2. What four changes occur in the circulation of the newborn?

   _____

   _____

   _____

3. Describe how cold stress can lead to respiratory distress for the infant.

   _____

   _____

   _____

4. List the four methods of heat loss for the newborn and identify two interventions to prevent heat loss with each.

   (1) _____

      (1) _____

      (2) _____

   (2) _____

      (1) _____

      (2) _____

   (3) _____

      (1) _____

      (2) _____

   (4) _____

      (1) _____

      (2) _____

5. As a student nurse, this was your first birth. "Congratulations!" you tell J.M. and T.M. after assisting with the difficult but rewarding vaginal birth of a baby boy. They have already named him M., since they have known for some time it was going to be a boy. You are working today with Jan, an experienced labor and delivery nurse who enjoys working with students. Jan has already started taking care of M.'s immediate needs after birth, including:

   (1) _____   (3) _____   (5) _____

   (2) _____   (4) _____   (6) _____.

   Jan tells you, "We will be giving the baby an injection of vitamin K because:

   _____."

   "We also need to use erythromycin ointment because:

   _____

   _____."

a. You help Jan by assessing M.'s vital signs. They are, T—99.1°F; HR—154; R—62. Which are not in the normal range for vital signs? _____

b. Together, you and Jan have completed M.'s first physical assessment, noting all of the following findings. Circle those that could be due to the difficult delivery.

Acrocyanosis	Epstein's pearls	Edematous scrotum	Nevus vascularis
Cephalhematoma	Facial petechiae	Milia	Strabismus
Cryptorchidism	Flexed extremities	Molding	Subconjunctival hemorrhage
Ecchymosis	Lanugo	Mongolian spots	Telangiectatic nevi

c. J.M. says, "Why is his head shaped so funny? Will it stay like that?" What will you tell the parents about molding?

_____

_____

d. You check M.'s reflexes and demonstrate three of them for T.M. and J.M. Describe how to elicit each of these reflexes:

Palmar grasp: _____

_____

Babinski's reflex:_____

_____

Moro reflex: _____

_____

Draw a line under the reflexes that will normally be gone by M.'s 6-month checkup. Circle those that Tyler will need for breastfeeding.

Babinski's	Gallant	Placing	Sucking
Blinking	Hiccupping	Plantar grasp	Swallowing
Crossed extension	Moro	Rooting	Tonic neck
Extrusion	Palmar grasp	Stepping	Yawning

e. It is time to estimate M's gestational age. You will be using the New Ballard Score for this, which you have found in your text. Jan has already completed the neuromuscular maturity section for a score of 20. You offer to complete the physical maturity section. Draw an X on each block on the following scale that corresponds to the physical assessment findings.

Copyright © 2011 Delmar Cengage Learning

	-1	0	1	2	3	4	5
Skin	sticky friable transparent	gelatinous red, translucent	smooth pink, visible veins	superficial peeling and or rash few veins	cracking pale areas rare veins	parchment deep cracking no vessels	feathery cracked wrinkled
Lanugo	none	sparse	abundant	thinning	bald areas	mostly bald	
Planiar Surface	heel-toe 40–50min: -1 <40min: -2	>50mm no crease	faint red marks	anterior transverse crease only	creases ant. 2/3	creases over entire sole	
Breast	imperceptible	barely imperceptible	flat areola no bud	stippled areola 1–2mm bud	raised areola 3–4mm bud	full areola 5–10mm bud	
Eye/Ear	lids fused loosely: -1 tightly: -2	lids open pinna flat stays folded	sl. curved pinna; soft slow recoil	well curved pinna; soft but ready recoil	formed and firm instant recoil	thick cartilage ear stiff	
Genitals Male	scrotum flat, smooth	scrotum empty faint rugae	testes in upper canal rare rugae	testes descending few rugae	testes down good rugae	testes pendulous deep rugae	
Genitals Female	clitoris prominant labia flat	prominant clitoris small labia minora	prominent clitoris enlarging minora	majora & minora equally prominent	majora large minora small	majora cover clitoris and minora	

He has some cracking on his skin, with rare veins.

Almost no lanugo remains.

Plantar creases cover the anterior two-thirds of the feet.

Breast tissue has a raised areola with a 4-mm bud.

The ears are formed and firm with in-stant recoil.

The testes are pendulous and have deep rugae.

Your total score for physical maturity is _____.

Added to Jan's neuromuscular maturity score of 20, this gives a total of_____.

Using the Maturity Rating scale in the text, what is his approximate gestational age based on this score? _____

Jan says that comparing his weight, length, and head circumference, M. is AGA. What does this mean?

_____

_____

f. Your instructor stops by and says you can give the baby his first bath. Why is a thorough cleans-ing of the infant important? How will you maintain M.'s temperature during the bath?

_____

_____

_____

g. You check on J.M. and the baby a few hours later. M. is quietly gazing into his mother's eyes and has very little body movement. He seems to be watching and listening to his mother in-tently. You realize that M. is exhibiting a behavioral state called _____.

h. J.M. and T.M. are considering circumcision for their baby. If M. is circumcised, what are your nursing responsibilities?

_____

_____

_____

i. During a final visit the next day, you find J.M., T.M., and M. together. J.M. is happy to see you because she needs some advice. The baby has been crying. J.M. says that a relative told her she ought to start feeding the baby formula instead of breast milk because he sounds hungry all the time. You remind J.M. that babies cry for other reasons, too, including:

_____

_____

You mention to J.M. some of the advantages of breastfeeding, including:

(1) _____   (5) _____

(2) _____   (6) _____

(3) _____   (7) _____

(4) _____   (8) _____

j. J.M. has a few more questions for you. Before you leave today, please go over them with her.

(1) "How often should M. breastfeed?"

(2) "How long should each feeding last?"

(3) "How can I tell if he is latched onto my breast properly?"

(4) "Since there is no 'air' in the breast, does M. need to be burped?"

(5) "How do I know if M. is getting enough milk?"

(6) "When do I take M. for his first doctor's appointment?"

_____

_____

_____

_____

_____

Self-Assessment Questions

Circle the letter that corresponds to the best answer.

1. A newborn has had difficulty maintaining its temperature within a normal range. The nurse recognizes that this can predispose the infant to
   a. cold stress.
   b. hyperglycemia.
   c. metabolic alkalosis.
   d. de-thermoregulation.

2. Which of the following physical assessment findings would the nurse observe in the preterm newborn with a gestational age of 35 weeks?
   a. Little or no lanugo
   b. Undescended testes
   c. Square window sign of 0°
   d. Creases on the anterior two-thirds of the sole

3. A nurse is caring for a new mother and infant. The nurse suspects transient tachypnea of the newborn because the infant is observed to have
   a. grade 0 on the Silverman-Anderson index.
   b. respiratory distress noted immediately after the birth.
   c. nasal flaring and a high respiratory rate several hours after birth.
   d. an irregular respiratory rate between 30 and 40 breaths per minute.

4. The nurse is caring for a new mother and infant after delivery. To facilitate mother–infant bonding and help initiate breastfeeding, the nurse will
   a. allow the infant to get hungry before beginning to breastfeed.
   b. leave the infant with its mother during the first period of reactivity.
   c. wait until the mother is fully rested after delivery to give her the infant.
   d. encourage mother–infant contact while the infant is in the active alert state.

5. The nursing instructor reminds the student to keep the newborn away from the cold window in the mother's room. This intervention will avoid heat loss in the newborn through
   a. radiation.
   b. convection.
   c. conduction.
   d. evaporation.

6. When an infant has nonshivering thermogenesis, it has:
   a. adequately raised its temperature.
   b. effectively increased its metabolism.
   c. now begun to metabolize brown fat.
   d. maintained heat retention.

7. A cold stethoscope is placed on an infant. The infant will have heat loss due to
   a. radiation.
   b. convection.
   c. conduction.
   d. evaporation.

8. A medication seldom used as an eye prophylaxis due to its lack of protection against chlamydial infection is:
   a. erythromycin.
   b. tetracycline.
   c. phytonadione.
   d. silver nitrate.

9. Bleeding from the cord is noted. The nurse should
   a. observe the cord bleeding for changes.
   b. check the clamp and apply a second clamp on the body side of the first one.
   c. clean the cord.
   d. check the clamp and apply a second clamp toward the outside of the first one.

10. Breast milk that has a higher fat content is called
    a. hindmilk.
    b. foremilk.
    c. colostrum.
    d. nutramigen.

Basics of Pediatric Care

Key Terms

Match the following terms with their correct definitions.

___ 1. Assent

___ 2. Child life specialist

___ 3. Emancipated minor

___ 4. Family-centered care

___ 5. Rooming-in

a. Health care professional with extensive knowledge of psychology and early childhood development.

b. Recognition that the family is the constant in a child's life, while the service systems and support personnel within those systems change (Shelton & Stepanek, 1994).

c. Voluntary agreement to participate in a research project or to accept treatment.

d. Practice of staying with the client 24 hours a day to provide care and comfort.

e. Child who has the legal competency of an adult because of circumstances involving marriage, divorce, parenting a child, living independently without parents, or enlistment in the armed services.

Abbreviation Review

Write the meaning or definition of the following abbreviations and acronyms.

1. BSA _____

2. DDST _____

3. EMLA _____

4. ID _____

5. IQ _____

6. NCHS _____

7. OBRA _____

Exercises and Activities

1. How does a child's developmental level affect the child's response to illness and health care?

_____

_____

2. Describe the nurse's role in supporting the child and caregivers. Why are prevention and teaching important aspects of this role?

   _____

   _____

   _____

3. List three factors or interventions that can help the caregiver feel prepared for the hospitalization of a child.

   (1) _____

   (2) _____

   (3) _____

4. How does rooming-in benefit the hospitalized child and caregiver?

   _____

   _____

   _____

5. Describe the role of a child life specialist in the health care setting.

   _____

   _____

   _____

6. What measurements are assessed in the child under 2 years of age?

   _____

   _____

   _____

7. What measurements are assessed in the child aged 2 years and older?

   _____

   _____

   _____

8. Describe how to correctly assess the blood pressure of a child.

   _____

   _____

   _____

9. Identify security measures used by health care agencies.

   _____

   _____

   _____

10. You are caring for a young child who may need to have an extremity immobilized for several hours. What interventions might prevent the need for a restraint?

   _____

   _____

   _____

11. If a restraint must be applied, what are your nursing responsibilities before and during its use? What documentation is needed?

   _____

   _____

   _____

12. You are administering an oral medication to an infant. How would you proceed?

   _____

   _____

   _____

13. During physical assessment of a child, several measurements are taken to ascertain normal growth and development.

   a. List the measurements in children under the age of 3.

   (1) _____

   (2) _____

   (3) _____

   (4) _____

   b. List the measurements for a child older than age 3.

   (1) _____

   (2) _____

14. You are caring for a 7-year-old child with a terminal illness. Identify two interventions that may be helpful for each of the following:

   The child: (1)_____

                       (2)_____

   Parents: (1)_____

                       (2)_____

   Siblings: (1)_____

                       (2)_____

   a. What support services might be helpful to the caregiver?

   _____

   _____

   b. How can the nurse deal with personal feelings of grief?

   _____

   _____

15. M. is the 3-year-old daughter of Y.T. and K.T. M. is scheduled to have heart surgery for the repair of an atrial septal defect (ASD) early next week. Other than concerns about the ASD, M. appears to be growing well and shows no developmental delays. She has not been hospitalized since birth. A quick recovery is anticipated.

   a. How can M. be prepared for the hospitalization and surgical experience?

   _____

   _____

b. Although Y.T. and K.T. have anticipated the surgery for some time, they are now anxious and have many questions. What resources can be offered or suggested to help them feel more comfortable with the experience?

_____

_____

c. What information will the nurse collect at the time of admission?

_____

_____

d. How can the caregivers be incorporated into the care of their daughter?

_____

_____

e. List specific safety measures that the nurse would incorporate for this toddler.

_____

_____

f. What are the advantages of discharging M. home as soon as possible after the surgery?

_____

_____

_____

_____

_____

16. At what age may a nurse begin using a radial pulse in the measurement of vital signs?

_____

17. How does the nurse measure urinary output on a child in diapers?

_____

_____

18. Explain the procedure for instilling ear drops in a child.

_____

_____

_____

Self-Assessment Questions

Circle the letter that corresponds to the best answer.

1. The most important aspect for preparation of a child for hospitalization is
   a. preparation of the caregiver.
   b. completing a developmental assessment.
   c. assigning a child life specialist to the care team.
   d. using age-specific books and pamphlets with the child.

2. The nurse is preparing medication to be administered to a young child. The most reliable method for determining the amount of medication to be used will be based on the child's
   a. age.
   b. weight.
   c. body surface area.
   d. degree of symptoms.

3. A nursing student is assisting in a well-baby clinic in the community. It is apparent that further instruction is needed when the student
   a. assesses the pulse apically for 1 full minute.
   b. compares the head and chest circumference in a 1-year-old.
   c. measures the height in the 1½-year-old in a recumbent position.
   d. measures the chest circumference 1 fingerbreadth below the nipple line.

4. The primary benefit of anxiety reduction for the child who is facing surgery is to reduce the
   a. anxiety of the parents.
   b. blood loss during surgery.
   c. preoperative medication needed.
   d. frequency of vital sign assessments.

5. A child is scheduled to have the Denver II performed. The caregiver asks the nurse what the purpose of this test is. The nurse responds by saying that the Denver II is a measurement tool that will determine
   a. whether any developmental delays exist.
   b. the child's IQ.
   c. how well the caregiver interacts with the child.
   d. whether the child's height and weight are within norms.

6. Federal guidelines state that children over 7 years of age have the right to give
   a. conscription.
   b. assent.
   c. informed consent.
   d. enlistment.

7. Normal vital signs for a 3-year-old could be
   a. temperature 98.8°F, pulse 160, respiratory rate 40, blood pressure 65/30.
   b. temperature 97.5°F, pulse 130, respiratory rate 36, blood pressure 70/46.
   c. temperature 97.5°F, pulse 120, respiratory rate 20, blood pressure 76/50.
   d. temperature 97.5°F, pulse 110, respiratory rate 14, blood pressure 90/60.

8. Normal vital signs for a 1-year-old could be:
   a. temperature 98.8°F, pulse 160, respiratory rate 40, blood pressure 65/30.
   b. temperature 97.5°F, pulse 130, respiratory rate 36, blood pressure 70/46.
   c. temperature 97.5°F, pulse 120, respiratory rate 20, blood pressure 76/50.
   d. temperature 97.5°F, pulse 110, respiratory rate 14, blood pressure 90/60.

Infants with Special Needs: Birth to 12 Months

Key Terms

Match the following terms with their correct definitions.

____ 1. Abduction

____ 2. Antipyretic

____ 3. Atresia

____ 4. Child abuse

____ 5. Circumoral cyanosis

____ 6. Colic

____ 7. Dislocation

____ 8. Dysplasia

____ 9. Erythematous

____10. Hypotonia

____11. Intussusception

____12. Jaundice

____13. Kernicterus

____14. Lecithin

____15. Meconium ileus

____16. Meningitis

____17. Milia

____18. Mongolian spots

a. Any intentional act of physical, emotional, or sexual abuse or neglect committed by a person responsible for the care of a child.

b. High-pitched, harsh sound heard on inspiration when the trachea or larynx is obstructed.

c. Surgical incision of the eardrum.

d. Abnormal development.

e. Yellow discoloration of the skin, sclera, mucous membranes, and body fluids that occurs when the liver is unable to fully remove bilirubin from the blood.

f. Lateral movement away from the body.

g. Severe itching.

h. Displacement of a bone from its normal position in a joint.

i. Impacted feces in the newborn, causing intestinal obstruction.

j. Large patches of bluish skin on the buttocks of dark-skinned infants.

k. Forceful ejection (up to 3 feet) of the contents of the stomach.

l. Lax muscle tone.

m. Saclike protrusion situated along the vertebral column and filled with spinal fluid, meninges, nerve roots, and spinal cord.

n. Major component of surfactant.

o. Telescoping of one part of the intestine into another.

p. Drug used to reduce an abnormally high temperature.

q. Characterized by reddishness of the skin.

r. Condition of sudden, recurrent attacks of abdominal pain.

___19. Myelomeningocele

s. Severe neurological damage resulting from a high level of bilirubin.

___20. Myringotomy

t. Absence or closure of a body orifice.

___21. Projectile vomiting

u. Bluish discoloration surrounding the mouth.

___22. Pruritus

v. Pearly white cysts on the face.

___23. Stridor

w. Inflammation of the meninges.

Abbreviation Review

Write the meaning or definition of the following abbreviations and acronyms.

1. AGE _____

2. ASD _____

3. BPD _____

4. CF _____

5. CFTR _____

6. CP _____

7. CPAP _____

8. CSF _____

9. DDH _____

10. FTT _____

11. GER _____

12. LTB _____

13. NGT _____

14. PDA _____

15. RDS _____

16. RSV _____

17. SCA _____

18. SIDS _____

19. TOF _____

20. VSD _____

21. WIC _____

Exercises and Activities

1. Why is it important to understand the differences in the systems of the infant versus the adult?

_____

_____

_____

2. List differences in the respiratory tract of the infant that increase the risk for obstruction and as-piration.

_____

_____

_____

3. Describe the signs and symptoms of pneumonia that might be noted in the infant.

_____

_____

_____

4. List several nursing interventions for the infant with pneumonia.

(1) _____   (4) _____

(2) _____   (5) _____

(3) _____   (6) _____

5. Describe signs and symptoms of respiratory distress syndrome.

_____

_____

_____

6. How would you explain the cause of cystic fibrosis to the caregivers of an infant with this disor-der? What symptoms would the infant or child experience?

_____

_____

_____

7. L. has just been diagnosed with her second ear infection in 3 months. What causes an infant to be susceptible to otitis media? What signs and symptoms should her caregivers watch for that would indicate an infection?

_____

_____

_____

8. What differences in the gastrointestinal (GI) system in infants increase their risk for GI disorders?

(1) _____   (5) _____

(2) _____   (6) _____

(3) _____   (7) _____

(4) _____

9. You are assessing for signs of dehydration in an infant with a GI disorder. What signs and symp-toms would you note?

_____

_____

_____

10. How can fluid intake be encouraged in the infant who is at risk of dehydration?

_____

_____

_____

11. W.'s caregiver tells you during her baby's 6-week checkup that he seems unusually colicky. She realizes that new babies cry a lot, but W. just cries for hours at a time. Nothing she does seems to help. What questions will you ask W.'s caregiver? What suggestions can you give that may alleviate his colic?

_____

_____

_____

12. Z. is being assessed at the pediatric clinic 2 days after his birth for his first well-baby visit. A right-sided hip click was noted at birth. What other findings might indicate hip dislocation? What would treatment for Z. include?

_____

_____

_____

13. What are signs of physical neglect and abuse in an infant?

_____

_____

_____

14. List several safety measures that are appropriate for the child's first year of life.

_____

_____

_____

_____

15. You are caring for A., the new daughter of J.T. and C.T. A. is a full-term infant weighing 7 lb, 8 oz and is 19 in. in length. However, A. was born with a cleft lip on the left side and a cleft palate. Although C.T. and J.T. are thrilled to be parents, they are visibly distressed about this congenital defect. They wonder how she will eat, how they will care for her, and when her lip and mouth can be repaired.

a. How will you support J.T. and C.T. following the birth of their infant?

_____

_____

b. Why is an interdisciplinary approach important to A.'s care?

_____

_____

c. Identify complications that A. is at risk for before her surgical repair.

_____

_____

d. C.T. asks you to help her feed A. with a special bottle and nipple. What suggestions will you make to help with the feeding?

_____

_____

e. When will the infant's cleft lip and palate be repaired?

_____

_____

f. List nursing interventions that will promote healing following the repair of her cleft palate.

(1) _____   (4) _____

(2) _____   (5) _____

(3) _____   (6) _____

16. Complete the following table regarding cardiac anomolies by describing each element.

	VSD	ASD	PDA	TOF
Condition				
Blood flow pattern				
Manifestations				
Treatment				

17. The client has sickle-cell disease. Explain the signs and symptoms of this condition.

_____

_____

a. Why is dehydration a serious problem for those with sickle-cell disease?

_____

_____

   b. Identify the 5 As of managing sickle-cell crisis?

    (1) _____

    (2) _____

    (3) _____

    (4) _____

    (5) _____

Self-Assessment Questions

Circle the letter that corresponds to the best answer.

1. The newborn who has a history of frank breech position, is large for gestational age, or is a twin is at greater risk for
   a. club foot.
   b. hypotonia.
   c. hip dysplasia.
   d. developmental delays.

2. A 10-month-old child is recovering from a sickle-cell crisis. To prevent a recurrence of a sickle-cell crisis for this child, the nurse encourages the caregiver to do all but which of the following?
   a. Delay immunizations.
   b. Avoid cold temperatures.
   c. Use prophylactic antibiotics.
   d. Maintain adequate hydration.

3. A 1-year-old has just experienced a febrile seizure. The nurse emphasizes to the caregiver that febrile seizures
   a. usually last for several minutes.
   b. do not cause neurological sequelae.
   c. increase the risk of seizure disorder in childhood.
   d. can be prevented by prompt administration of aspirin for fever.

4. When caring for an infant with acute gastroenteritis, it is most important for the nurse to assess the infant for
   a. dehydration.
   b. abdominal pain.
   c. intake and output.
   d. number of diarrheal stools.

5. An infant arrives at the community clinic with signs of an upper respiratory illness. The infant has mild stridor when active, a barking cough, and hoarseness. The temperature is 99.6°F, and there is a nasal discharge. It is most important to instruct the caregiver to
   a. increase fluid intake.
   b. maintain a humid environment.
   c. watch for signs of respiratory distress.
   d. suction the mouth and nose for mucus.

6. What is *not* considered a clinical manifestation of abuse?
    a. Bruises on the abdomen
    b. Multiple bone fractures at various stages of healing
    c. Withdrawal
    d. Mongolian spots

7. A clinical manifestation present in ventricular septal defect is
    a. delayed growth and development.
    b. dysrhythmias.
    c. increased respiratory infections.
    d. a machine-like murmur.

8. A clinical manifestation present in tetralogy of fallot is
    a. delayed growth and development.
    b. dysrhythmia.
    c. increased respiratory infection.
    d. a machine-like murmur.

Common Problems: 1–18 Years

Key Terms

Match the following terms with their correct definitions.

___ 1. Acanthesis nigricans

___ 2. Comedone

___ 3. Encopresis

___ 4. Epistaxis

___ 5. Gowers' sign

___ 6. Rhinorrhea

a. Watery nasal discharge.

b. Passage of watery colonic contents around a hard fecal mass.

c. Whitehead or blackhead.

d. Hemorrhage of the nares or nostrils; also known as nosebleed.

e. Walking the hands up the legs to get from a sitting to a standing position (as in Duchenne muscular dystrophy).

f. A velvety hyperpigmented patch on the back of the neck, axilla, or antecubital area.

Abbreviation Review

Write the meaning or definition of the following abbreviations and acronyms.

1. AAP _____
2. ACIP _____
3. ADHD _____
4. ALL _____
5. APSGN _____
6. ASO _____
7. BMI _____
8. CPT _____
9. DMD _____
10. DTaP _____
11. ESR _____
12. FPG _____
13. HBV _____
14. HSV _____
15. IPV _____

16. ITP _____

17. JA _____

18. MCNS _____

19. MDI _____

20. MMR _____

21. OPV _____

22. PCOS _____

23. RAD _____

24. TIG _____

Exercises and Activities

1. What factors put children at greater risk for parasitic infections than adults?

   _____
   _____
   _____

2. How would you differentiate pharyngitis from influenza? Are there differences in the treatment?

   _____
   _____
   _____

3. What are early signs and symptoms of asthma? What assessment findings might be noted in children with chronic asthma?

   _____
   _____
   _____

4. J., a 6-year-old boy in your pediatric clinic, has been recently diagnosed with asthma. What information will you give to J.'s caregiver about ways to manage his asthma at home?

   _____
   _____
   _____

5. Describe the pharmacological treatment for asthma.

   _____
   _____
   _____

6. List signs and symptoms and the medical–nursing management for each of the following common pediatric disorders.

	Signs and Symptoms	*Treatment*
Impetigo		
Pediculosis		
Acne		

7. How would you detect scoliosis during a routine screening of adolescents?

8. Describe symptoms that might be noted in a child with ADHD. What are the goals for nursing care for a child with ADHD?

9. Identify several risk factors for suicide.

   (1) _____   (5) _____

   (2) _____   (6) _____

   (3) _____   (7) _____

   (4) _____   (8) _____

10. What behaviors might indicate to you that an individual is considering suicide?

11. Of the following communicable diseases, underline those for which there is a vaccine. Circle those that are transmitted by way of respiratory droplets.

Chickenpox	Hepatitis B	Mumps	Roseola
Diphtheria	Measles	Pertussis	Rubella
Fifth disease	Mononucleosis	Poliomyelitis	Scarlet fever
			Tetanus

12. Identify four barriers to immunization.

   (1) _____   (3) _____

   (2) _____   (4) _____

13. The caregiver of a newborn tells you that she is concerned about having her baby immunized. She has heard that some immunizations can have serious side effects and cause long-term complications. What would you tell her?

_____

_____

_____

14. What is the nurse's responsibility related to immunizations and documentation?

_____

_____

_____

15. D., who is 9 years old, was brought in to the pediatric office by his caregiver. She tells you that he had a fever at home of 101°F, pain in his joints, and a pinkish rash. During the health history, his caregiver reveals that D. had an untreated upper respiratory infection with a bad sore throat about a month ago. He seemed to get over it at the time without too much trouble. D. is now suspected of having rheumatic fever.

a. List laboratory test results that might confirm this diagnosis.

_____

_____

b. What other signs and symptoms might D. exhibit with rheumatic fever?

_____

_____

c. Identify the goals of medical management.

(1) _____

(2) _____

(3) _____

d. What will D.'s treatment include?

_____

_____

_____

e. List long-term complications that can result from rheumatic fever.

_____

_____

_____

f. D.'s caregiver wants to know if he can ever get rheumatic fever again. What will you tell her?

_____

_____

_____

16. V., age 6, has tonsillitis again. Identify the symptoms of tonsillitis.

_____

_____

   a. The surgeon performed a tonsillectomy and adenoidectomy. Describe this surgery in terms that V.'s caregiver might understand.

_____

_____

   b. What actions should the nurse take when caring for V. in the postoperative phase?

_____

_____

   c. Explain why the caregiver should avoid giving V. red or brown liquids immediately postoperatively.

_____

_____

17. Complete the following table regarding communicable diseases in children.

Disease	Transmission	Signs	Treatment
Chicken pox			
Diptheria			
Fifth disease			
Measles			
Mononucleosis			
Mumps			
Pertussis			
Roseola			
Rubella			

Self-Assessment Questions

Circle the letter that corresponds to the best answer for each question.

1. The nurse is caring for a child diagnosed with asthma. To reduce mucosal edema and improve the effect of a bronchodilator, the physician orders
   a. Alupent.
   b. Brethine.
   c. prednisone.
   d. theophylline.

2. Laboratory test results show that a young child has ITP. The nurse recalls that ITP is
   a. most common in school-aged children.
   b. cured with antibiotics if diagnosed early.
   c. a complication of a streptococcus infection.
   d. an autoimmune disorder that destroys platelets.

3. The nurse is performing an assessment on a child who is ill with rheumatic fever. All but which of the following findings might the nurse anticipate?
   a. Chorea
   b. Polyarthritis
   c. Strawberry tongue
   d. Subcutaneous nodules

4. A child with fever, headache, sore throat, and rash has just been diagnosed with scarlet fever. You explain to the caregiver that the child
   a. will be treated with penicillin.
   b. will have lifelong immunity after recovery.
   c. may have complications such as meningitis.
   d. is not contagious after symptoms have begun.

5. Home treatment for asthma may include all but which of the following interventions?
   a. Family education
   b. Chest physiotherapy
   c. Use of a peak flowmeter
   d. Restriction of physical activity

6. An elevated _____ is indicative of a recent streptococcal infection.
   a. ASO
   b. ESR
   c. C-reactive protein
   d. leukocyte

7. Mild hemophilia may
   a. be detected from bleeding from the umbilical cord.
   b. not be detected until a toddler becomes mobile.
   c. not ever show any clinical manifestations.
   d. be detected from bleeding from a circumcision site.

8. Itching around the anus may indicate which common intestinal parasite?
    a. Giardiasis
    b. Roundworm
    c. Pinworm
    d. Hookworm

Answer Key

Chapter 1 Student Nurse Skills for Success

Key Terms
1. o
2. s
3. d
4. t
5. n
6. h
7. j
8. q
9. u
10. m
11. p
12. c
13. i
14. l
15. b
16. g
17. k
18. f
19. r
20. e
21. a

Abbreviation Review
1. blood pressure
2. computer-assisted instruction
3. National Council Licensure Examination–Practical Nursing
4. Authorization to Test
5. Unlicensed Assistive Personnel
6. The National Council of State Boards of Nursing
7. Certified Nurse Assistant

Self-Assessment Questions
1. c
2. d
3. c
4. a
5. b
6. c
7. d
8. b
9. b
10. d

Chapter 2 Holistic Care

Key Terms
1. e
2. i
3. h
4. m
5. p
6. c
7. g
8. l
9. d
10. k
11. b
12. f
13. j
14. n
15. a
16. o

Abbreviation Review
1. American Holistic Nurses' Association
2. Centers for Disease Control and Prevention
3. National Institutes of Health
4. Office of Alternative Medicine

5. World Health Organization
6. National Center for Complementary and Alternative Medicine

Self-Assessment Questions

1. c
2. a
3. d
4. a
5. b
6. d
7. c
8. b
9. a
10. c

Chapter 3 Nursing History, Education, and Organizations

Key Terms

1. b
2. k
3. h
4. a
5. l
6. e
7. g
8. d
9. j
10. i
11. c
12. f

Abbreviation Review

1. associate degree nurse (nursing)
2. *American Journal of Nursing*
3. American Nursing Association
4. advance practice registered nurse
5. bachelor of science in nursing
6. Certification Examination for Practical and Vocational Nurses in Long-Term Care
7. continuing education unit
8. certified in long term care
9. Council of Practical Nursing Programs
10. general education development

11. health maintenance organization
12. International Council of Nurses
13. Joint Commission on Accreditation of Healthcare Organizations
14. licensed practical nurse
15. licensed practical/vocational nurse
16. licensed vocational nurse
17. National Association of Practical Nurse Education and Service Inc.
18. National Council Licensure Examination
19. National Council of State Boards of Nursing
20. National Federation of Licensed Practical Nurses, Inc.
21. National League for Nursing
22. National League for Nursing Accrediting Commission
23. Omnibus Budget Reconciliation Act
24. registered nurse
25. Tax Equity Fiscal Responsibility Act
26. U.S. Department of Health and Human Services

Self-Assessment Questions

1. c
2. d
3. a
4. b
5. c
6. b
7. d
8. a
9. c
10. b

Chapter 4 Legal and Ethical Responsibilities

Key Terms

1. ss
2. d
3. g
4. n
5. ww
6. aaa
7. t
8. xx
9. mm
10. vv

11. x
12. cc
13. hh
14. m
15. u
16. ee
17. bbb
18. c
19. qq
20. ddd
21. nn
22. tt
23. eee
24. w
25. h
26. v
27. hhh
28. o
29. b
30. l
31. dd
32. e
33. q
34. p
35. uu
36. gg
37. f
38. bb
39. kk
40. i
41. fff
42. y
43. jj
44. iii
45. j
46. ggg
47. ff
48. jjj
49. r
50. ii
51. z
52. s
53. aa
54. rr
55. a
56. k
57. zz
58. ll
59. oo

60. yy
61. ccc
62. pp

Abbreviation Review

1. Americans with Disabilities Act
2. Americans Hospital Association
3. against medical advice
4. American Nurses Association
5. cardiopulmonary resuscitation
6. do not resuscitate
7. durable power of attorney for health care
8. Emergency Department
9. False Claims Act
10. Health Insurance Portability and Accountability Act
11. Health Care Integrity and Protection Data Bank
12. human immunodeficiency virus
13. International Council of Nurses
14. intramuscular
15. Joint Commission on Accreditation of Healthcare Organizations
16. licensed practical/vocational nurse
17. National Council Licensure Exam
18. National Federation of Licensed Practical Nurses
19. Protected Health Information
20. registered nurse
21. Veterans Affairs

Self-Assessment Questions

1. c
2. d
3. b
4. a
5. b
6. d
7. a
8. b
9. a
10. b

Chapter 5 The Health Care Delivery System

Key Terms

1. d
2. a

3. e
4. j
5. p
6. i
7. b
8. t
9. k
10. n
11. u
12. q
13. l
14. c
15. f
16. o
17. g
18. m
19. h
20. r
21. s

Abbreviation Review

1. Alcohol, Drug Abuse, and Mental Health Administration
2. Agency for Health Care Policy and Research
3. Agency for Health Care Research and Quality
4. acquired immunodeficiency syndrome
5. American Medical Association
6. American Nurses Association
7. advanced practice registered nurse
8. Agency for Toxic Substances and Disease Registry
9. Centers for Disease Control and Prevention
10. Children's Health Insurance Program
11. certified nurse midwife
12. community nursing organization
13. clinical nurse specialist
14. doctor of dental surgery
15. doctor of dental medicine
16. diagnosis-related group
17. exclusive provider organization
18. Food and Drug Administration
19. Health Care Financing Administration
20. health maintenance organization
21. Health Resources and Services Administration
22. Indian Health Service

23. licensed practical/vocational nurse
24. medical doctor
25. National Federation of Licensed Practical Nurses
26. National Institutes of Health
27. National League for Nursing
28. nurse practitioner
29. occupational therapist
30. physician's assistant
31. primary care provider
32. preferred provider organization
33. physical therapist
34. registered dietician
35. registered nurse
36. registered pharmacist
37. respiratory therapist
38. social worker
39. U.S. Department of Health & Human Services
40. U.S. Public Health Service
41. Veterans Administration

Self-Assessment Questions

1. a
2. d
3. c
4. c
5. a
6. b
7. d
8. b
9. d
10. a

Chapter 6 Arenas of Care

Key Terms

1. b.
2. i
3. g
4. a
5. f
6. c
7. h
8. d
9. e
10. j

Abbreviation Review

1. Activities of Daily Living
2. American Health Care Association
3. Acquired Immunodeficiency Syndrome
4. Assisted Living Federation of America
5. Advanced Practice Registered Nurse
6. Commission on Accreditation of Rehabilitation Facilities
7. continuing care retirement community
8. Coronary Care Unit
9. Certification Examination for Practical and Vocational Nurses in Long-Term Care
10. community health accreditation program
11. certified in long-term care
12. computed tomography
13. extended care facility
14. Electrocardiogram
15. Emergency Department
16. Electroencephalography
17. Electromyogram
18. Health Care Finance Administration
19. health maintenance organization
20. instrumental activities of daily living
21. intermediate care facility
22. Intensive Care Unit
23. interdisciplinary health care team
24. Joint Commission on Accreditation of Healthcare Organizations
25. Magnetic Resonance Imaging
26. Omnibus Budget Reconciliation Act
27. Operating Room
28. Rural Primary Care Hospital
29. Recovery Room
30. School-Based Clinic
31. skilled nursing facility

Self-Assessment Questions

1. c
2. a
3. d
4. b
5. c
6. c
7. a
8. b
9. d
10. c

Chapter 7 Communication

Key Terms

1. g
2. p
3. m
4. q
5. e
6. l
7. r
8. f
9. o
10. v
11. u
12. j
13. d
14. a
15. n
16. k
17. s
18. h
19. b
20. t
21. c
22. i

Abbreviation Review

1. American Nurses Association
2. computerized patient record
3. human immunodeficiency virus
4. Institute of Medicine
5. words per minute

Self-Assessment Questions

1. c
2. a
3. b
4. d
5. a
6. d
7. d
8. b
9. c
10. a

Chapter 8 Client Teaching

Key Terms

1. g
2. k
3. m
4. h
5. c
6. l
7. n
8. i
9. p
10. q
11. d
12. o
13. f
14. j
15. a
16. b
17. e

Abbreviation Review

1. as evidenced by
2. Joint Commission on Accreditation of Healthcare Organizations
3. *nil per os*, Latin for "nothing by mouth"
4. related to

Self-Assessment Questions

1. d
2. c
3. c
4. a
5. b
6. a
7. d
8. b
9. d
10. b

Chapter 9 Nursing Process/ Documentation/ Informatics

Key Terms

1. o
2. mm
3. u
4. n
5. rr
6. ff
7. w
8. c
9. bb
10. x
11. p
12. oo
13. d
14. i
15. gg
16. xx
17. s
18. hh
19. b
20. m
21. qq
22. nn
23. ee
24. q
25. iii
26. jj
27. h
28. ccc
29. e
30. j
31. cc
32. ww
33. aa
34. pp
35. ll
36. r
37. v
38. a
39. yy
40. t
41. vv
42. y
43. ss
44. ii
45. l
46. z
47. aaa
48. zz
49. f
50. dd
51. kk
52. g
53. uu

54. tt
55. k

Abbreviation Review
1. as evidenced by
2. American Nurses Association
3. charting by exception
4. document, action, response
5. do not resuscitate
6. diagnosis-related group
7. hospital information system
8. Joint Commission on Accreditation of Healthcare Organizations
9. liter
10. medication administration record
11. North American Nursing Diagnosis Association
12. Nursing Interventions Classification
13. nursing information system
14. nursing minimum data set
15. Nursing Outcomes Classification
16. problem, implementation, evaluation
17. problem-oriented medical record
18. prospective payment system
19. peer review organization
20. registered nurse
21. range of motion
22. related to
23. subjective data, objective data, assessment plan
24. subjective data, objective data, assessment plan, implementation, evaluation
25. subjective data, objective data, assessment plan, implementation, evaluation, revision
26. telephone order
27. Universal Medical Language System

Self-Assessment Questions
1. a
2. a
3. d
4. c
5. b
6. b
7. a
8. b
9. d
10. c

Chapter 10 Life Span Development

Key Terms
1. b
2. h
3. v
4. c
5. aa
6. i
7. x
8. n
9. d
10. y
11. o
12. r
13. j
14. bb
15. z
16. a
17. g
18. m
19. p
20. dd
21. ff
22. s
23. q
24. f
25. t
26. w
27. l
28. ee
29. u
30. cc
31. k
32. e

Abbreviation Review
1. acquired immunodeficiency syndrome
2. breast self-exam
3. Centers for Disease Control and Prevention
4. central nervous system
5. fetal alcohol syndrome
6. phenylketonuria
7. sexually transmitted disease
8. tetanus/diphtheria
9. testicular self-exam

Self-Assessment Questions

1. d
2. c
3. b
4. a
5. c
6. b
7. d
8. c
9. d
10. a

Chapter 11 Cultural Considerations

Key Terms

1. d
2. j
3. n
4. e
5. k
6. f
7. o
8. c
9. g
10. l
11. h
12. p
13. b
14. i
15. m
16. q
17. a

Abbreviation Review

1. White, Anglo-Saxon, Protestant
2. World Health Organization

Self-Assessment Questions

1. c
2. a
3. d
4. b
5. b
6. d
7. b
8. d
9. c
10. a

Chapter 12 Stress, Adaptation, and Anxiety

Key Terms

1. b
2. f
3. k
4. o
5. a
6. p
7. r
8. c
9. e
10. x
11. j
12. l
13. q
14. u
15. s
16. w
17. g
18. m
19. t
20. v
21. i
22. d
23. n
24. h

Abbreviation Review

1. cerebral vascular accident
2. general adaptation syndrome
3. local adaptation syndrome
4. North American Nursing Diagnosis Association

Self-Assessment Questions

1. a
2. c
3. a
4. b
5. d
6. b
7. b
8. a
9. c
10. d

Chapter 13 End-of-Life Care

Key Terms

1. cc
2. i
3. m
4. v
5. f
6. p
7. a
8. j
9. w
10. q
11. b
12. bb
13. aa
14. r
15. x
16. d
17. k
18. u
19. e
20. l
21. z
22. n
23. g
24. s
25. o
26. h
27. y
28. c
29. t

Abbreviation Review

1. American Nurses Association
2. do not resuscitate
3. health maintenance organization
4. intramuscular
5. morphine sulfate
6. North American Nursing Diagnosis Association
7. Omnibus Budget Reconciliation Act
8. Patient Self-Determination Act
9. post-traumatic stress disorder
10. sudden infant death syndrome
11. tuberculosis

Self-Assessment Questions

1. c
2. a
3. b
4. d
5. c
6. c
7. a
8. d
9. c
10. b

Chapter 14 Wellness Concepts

Key Terms

1. g
2. c
3. d
4. f
5. a
6. e
7. b

Abbreviation Review

1. acquired immunodeficiency syndrome
2. Body Mass Index
3. Centers for Disease Control and Prevention
4. electrocardiogram
5. electrocardiogram
6. hemoglobin
7. human immunodeficiency virus
8. low density lipoprotein
9. papanicolau test
10. Public Health Service
11. sun protection factor
12. United States Department of Health and Human Services
13. World Health Organization

Self-Assessment Questions

1. c
2. b
3. a
4. b
5. c
6. b
7. d
8. d
9. c
10. d

Chapter 15 Self-Concept

Key Terms

1. a
2. e
3. i
4. k
5. b
6. a
7. h
8. g
9. c
10. f
11. j

Abbreviation Review

1. North American Nursing Diagnosis Association

Self-Assessment Questions

1. b
2. a
3. a
4. c
5. d

Chapter 16 Spirituality

Key Terms

1. h
2. e
3. c
4. b
5. g
6. d
7. i
8. a
9. f

Abbreviation Review

1. American Nurses Association
2. North American Nursing Diagnosis Association

Self-Assessment Questions

1. b
2. b
3. d
4. b
5. c

Chapter 17 Complementary/ Alternative Therapies

Key Terms

1. f
2. m
3. z
4. d
5. w
6. l
7. g
8. n
9. k
10. a
11. x
12. r
13. y
14. h
15. b
16. j
17. i
18. o
19. t
20. e
21. p
22. c
23. v
24. q
25. s
26. u

Abbreviation Review

1. Animal-Assisted therapy
2. Complementary/alternative
3. Food and Drug Administration
4. National Center for Complementary and Alternative Medicine
5. National Institutes of Health
6. progressive muscle relaxation
7. psychoneuroimmunoendocrinology

Self-Assessment Questions

1. a
2. d
3. a
4. b
5. c
6. c

7. b
8. a
9. c
10. c

Chapter 18 Basic Nutrition

Key Terms

1. h
2. a
3. m
4. gg
5. x
6. d
7. hh
8. mm
9. oo
10. cc
11. e
12. n
13. r
14. ee
15. jj
16. pp
17. vv
18. uu
19. s
20. tt
21. aa
22. ll
23. b
24. t
25. l
26. nn
27. qq
28. v
29. bb
30. ff
31. kk
32. xx
33. c
34. rr
35. zz
36. ii
37. i
38. w
39. aaa
40. k
41. ww
42. q
43. bbb
44. o
45. y
46. dd
47. ss
48. f
49. u
50. ccc
51. z
52. yy
53. g
54. p
55. ddd
56. j

Abbreviation Review

1. adequate intake
2. body mass index
3. carbohydrate (carbon, hydrogen, oxygen)
4. protein (carbon, hydrogen, oxygen, nitrogen)
5. chloride
6. central nervous system
7. deciliter
8. deoxyribonucleic acid
9. dietary reference intake
10. estimated average requirement
11. extracellular fluid
12. Food and Drug Administration
13. Iron
14. foot
15. gram
16. gastrointestinal
17. intake and output
18. intracellular fluid
19. inch
20. Potassium
21. kilocalorie
22. kilogram
23. pound
24. Magnesium
25. milligram
26. milliliter
27. Sodium
28. nasogastric
29. Nutrition, Labeling, and Education Act
30. *nil per os,* Latin for "nothing by mouth"
31. ounce

32. Phosphorus
33. red blood cell
34. recommended dietary allowances
35. ribonucleic acid
36. Sulfur
37. tube feeding
38. total parental nutrition
39. upper intake level
40. U.S. Department of Agriculture
41. white blood cell
42. Zinc

Self-Assessment Questions
1. a
2. d
3. b
4. a
5. c
6. d
7. b
8. d
9. c
10. a

Chapter 19 Rest and Sleep

Key Terms
1. n
2. d
3. m
4. g
5. l
6. a
7. h
8. i
9. b
10. j
11. f
12. k
13. c
14. e
15. p
16. q
17. r
18. o

Abbreviation Review
1. continuous positive airway pressure
2. electroencephalograph

3. North American Nursing Diagnosis
4. non-rapid eye movement
5. National Sleep Foundation
6. Nocturnal Sleep-Related Eating Disorder
7. periodic limb movement in sleep
8. premenstrual syndrome
9. rapid eye movement
10. restless leg syndrome

Self Assessment Questions
1. c
2. d
3. b
4. a
5. d
6. b
7. b
8. d
9. c
10. a

Chapter 20 Safety/Hygiene

Key Terms
1. d
2. j
3. c
4. e
5. h
6. b
7. k
8. n
9. g
10. a
11. l
12. i
13. f
14. m

Abbreviation Review
1. activities of daily living
2. Centers for Disease Control and Prevention
3. coronary heart disease
4. Centers for Medicare and Medicaid Services
5. cardiopulmonary resuscitation
6. Food and Drug Administration
7. Glasgow Coma Scale

8. high density lipoprotein
9. identification
10. Joint of Accreditation of Healthcare Organizations
11. material safety data sheet
12. North American Nursing Diagnosis Association
13. Omnibus Budget Reconciliation Act
14. Occupational Safety and Health Administration
15. patient-controlled analgesia

Self-Assessment Questions

1. a
2. d
3. c
4. d
5. b
6. c
7. d
8. b
9. a
10. c

Chapter 21 Infection Control/ Asepsis

Key Terms

1. d
2. oo
3. x
4. ii
5. tt
6. rr
7. z
8. aaa
9. qq
10. k
11. pp
12. q
13. hh
14. w
15. u
16. r
17. y
18. e
19. ff
20. ss
21. zz
22. jj
23. xx
24. c
25. j
26. v
27. p
28. bbb
29. aa
30. kk
31. gg
32. ccc
33. f
34. mm
35. vv
36. cc
37. b
38. ll
39. l
40. s
41. ww
42. yy
43. i
44. nn
45. dd
46. o
47. ee
48. g
49. t
50. uu
51. m
52. bb
53. a
54. h
55. n

Abbreviation Review

1. acquired immunodeficiency syndrome
2. Association for Professionals in Infection Control and Epidemiology
3. Centers for Disease Control and Prevention
4. deoxyribonucleic acid
5. Environmental Protection Agency
6. erythrocyte sedimentation rate
7. hepatitis B virus
8. hepatitis C virus
9. human immunodeficiency virus
10. North American Nursing Disgnosis Association

11. operating room
12. Occupational Safety and Health Administration
13. potential hydrogen
14. ribonucleic acid
15. tuberculosis
16. white blood cell, white blood count

Self-Assessment Questions
1. d
2. b
3. c
4. a
5. d
6. a
7. d
8. c
9. b
10. a

Chapter 22 Standard Precautions and Isolation

Key Terms

1. c
2. i
3. k
4. d
5. f
6. h
7. l
8. g
9. a
10. b
11. j
12. e

Abbreviation Review
1. acquired immunodeficiency syndrome
2. body substance isolation
3. Centers for Disease Control and Prevention
4. Department of Health and Human Services
5. hepatitis B virus

6. Hospital Infection Control Practices Advisory Committee
7. human immunodeficiency virus
8. multidrug-resistant
9. Occupational Safety and Health Administration
10. tuberculosis

Self-Assessment Questions
1. b
2. c
3. d
4. a
5. b
6. c
7. b
8. a
9. c
10. d

Chapter 23 Bioterrorism

Key Terms
1. c
2. m
3. l
4. g
5. k
6. d
7. i
8. j
9. n
10. f
11. e
12. h
13. a
14. b
15. o

Abbreviation Review
1. Centers for Disease Control and Prevention
2. Chemical, Biological, Radiological/Nuclear, and Explosive Enhanced Response Force Package
3. Expeditionary Medical Support
4. Emergency operations plan
5. Federal Emergency Management Agency

6. potassium iodide
7. Strategic National Stockpile
8. Vendor-managed inventory
9. Nerve agents

Self-Assessment Questions

1. a
2. b
3. b
4. a
5. a

Chapter 24 Fluid, Electrolyte, and Acid-Base Balance

Key Terms

1. oo
2. t
3. cc
4. pp
5. e
6. dd
7. s
8. f
9. bb
10. qq
11. g
12. rr
13. h
14. r
15. u
16. ee
17. v
18. tt
19. kk
20. gg
21. n
22. m
23. b
24. ss
25. ff
26. a
27. i
28. p
29. w
30. ll
31. o
32. uu
33. c
34. x
35. aa
36. d
37. mm
38. q
39. z
40. hh
41. j
42. ii
43. nn
44. vv
45. y
46. k
47. jj
48. l

Fill in the Blank

1. anion
2. cation
3. ion
4. atom

Abbreviation Review

1. arterial blood gases
2. antidiuretic hormone
3. adenosine triphosphatase
4. blood pressure
5. blood urea nitrogen
6. calcium ion
7. complete blood count
8. chloride ion
9. carbon dioxide ion
10. carboxyl group
11. central nervous system
12. dextrose 5% in water
13. deciliter
14. extracellular fluid
15. gastrointestinal
16. hydrogen ion
17. carbonic acid
18. water
19. hydrochloric acid
20. bicarbonate ion
21. hematocrit
22. hemoglobin
23. intake and output

24. intracellular fluid
25. intravenous
26. potassium ion
27. potassium chloride
28. kilogram
29. liter
30. pound
31. milliequivalent
32. milligram
33. magnesium ion
34. milliliter
35. millimeters of mercury
36. Milk of Magnesia
37. milliosmoles/kilogram
38. sodium ion
39. sodium chloride
40. sodium dihydrogen phosphate
41. sodium bicarbonate
42. sodium monohydrogen phosphate
43. sodium hydroxide
44. amino group
45. nothing by mouth
46. oxygen
47. hydroxyl
48. partial pressure of carbon dioxide
49. potential hydrogen
50. partial pressure of oxygen
51. phosphate ion
52. oxygen saturation
53. total parenteral nutrition
54. temperature, pulse, respirations
55. weight

Self-Assessment Questions

1. d
2. a
3. b
4. a
5. c
6. a
7. b
8. b
9. c
10. d

Chapter 25 Medication Administration and IV Therapy

Key Terms

1. n
2. v
3. g
4. ee
5. u
6. o
7. kk
8. a
9. ff
10. i
11. jj
12. t
13. ii
14. pp
15. oo
16. gg
17. bb
18. b
19. s
20. j
21. c
22. f
23. w
24. dd
25. ll
26. mm
27. p
28. e
29. x
30. cc
31. y
32. m
33. d
34. z
35. l
36. q
37. h
38. aa
39. nn
40. hh
41. k
42. r

Fill in the Blank
1. *United States Pharmacopia/National Formulary*
2. generic
3. parenteral route
4. absorption

Abbreviation Review
1. acquired immunodeficiency syndrome
2. body surface area
3. cup
4. cubic centimeter
5. centimeter
6. central venous catheter
7. dextrose 5% in water
8. Drug Enforcement Agency
9. dram, or ʒ
10. Food and Drug Administration
11. fluid
12. gram
13. gastrointestinal
14. grain
15. drops
16. intradermal
17. intramuscular
18. intravenous
19. intravenous piggyback
20. kilogram
21. keep vein open
22. liter
23. pound
24. ℔
25. medication administration record
26. microgram, or μg
27. milligram
28. minute
29. milliliter
30. *National Formulary*
31. nasogastric
32. nothing by mouth
33. nitroglycerin
34. ounce or ʒ?
35. *per os*, Latin for "by mouth"
36. Latin for "as needed"
37. pint
38. prothrombin time
39. partial thromboplastin time
40. everyday
41. quart
42. red blood cell, red blood count
43. subcutaneous
44. teaspoon
45. tablespoon
46. *United States Pharmacopeia*
47. vascular access device

Self-Assessment Questions
1. b
2. c
3. a
4. b
5. a
6. b
7. c
8. d
9. b
10. c

Chapter 26 Assessment

Key Terms
1. i
2. u
3. l
4. a
5. m
6. v
7. dd
8. s
9. j
10. d
11. cc
12. t
13. k
14. ff
15. z
16. w
17. ee
18. b
19. n
20. f
21. bb
22. o
23. e
24. p
25. r
26. y
27. q

28. h
29. c
30. x
31. g
32. aa

Abbreviation Review

1. blood pressure
2. centimeter
3. left lower quadrant
4. level of consciousness
5. left upper quadrant
6. pulse
7. pupils equal, round, reactive to light and accommodation
8. respiration
9. right lower quadrant
10. review of systems
11. right upper quadrant
12. temperature

Self-Assessment Questions

1. b
2. c
3. d
4. a
5. c
6. b
7. d
8. c
9. a
10. b

Chapter 27 Pain Management

Key Terms

1. hh
2. a
3. g
4. bb
5. aa
6. ii
7. rr
8. kk
9. b
10. gg
11. jj
12. h
13. y
14. j
15. c
16. z
17. i
18. ll
19. k
20. cc
21. t
22. f
23. o
24. mm
25. p
26. dd
27. n
28. e
29. u
30. ff
31. v
32. d
33. m
34. w
35. l
36. x
37. oo
38. qq
39. ee
40. s
41. r
42. q
43. nn
44. pp

Abbreviation Review

1. American Pain Society
2. Agency for Health Care Policy and Research
3. around the clock
4. eutectic (cream) mixture of local anesthetics
5. International Association for the Study of Pain
6. magnetic resonance imaging
7. *nil per os*, Latin for "nothing by mouth"
8. nonsteroidal anti-inflammatory drug
9. patient-controlled analgesic
10. *pro re nata*, Latin for "as required"

11. tetracaine, adrenaline, cocaine
12. transcutaneous electrical nerve stimulation
13. temporomandibular joint
14. Visual Analog Scale
15. World Health Organization

Self-Assessment Questions
1. a
2. b
3. b
4. c
5. d
6. b
7. a
8. c
9. d
10. a

Chapter 28 Diagnostic Tests

Key Terms
1. l
2. x
3. k
4. tt
5. kk
6. a
7. m
8. n
9. vv
10. jj
11. y
12. ss
13. d
14. o
15. e
16. ff
17. i
18. w
19. ll
20. qq
21. j
22. mm
23. uu
24. oo
25. b
26. ii
27. c
28. aa
29. p
30. rr
31. q
32. aaa
33. z
34. gg
35. ee
36. h
37. u
38. dd
39. v
40. ww
41. hh
42. g
43. t
44. cc
45. xx
46. zz
47. s
48. nn
49. yy
50. f
51. bb
52. pp
53. r

Abbreviation Review
1. arterial blood gas
2. culture and sensitivity
3. cerebrospinal fluid
4. computed tomography
5. electrocardiogram
6. electroencephalogram
7. intravenous pyelogram
8. partial pressure of carbon dioxide
9. partial pressure of oxygen
10. red blood cell, red blood count
11. white blood cell, white blood count

Self-Assessment Questions
1. c
2. a
3. b
4. d
5. c
6. d
7. b
8. b

9. d
10. c

Chapter 29 Basic Procedures

Key Terms
1. e
2. m
3. k
4. c
5. d
6. a
7. f
8. b
9. i
10. j
11. h
12. g
13. l

Abbreviation Review
1. Airway, breathing, circulation, defibrillation
2. Automated External Defibrillator
3. Centers for Disease Control and Prevention
4. Cardiopulmonary resuscitation
5. Emergency Medical System
6. Intake and Output
7. Point of maximal impulse
8. Passive range of motion
9. Range of motion
10. Vancomycin-resistant enterococci

Self-Assessment Questions
1. d
2. d
3. b
4. a
5. c
6. b
7. c
8. a

Chapter 30 Intermediate Procedures

Key Terms
1. d
2. b
3. c
4. i
5. g
6. j
7. a
8. f
9. h
10. e

Abbreviation Review
1. Arterial blood gas
2. Chronic obstructive pulmonary disease
3. Fraction of inspired oxygen
4. Gastrointestinal
5. Intravenous
6. Medication administration record
7. Nasogastric
8. Right eye
9. Operating room
10. Left eye
11. Occupational Safety and Health Administration
12. Over-the-counter
13. Both eyes
14. Percutaneous endoscopic gastrostomy
15. Arterial blood oxygen saturation
16. Sustained maximum inspiration

Self -Assessment Questions
1. d
2. b
3. a
4. c
5. d

Chapter 31 Advanced Procedures

Key Terms
1. c
2. a
3. d
4. e
5. b

Abbreviation Review
1. Centers for Disease Control and Prevention
2. Intravenous
3. Medication administration record
4. Nasogastric
5. Nothing by mouth
6. Over-the-needle catheter
7. Occupational Safety and Health Administration

Self-Assessment Questions
1. b
2. d
3. b
4. c

Chapter 32 Anesthesia
Key Terms
1. b
2. g
3. i
4. h
5. f
6. k
7. a
8. d
9. c
10. j
11. e

Abbreviation Review
1. blood pressure
2. central nervous system
3. certified registered nurse anesthetist
4. cerebrospinal fluid
5. electrocardiogram
6. endotracheal tube
7. heart rate
8. patient-controlled analgesia
9. postdural puncture headache
10. respiratory rate

Self-Assessment Questions
1. d
2. a
3. b
4. b

5. a
6. d
7. b
8. c
9. d
10. c

Chapter 33 Surgery
Key Terms
1. l
2. g
3. r
4. o
5. d
6. i
7. n
8. a
9. j
10. b
11. m
12. c
13. p
14. f
15. k
16. q
17. e
18. h

Abbreviation Review
1. Association of Operating Room Nurses
2. eyes, ears, nose, and throat
3. nothing by mouth
4. operating room
5. postanesthesia care unit
6. patient-controlled analgesia

Self-Assessment Questions
1. a
2. c
3. d
4. b
5. d
6. a
7. d
8. b
9. b
10. a

Chapter 34 Oncology

Key Terms
1. h
2. d
3. q
4. g
5. p
6. a
7. i
8. w
9. r
10. o
11. e
12. j
13. n
14. f
15. b
16. s
17. k
18. m
19. v
20. t
21. x
22. l
23. y
24. z
25. u
26. c
27. aa
28. bb

Abbreviation Review
1. American Cancer Society
2. Agency for Health Care Policy and Research
3. *bacillus Calmette-Guérin*
4. bone marrow transplantation
5. cell-cycle nonspecific
6. cell-cycle specific
7. central nervous system
8. computed tomography
9. deoxyribonucleic acid
10. Environmental Protection Agency
11. transcutaneous electrical nerve stimulation
12. tumor, node, metastasis

Fill in the Blank
1. lymphomas
2. leukemias
3. sarcomas
4. carcinomas

Self-Assessment Questions
1. c
2. b
3. b
4. d
5. c
6. d
7. c
8. a
9. c
10. d

Chapter 35 Respiratory System

Key Terms
1. g
2. e
3. w
4. x
5. gg
6. m
7. y
8. l
9. z
10. aa
11. f
12. bb
13. hh
14. a
15. cc
16. n
17. dd
18. jj
19. b
20. o
21. q
22. v
23. ff
24. i
25. u
26. t
27. h
28. d

29. s
30. j
31. ee
32. r
33. c
34. kk
35. k
36. p
37. ii

Abbreviation Review

1. arterial blood gas
2. American Cancer Society
3. acid-fast bacillus
4. activated partial thromboplastin time
5. adult respiratory distress syndrome
6. antireptolysin O
7. *bacillus Calmette-Guérin*
8. computerized axial tomography
9. congestive heart failure
10. carbon dioxide
11. chronic obstructive lung disease
12. chronic obstructive pulmonary disease
13. human immunodeficiency virus
14. multidrug-resistant TB
15. minute
16. pulmonary embolism
17. pulmonary function test
18. purified protein derivative
19. prothrombin time
20. oxygen saturation
21. severe acute respiratory syndrome
22. tuberculosis
23. upper respiratory infection

Self-Assessment Questions

1. d
2. b
3. d
4. c
5. b
6. c
7. c
8. d
9. b
10. a

Chapter 36 Cardiovascular System

Key Terms

1. k
2. jj
3. w
4. ii
5. l
6. hh
7. m
8. v
9. oo
10. u
11. a
12. ff
13. t
14. b
15. n
16. gg
17. dd
18. c
19. s
20. ee
21. q
22. j
23. x
24. d
25. i
26. p
27. y
28. e
29. o
30. qq
31. f
32. rr
33. z
34. cc
35. g
36. aa
37. r
38. bb
39. h
40. kk
41. nn
42. ll
43. pp
44. mm

Anatomy and Physiology
Key Terms
   1. g
   2. d
   3. c
   4. j
   5. a
   6. i
   7. f
   8. b
   9. e
   10. k
   11. h

Abbreviation Review
   1. arterial blood gas
   2. angiotensin-converting enzyme
   3. antilymphocytic globulin
   4. activated partial thromboplastin time
   5. aspartate aminotransferase
   6. antihymocytic globulin
   7. atrioventricular
   8. coronary artery bypass graft
   9. coronary artery disease
   10. complete blood count
   11. congestive heart failure
   12. creatine kinase or creatine phosphokinase
   13. cardiopulmonary resuscitation
   14. deep vein thrombosis
   15. electrocardiogram
   16. erythrocyte sedimentation rate
   17. hematocrit
   18. high density lipoprotein
   19. hemoglobin
   20. hypertension
   21. intra-aortic balloon pump
   22. implantable cardioverter-defibrillator
   23. intensive care unit
   24. International Normalized Ration
   25. left anterior descending
   26. lactic dehydrogenase
   27. low density lipoprotein
   28. myocardial infarction
   29. magnetic resonance imaging
   30. multigated acquisition
   31. premature atrial contraction
   32. paroxysmal atrial tachycarida
   33. paroxysmal supraventricular tachycardia
   34. prothrombin time
   35. percutaneous transluminal coronary angioplasty
   36. partial thromboplastin time
   37. premature ventricular contraction
   38. sinoatrial
   39. transesophageal echocardiography
   40. ventricular fibrillation
   41. very low-density lipoprotein
   42. ventricular tachycardia

Self-Assessment Questions
   1. b
   2. c
   3. a
   4. b
   5. d
   6. a
   7. d
   8. b
   9. c
   10. b

Chapter 37 Hematologic and Lymphatic Systems

Key Terms
   1. c
   2. h
   3. v
   4. n
   5. b
   6. j
   7. a
   8. m
   9. i
   10. o
   11. u
   12. g
   13. p
   14. f
   15. k
   16. t
   17. e
   18. s
   19. q
   20. l
   21. r
   22. d

Abbreviation Review

1. a combination of chemotherapy drugs: doxorubicin (Adriamycin), bleomycin sulfate (Blenoxane), vinblastine (Velban), dacarbazine (DTIC-Dome)
2. acute lymphocytic leukemia
3. acute myelocytic leukemia
4. activated partial thomboplastin time
5. antihymocyte globulin
6. a combination of chemotherapy drugs: cyclophosphamide (Cytoxan), doxorubin (Adriamycin), vincristine (Oncovin), prednisone (Deltasone)
7. chronic lymphocytic leukemia
8. chronic myelocytic leukemia
9. a combination of chemotherapy drugs: cyclophosphamide (Cytoxan), vincristine (Oncovin), procarbazine (Matulanel), predisone (Deltasone)
10. a combination of chemotherapy drugs: cyclophosphamide (Cytoxan), vincristine (Oncovin), prednisone (Deltasone)
11. disseminated intravascular coagulation
12. erythrocyte sedimentation rate
13. hematocrit
14. hemoglobin
15. human leukocyte antigen
16. idiopathic thrombocytopenic purpura
17. lactic dehydrogenase
18. a combination of chemotherapy drugs: mechlorethamine or nitrogen mustard (Mustargen), vincristine (Oncovin), procarbazine hydrochloric (Matulane), prednisone (Deltasone)
19. non-Hodgkin's lymphoma
20. patient-controlled analgesia
21. polymorphonuclear leukocyte
22. prothrombin time
23. partial thromboplastin time
24. red blood cell
25. total iron binding capacity
26. white blood cell

Self-Assessment Questions

1. c
2. b
3. c
4. a
5. d
6. a
7. a
8. b
9. c
10. c

Chapter 38 Gastrointestinal System

Key Terms

1. f
2. g
3. l
4. m
5. z
6. y
7. q
8. a
9. r
10. h
11. k
12. s
13. j
14. o
15. v
16. n
17. aa
18. b
19. t
20. c
21. i
22. d
23. p
24. w
25. u
26. e
27. x

Key Terms: Inflammatory Conditions of the Gastrointestinal System

1. e
2. f
3. b
4. a
5. h
6. g
7. c
8. d

Abbreviation Review

1. alanine aminotransferase
2. aspartate aminotransferase
3. common bile duct
4. carcinoembryonic antigen
5. esophagogastroduodenoscopy
6. endoscopic retrograde cholangiopancreatogram
7. enterostomal
8. gastroesophageal reflux disease
9. gammaglutamy transpeptidase
10. hepatitis A virus
11. hepatitis B immune globulin
12. hydrochloric acid
13. hepatitis C virus
14. hepatitis D virus
15. inflammatory bowel disease
16. lactate dehydrogenase
17. lower esophageal sphincter
18. nasogastric
19. *nil per os*, Latin for "nothing by mouth"
20. nonsteroidal anti-inflammatory drug
21. prothrombin time
22. partial thromboplastin time
23. right lower quadrant
24. transjugular intrahepatic portosystematic shunt
25. ulcerative colitis
26. upper gastrointestinal tract

Self-Assessment Questions

1. b
2. a
3. b
4. c
5. d
6. c
7. c
8. d
9. c
10. a

Chapter 39 Urinary System

Key Terms

1. f
2. i
3. r
4. n

5. aa
6. t
7. j
8. e
9. h
10. y
11. cc
12. dd
13. k
14. c
15. p
16. g
17. o
18. bb
19. ee
20. s
21. v
22. ff
23. q
24. b
25. m
26. w
27. l
28. u
29. a
30. gg
31. x
32. z
33. d

Abbreviation Review

1. acquired cystic kidney disease
2. American Cancer Society
3. amyotrophic lateral sclerosis
4. acute renal failure
5. acute tubular necrosis
6. arteriovenous
7. benign prostatic hypertrophy
8. blood urea nitrogen
9. culture and sensitivity
10. continuous ambulatory peritoneal dialysis
11. effective arterial blood volume
12. erythrocyte sedimentation rate
13. end-stage renal disease
14. extracorporeal shock wave lithotripsy
15. glomerular filtration rate
16. intravenous pyelogram
17. kidneys, ureters, and bladder

18. National Institute of Diabetes and Digestive and Kidney Diseases
19. nonsteroidal anti-inflammatory drug
20. polycystic kidney disease
21. urinary tract infection

Self-Assessment Questions

1. d
2. b
3. a
4. c
5. a
6. b
7. d
8. a
9. c
10. b

Chapter 40 Musculoskeletal System

Key Terms

1. b
2. u
3. i
4. q
5. a
6. v
7. j
8. o
9. c
10. r
11. w
12. aa
13. k
14. d
15. n
16. h
17. e
18. x
19. l
20. s
21. g
22. t
23. y
24. z
25. m
26. p
27. f

Abbreviation Review

1. bone mineral density
2. circulation, movement, sensation
3. continuous passive motion
4. c-reactive protein
5. dual energy x-ray
6. enzyme-linked immunosorbent assay
7. electromyography
8. National Institute of Arthritis and Musculoskeletal and Skin Diseases
9. National Osteoporosis Foundation
10. osteoarthritis
11. open reduction internal fixation
12. rheumatoid factor
13. range of motion
14. sequential compression device
15. single energy x-ray absorptiometry
16. temporomandibular joint disease/disorder
17. temporomandibular joint

Self-Assessment Questions

1. a
2. b
3. b
4. d
5. c
6. a
7. d
8. c
9. c
10. d

Chapter 41 Neurological System

Key Terms

1. aa
2. f
3. l
4. r
5. hh
6. bb
7. a
8. ee
9. e
10. uu
11. s
12. j
13. q

14. rr
15. i
16. ss
17. x
18. d
19. ff
20. jj
21. mm
22. h
23. w
24. oo
25. m
26. pp
27. y
28. cc
29. b
30. ii
31. qq
32. ll
33. dd
34. o
35. z
36. kk
37. c
38. nn
39. tt
40. gg
41. u
42. p
43. g
44. k
45. n
46. vv
47. v
48. t

Abbreviation Review
1. arterial blood gas
2. American Council for Headache Education
3. adrenocorticotropic hormone
4. Alzheimer's disease
5. activities of daily living
6. amyotrophic lateral sclerosis
7. autonomic nervous system
8. cranial nerve
9. central nervous system
10. cerebrospinal fluid
11. computerized tomography

12. cerebrovascular accident
13. diffuse axonal injury
14. electroencephalogram
15. electromyogram
16. γ-aminobutyric acid
17. immunoglobulin
18. lumbar puncture
19. monoamine oxidase
20. mean arterial pressure
21. magnetic resonance imaging
22. multiple sclerosis
23. monosodium glutamate
24. National Stroke Association
25. nonsteroidal anti-inflammatory drug
26. partial pressure of carbon dioxide
27. pupils equal, round, reactive to light and accommodation
28. positron emission tomography
29. peripheral nervous system
30. prothrombin time
31. range of motion
32. spinal cord injury
33. single photon emission computed tomography
34. transient ischemic attack

Self-Assessment Questions
1. b
2. a
3. c
4. b
5. a
6. d
7. b
8. c
9. d
10. a

Chapter 42 Sensory System
Key Terms
1. a
2. u
3. bb
4. n
5. q
6. w
7. cc
8. p

9. b
10. m
11. i
12. t
13. l
14. v
15. x
16. j
17. c
18. ee
19. r
20. g
21. y
22. dd
23. k
24. ff
25. s
26. d
27. e
28. z
29. o
30. aa
31. h
32. gg
33. hh
34. f

Abbreviation Review
1. autonomic nervous system
2. brainstem auditory evoked response
3. central nervous system
4. computerized tomography
5. electroretinogram
6. intraocular lens
7. intraocular pressure
8. level of consciousness
9. magnetic resonance imaging
10. peripheral nervous system
11. telecommunication device for the deaf
12. University of Pennsylvania Smell Identification Test

Self-Assessment Questions
1. b
2. c
3. d
4. a
5. d

6. c
7. c
8. b
9. a
10. d

Chapter 43 Endocrine System
Key Terms
1. c
2. m
3. t
4. n
5. a
6. o
7. b
8. e
9. u
10. x
11. l
12. p
13. d
14. v
15. f
16. z
17. h
18. i
19. w
20. aa
21. cc
22. q
23. g
24. bb
25. y
26. j
27. r
28. k
29. s

Abbreviation Review
1. adrenocorticotropic hormone
2. American Diabetes Association
3. antidiuretic hormone
4. computerized axialtransverse tomography
5. cerebrovascular accident
6. diabetic ketoacidosis
7. fasting blood sugar
8. follicle-stimulating hormone

9. gestational diabetes mellitus
10. growth hormone
11. glucose tolerance test
12. hyperosmolar hyperglycemic nonketotic syndrome
13. insulin-dependent diabetes mellitus
14. impaired fasting glucose
15. impaired glucose tolerance
16. luteinizing hormone
17. melanocyte-stimulating hormone
18. non-insulin-dependent diabetes mellitus
19. parathyroid hormone
20. propylthiouracil
21. peripheral vascular disease
22. radioactive iodine uptake
23. syndrome of inappropriate antidiuretic hormone
24. thyroid-stimulating hormone
25. vanilly/mandelic acid

Self-Assessment Questions
1. a
2. b
3. c
4. a
5. c
6. d
7. b
8. c
9. d
10. a

Chapter 44 Reproductive System

Key Terms
1. c
2. j
3. q
4. i
5. t
6. a
7. o
8. u
9. k
10. w
11. b
12. l
13. v

14. p
15. f
16. x
17. z
18. d
19. y
20. m
21. r
22. aa
23. e
24. s
25. g
26. n
27. h

Abbreviation Review
1. American Cancer Society
2. alpha-fetoprotein
3. anterior/posterior
4. belladonna and opium
5. benign prostatic hypertrophy
6. breast self-examination
7. carcinoma *in situ*
8. continuous positive airway pressure
9. dilation and curettage
10. diethylstilbestrol
11. dynamic infusion cavernosometry and cavernosography
12. estrogen replacement therapy
13. fibrocystic breast disease
14. follicle-stimulating hormone
15. gamete-intrafallopian transfer
16. human chorionic gonadatropin
17. *in vitro* fertilization and embryo replacement
18. intrauterine device
19. intravenous pyelogram
20. kidneys/ureters/bladder
21. luteinizing hormone
22. nurse practitioner
23. Papanicolaou
24. pelvic inflammatory disease
25. premenstrual syndrome
26. prostate specific antigen
27. sexually transmitted disease
28. testicular self-examination
29. toxic shock syndrome

30. transurethral ultrasound-guided laser-induced prostatectomy
31. transurethral resection of the prostate
32. urinary tract infection
33. vacuum constriction device
34. zygote-intra-fallopian transfer

Self-Assessment Questions

1. b
2. a
3. c
4. b
5. a
6. d
7. b
8. b
9. c
10. a

Chapter 45 Sexually Transmitted Infections

Key Terms

1. e
2. f
3. b
4. c
5. a
6. d

Abbreviation Review

1. acquired immunodeficiency syndrome
2. cytomegalovirus
3. enzyme-linked immunosorbent assay
4. hepatitis B virus
5. human immunodeficiency virus
6. human papillomavirus
7. herpes simplex virus
8. National Institute of Allergy and Infectious Diseases
9. pelvic inflammatory disease
10. rapid plasma regain
11. sexually transmitted infection
12. venereal disease research laboratory

Self-Assessment Questions

1. a
2. b
3. a
4. d
5. a
6. c
7. a
8. a
9. c
10. c

Chapter 46 Integumentary System

Key Terms

1. e
2. n
3. t
4. u
5. o
6. d
7. m
8. v
9. cc
10. jj
11. s
12. gg
13. dd
14. b
15. f
16. w
17. l
18. i
19. r
20. p
21. x
22. bb
23. ee
24. a
25. c
26. g
27. y
28. ii
29. k
30. aa
31. h
32. ff
33. hh
34. q
35. z
36. j

Abbreviation Review

1. asymmetry, border, color, diameter
2. angiogenesis factor
3. fibroblast activating factor
4. methicillin-resistant *Staphylococcus aureus*
5. maggot debridement therapy
6. National Pressure Ulcer Advisory Panel
7. range of motion
8. sun protection factor
9. total parenteral nutrition
10. U.S. Department of Health and Human Services
11. vacuum-assisted closure

Self-Assessment Questions

1. a
2. b
3. a
4. c
5. b
6. d
7. a
8. c
9. b
10. d

Chapter 47 Immune System

Key Terms

1. g
2. e
3. q
4. k
5. r
6. t
7. w
8. d
9. l
10. b
11. s
12. j
13. x
14. m
15. y
16. z
17. u
18. c

19. n
20. f
21. q
22. aa
23. h
24. o
25. bb
26. p
27. i
28. v

Abbreviation Review

1. AIDS dementia complex
2. acid-fast bacillus
3. cervical intraepithelial neoplasia
4. cytomegalovirus
5. disease-modifying antirheumatic drug
6. enzyme-linked immonosorbent assay
7. electromyogram
8. erythrocyte sedimentation rate
9. highly active antiretroviral therapy
10. hepatitis B virus
11. hepatitis C virus
12. hepatitis D virus
13. human immunodeficiency virus
14. human papilloma virus
15. immunoglobulin G
16. immunoglobulin M
17. Kaposi's sarcoma
18. lupus erythematosus
19. *Mycobacterium avium* complex
20. multi-drug-resistant tuberculosis
21. myasthenia gravis
22. non-Hodgkin's lymphoma
23. National Institute of Allergy and Infectious Diseases
24. nonnucleoside reverse transcriptase inhibitor
25. nucleoside analog reverse transcriptase inhibitor
26. oral hairy leukoplakia
27. *Pneumocystis carinii* pneumonia
28. polymerase chain reaction
29. purified protein derivative
30. rheumatoid arthritis
31. rheumatoid factor
32. ribonucleic acid
33. range of motion

34. systemic lupus erythematosus
35. sun protection factor
36. white blood cells

Self-Assessment Questions
1. a
2. c
3. a
4. b
5. a
6. c
7. c
8. d
9. a
10. b

Chapter 48 Mental Illness

Key Terms
1. l
2. z
3. gg
4. jj
5. w
6. b
7. j
8. r
9. k
10. bb
11. e
12. ff
13. kk
14. p
15. y
16. h
17. x
18. mm
19. n
20. pp
21. s
22. c
23. o
24. t
25. ee
26. f
27. hh
28. ss
29. ii

30. v
31. i
32. m
33. ll
34. d
35. g
36. aa
37. dd
38. a
39. cc
40. nn
41. u
42. oo
43. qq
44. q
45. rr

Abbreviation Review
1. American Bar Association
2. attention deficit hyperactivity disorder
3. American Psychiatric Association
4. Adult Protective Services
5. Child Protective Services
6. Depression and Bipolar Support Alliance
7. *Diagnostic and Statistical Manual of Mental Disorders*, 4th edition
8. electroconvulsive therapy
9. extrapyramidal symptom
10. Family Violence Prevention Fund
11. generalized anxiety disorder
12. intensive care unit
13. monoamine oxidase inhibitor
14. National Coalition Against Domestic Violence
15. neuroleptic malignant syndrome
16. obsessive compulsive disorder
17. over-the-counter
18. phencyclidine
19. post-traumatic stress disorder
20. selective serotonin reuptake inhibitor
21. tardive dyskinesia

Self-Assessment Questions
1. d
2. a
3. b
4. a
5. d

6. d
7. a
8. c
9. b
10. c

Chapter 49 Substance Abuse

Key Terms
1. d
2. a
3. h
4. j
5. m
6. b
7. n
8. l
9. t
10. i
11. p
12. c
13. o
14. k
15. e
16. g
17. q
18. s
19. r
20. f

Abbreviation Review
1. Alcoholics Anonymous
2. attention deficit hyperactivity disorder
3. alcohol withdrawal syndrome
4. central nervous system
5. Drug Enforcement Agency
6. diethyltriptamine
7. detoxification
8. dimethyltryptamine
9. Diagnostic and Statistical Manual of Mental Health Disorders, 4th edition
10. fetal alcohol effects
11. fetal alcohol syndrome
12. lysergic acid diethylamide
13. Mothers Against Drunk Driving
14. monoamine oxidase inhibitor
15. methylenedioxyamphetamine
16. Narcotics Anonymous

17. National Institute on Alcohol Abuse and Alcoholism
18. National Institute on Drug Abuse
19. phencyclidine
20. range of motion
21. Students Against Drunk Driving
22. sudden infant death syndrome

Self-Assessment Questions
1. b
2. c
3. a
4. c
5. b
6. c
7. a
8. d
9. a
10. b

Chapter 50 The Older Adult

Key Terms
1. b
2. h
3. e
4. g
5. a
6. f
7. d
8. c

Abbreviation Review
1. American Association of Retired Persons
2. Alzheimer's disease
3. American Nurses Association
4. Balanced Budget Act
5. benign prostatc hypertrophy
6. congestive heart failure
7. Centers for Medicare and Medicaid Services
8. chronic obstructive pulmonary disease
9. estrogen replacement therapy
10. Health Care Financing Agency
11. National Council of Aging
12. Omnibus Reconciliation Act
13. open reduction/internal fixation
14. prospective payment system
15. prostate specific antigen

16. peripheral vascular disease
17. respiratory tract infection
18. resource utilization group system
19. skilled nursing facility
20. social security administration
21. total hip arthoplasty
22. urinary tract infection

Self-Assessment Questions
1. b
2. d
3. b
4. c
5. a
6. a
7. d
8. d
9. a
10. b

Chapter 51 Ambulatory, Restorative, and Palliative Care in Community Settings

Key Terms
1. c
2. f
3. j
4. o
5. a
6. b
7. m
8. d
9. e
10. g
11. l
12. h
13. p
14. i
15. k
16. t
17. r
18. n
19. q
20. s

Abbreviation Review
1. activities of daily living
2. Centers for Medicare and Medicaid Services
3. extended-care facility
4. Functional Assessment Measure
5. Functional Independence Measure
6. Health Insurance Portability and Accountability Act
7. Minimum data set
8. Outcomes and Assessment Information Set
9. Omnibus Budget Reconciliation Act of 1987
10. State Health Insurance Assistance Program
11. Uniform Data System for Medical Rehabilitation

Self-Assessment Questions
1. a
2. c
3. d
4. d
5. d

Chapter 52 Responding to Emergencies

Key Terms
1. c
2. j
3. a
4. f
5. h
6. b
7. g
8. d
9. i
10. e

Abbreviation Review
1. airway, breathing, circulation
2. Acute Radiation Syndrome
3. Centers for Disease Control and Prevention
4. cardiopulmonary resuscitation
5. emergency department
6. emergency medical services

7. emergency medical technician
8. level of consciousness
9. motor vehicle collision
10. Radiation Dispersal Device
11. rest, ice, compression, elevation
12. standard operating procedure
13. Viral Hemorrhagic Fever

Self-Assessment Questions
1. a
2. d
3. b
4. d
5. a
6. b
7. d
8. b
9. c
10. a

Chapter 53 Integration

Note: Answers will be individualized.

Chapter 54 Prenatal Care

Key Terms
1. j
2. d
3. i
4. t
5. l
6. f
7. gg
8. aa
9. cc
10. m
11. z
12. c
13. tt
14. u
15. aaa
16. dd
17. fff
18. g
19. qq
20. bbb
21. v
22. ll

23. ccc
24. vv
25. yy
26. ee
27. xx
28. ss
29. uu
30. kk
31. mm
32. n
33. ggg
34. pp
35. rr
36. ddd
37. ww
38. eee
39. zz
40. hh
41. o
42. ii
43. hhh
44. p
45. y
46. a
47. r
48. w
49. b
50. bb
51. ff
52. jj
53. s
54. nn
55. e
56. h
57. oo
58. k
59. x
60. q

Abbreviation Review
1. American Society for Psychoprophylaxis in Obstetrics
2. Association of Women's Health, Obstetric, and Neonatal Nurses
3. bag of water
4. biparietal diameter
5. crown-heel
6. crown-rump
7. diethylstilbestrol

8. estimated date of birth
9. estimated date of delivery
10. gravid, para/term, preterm, abortions, living
11. glomerular filtration rate
12. human chorionic gonadotropin
13. Fetal hemoglobin
14. human placental lactogen
15. International Childbirth Education Association
16. last menstrual period
17. Nurses Association of the American College of Obstetricians and Gynecologists
18. over-the-counter
19. protein bound iodine

Self-Assessment Questions
1. a
2. d
3. c
4. b
5. d
6. a
7. a
8. d
9. b
10. d

Chapter 55 Complications of Pregnancy

Key Terms
1. d
2. l
3. e
4. c
5. h
6. m
7. a
8. k
9. n
10. f
11. r
12. p
13. s
14. u
15. b
16. i

17. o
18. w
19. g
20. q
21. t
22. v
23. j

Abbreviation Review
1. cytomegalovirus
2. contraction stress test
3. chorionic villi sampling
4. dilatation and curettage
5. disseminated intravascular coagulation
6. estimated date of birth
7. electronic fetal monitoring
8. fetal acoustic stimulation test
9. fetal biophysical profile
10. fetal heart rate
11. fetal heart tones
12. gestational diabetes mellitus
13. human chorionic gonadotrophin
14. hemolysis, elevated liver enzymes, low platelet count
15. human placental lactogen
16. herpes simplex virus type 2
17. intrauterine growth retardation
18. lecithin/sphingomyelin
19. magnesium sulfate
20. maternal serum alpha-fetoprotein
21. nonstress test
22. phosphatidyglycerol
23. pregnancy-induced hypertension
24. phenylketonuria
25. Rh immune globulin
26. small for gestational age
27. toxoplasmosis, rubella, cytomegalovirus, herpes virus type 2
28. vibroacoustic stimulation test

Self-Assessment Questions
1. a
2. d
3. a
4. b
5. c
6. a
7. d

8. c
9. b
10. a

Chapter 56 The Birth Process

Key Terms

1. t
2. x
3. ll
4. i
5. y
6. e
7. dd
8. mm
9. oo
10. qq
11. b
12. h
13. o
14. w
15. aa
16. q
17. z
18. f
19. v
20. a
21. ee
22. k
23. bb
24. nn
25. l
26. kk
27. r
28. ff
29. u
30. cc
31. pp
32. rr
33. gg
34. vv
35. m
36. ss
37. hh
38. jj
39. uu
40. n
41. ii
42. d
43. p
44. ww
45. j
46. c
47. s
48. g

Abbreviation Review

1. passage, passenger, powers, psyche
2. artificial rupture of membranes
3. certified nurse midwife
4. cephalopelvic disproportion
5. fetal heart rate
6. labor, delivery, recovery, postpartum
7. left mentum anterior
8. left mentum posterior
9. left mentum transverse
10. left occiput anterior
11. left occiput posterior
12. left occiput transverse
13. left sacrum anterior
14. left sacrum posterior
15. left sacrum transverse
16. premature rupture of membranes
17. right mentum anterior
18. right mentum posterior
19. right mentum transverse
20. right occiput anterior
21. rupture of membranes
22. right occiput posterior
23. right occiput transverse
24. right sacrum anterior
25. right sacrum posterior
26. right sacrum transverse
27. spontaneous rupture of membranes
28. vaginal birth after cesarean

Self-Assessment Questions

1. a
2. b
3. d
4. c
5. b
6. c
7. b
8. c
9. a
10. d

Chapter 57 Postpartum Care

Key Terms

1. i
2. e
3. n
4. s
5. u
6. m
7. d
8. l
9. w
10. y
11. f
12. b
13. g
14. q
15. x
16. h
17. t
18. v
19. z
20. p
21. r
22. j
23. a
24. o
25. c
26. k

Abbreviation Review

1. breasts, uterus, bladder, bowel, lochia, and episiotomy
2. certified nurse midwife
3. disseminated intravascular coagulation
4. deep vein thrombosis
5. human chorionic gonadotropin
6. human placental lactogen
7. melanocyte-stimulating hormone
8. postpartum depression
9. Rh immune globulin

Self-Assessment Questions

1. c
2. b
3. a
4. d
5. c
6. d
7. b
8. c
9. b
10. a

Chapter 58 Newborn Care

Key Terms

1. p
2. l
3. o
4. w
5. aa
6. u
7. ee
8. d
9. hh
10. jj
11. k
12. c
13. dd
14. q
15. m
16. v
17. ff
18. x
19. gg
20. h
21. t
22. e
23. n
24. g
25. i
26. r
27. y
28. cc
29. z
30. j
31. bb
32. ii
33. s
34. f
35. a
36. b

Key Terms Regarding Physical Characteristics of Newborns

1. h
2. f
3. i
4. k
5. g
6. a
7. b
8. d
9. c
10. e
11. j

Abbreviation Review

1. American Academy of Family Physicians
2. American Academy of Pediatrics
3. Advisory Committee on Immunization Practices
4. appropriate for gestational age
5. continuous positive airway pressure
6. fetal alcohol syndrome
7. hepatitis B immune globulin
8. hepatitis B
9. infant of diabetic mother
10. infant of substance abusing mother
11. large for gestational age
12. phenylketonuria
13. respiratory distress syndrome
14. rapid eye movement
15. sudden infant death syndrome
16. small for gestational age
17. transient tachypnea of the newborn

Self-Assessment Questions

1. a
2. b
3. c
4. b
5. a
6. c
7. c
8. d
9. b
10. a

Chapter 59 Basics of Pediatric Care

Key Terms

1. c
2. a
3. e
4. b
5. d

Abbreviation Review

1. body surface area
2. Denver Development Screening Test
3. eutectic (cream) mixture of local anesthetics
4. identification
5. intelligence quotient
6. National Center for Health Services
7. Omnibus Budget Reconciliation Act

Self-Assessment Questions

1. a
2. b
3. d
4. c
5. a
6. b
7. c
8. b

Chapter 60 Infants with Special Needs: Birth to 12 Months

Key Terms

1. f
2. p
3. t
4. a
5. u
6. r
7. h
8. d
9. q
10. l
11. o
12. e
13. s

14. n
15. i
16. w
17. v
18. j
19. m
20. c
21. k
22. g
23. b

Abbreviation Review

1. acute gastroenteritis
2. atrial septal defect
3. bronchopulmonary dysplasia
4. cystic fibrosis
5. cystic fibrosis transmembrane regulator
6. cerebral palsy
7. continuous positive airway pressure
8. cerebrospinal fluid
9. developmental dysplasia of the hip
10. failure to thrive
11. gastroesophageal reflux
12. laryngotracheobronchitis
13. nasogastric tube
14. patent ductus arteriosis
15. respiratory distress syndrome
16. respiratory syncytial virus
17. sickle-cell anemia
18. sudden infant death syndrome
19. tetralogy of Fallot
20. ventricular septal defect
21. Women, Infants, and Children

Self-Assessment Questions

1. c
2. a
3. b
4. a
5. c
6. d
7. c
8. a

Chapter 61 Common Problems: 1-18 Years

Key Terms

1. f
2. c
3. b
4. d
5. e
6. a

Abbreviation Review

1. American Academy of Pediatrics
2. Advisory Committee on Immunization Practices
3. attention deficit hyperactivity disorder
4. acute lymphocytic leukemia
5. acute poststreptococcal glomerulonephritis
6. antistreptolysin-O
7. body mass index
8. chest physiotherapy
9. Duchenne muscular dystrophy
10. diphtheria, tetanus, acellular pertussis
11. erythrocyte sedimentation rate
12. fasting plasma glucose
13. hepatitis B virus
14. herpes simplex virus
15. inactivated polio vaccine
16. idiopathic thrombocytopenic purpura
17. juvenile arthritis
18. minimal change nephrotic syndrome
19. metered-dose inhaler
20. measles, mumps, rubella
21. oral polio vaccine
22. polycystic ovarian syndrome
23. reactive airway disease
24. tetanus immune globulin

Self-Assessment Questions

1. c
2. d
3. c
4. a
5. d
6. a
7. b
8. c